Prenatal Care

Guest Editor

DAVID R. HARNISCH Sr, MD

PRIMARY CARE: CLINICS IN OFFICE PRACTICE

www.primarycare.theclinics.com

Consulting Editor

JOEL J. HEIDELBAUGH, MD

March 2012 • Volume 39 • Number 1

SAUNDERS an imprint of ELSEVIER, Inc.

W.B. SAUNDERS COMPANY
A Division of Elsevier Inc.

1600 John F. Kennedy Boulevard, Suite 1800 ● Philadelphia, PA 19103-2899

http://www.theclinics.com

PRIMARY CARE: CLINICS IN OFFICE PRACTICE Volume 39, Number 1
March 2012 ISSN 0095-4543, ISBN-13: 978-1-4557-3923-3

Editor: Yonah Korngold

Primary Care: Clinics in Office Practice (ISSN: 0095–4543) is published quarterly by Elsevier Inc., 360 Park Avenue South, New York, NY 10010-1710. Months of issue are March, June, September, and December. Periodicals postage paid at New York, NY and additional mailing offices. Subscription prices are $216.00 per year (US individuals), $353.00 (US institutions), $108.00 (US students), $264.00 (Canadian individuals), $415.00 (Canadian institutions), $169.00 (Canadian students), $329.00 (international individuals), $415.00 (international institutions), and $169.00 (international students). Foreign air speed delivery is included in all _Clinics_ subscription prices. All prices are subject to change without notice. POSTMASTER: Send address changes to _Primary Care: Clinics in Office Practice_, Elsevier Periodicals Customer Service, 11830 Westline Industrial Drive, St. Louis, MO 63146. Customer Service Health Sciences Division, Subscription Customer Service, 3251 Riverport Lane, Maryland Heights, MO 63043. **Customer Service: 1-800-654-2452 (U.S. and Canada); 314-447-8871 (outside U.S. and Canada). Fax: 314-447-8029. E-mail: journalscustomerservice-usa@elsevier.com (for print support); journalsonlinesupport-usa@elsevier.com (for online support).**

Reprints. For copies of 100 or more, of articles in this publication, please contact the Commercial Reprints Department, Elsevier Inc., 360 Park Avenue South, New York, NY 10010-1710. Tel. (212) 633-3812; Fax: (212) 482-1935; E-mail: reprints@elsevier.com.

Primary Care: Clinics in Office Practice is covered in _MEDLINE/PubMed (Index Medicus)_ and _EMBASE/Excerpta Medica, Current Contents/Clinical Medicine,_ and _ISI/BIOMED._

Contributors

CONSULTING EDITOR

JOEL J. HEIDELBAUGH, MD
Clinical Assistant Professor and Clerkship Director, Department of Family Medicine;
Clinical Assistant Professor, Department of Urology, University of Michigan Medical
School, Ann Arbor, Michigan

GUEST EDITOR

DAVID R. HARNISCH Sr, MD, FAAFP, FACOG
Staff Physician, Clarkson Family Medicine Residency, The Nebraska Medical Center,
Omaha, Nebraska

AUTHORS

JANE E. ANDERSON, MD, MS
Assistant Professor of Family Medicine, Department of Family Medicine, University
of Wisconsin School of Medicine and Public Health, Verona, Wisconsin

K.M. RODNEY ARNOLD, MD
Assistant Professor of Clinical Family Medicine, University of Tennessee College
of Medicine Chattanooga, Chattanooga, Tennessee

ERIN KATE DOOLEY, MD, MPH
FM/Ob Fellow, Médicos Para La Familia, Department of Surgical Family Medicine,
Memphis, Tennessee

LEE T. DRESANG, MD
Professor, Department of Family Medicine, University of Wisconsin School of Medicine
and Public Health, Madison, Wisconsin

ANN E. EVENSEN, MD, FAAFP
Assistant Professor, Department of Family Medicine, University of Wisconsin School
of Medicine and Public Health, Madison, Wisconsin

DAVID R. HARNISCH Sr, MD, FAAFP, FACOG
Staff Physician, Clarkson Family Medicine Residency, The Nebraska Medical Center,
Omaha, Nebraska

JEAN M. HARNISCH, BS, RD
Chief Nutrition and Food Service, Central Alabama Veterans Health Care System,
Montgomery, Alabama

PATRICIA H. HARNISCH, BS, MEd, RD
Registered Dietitian, Papillion, Nebraska

BENJAMIN J.F. HUNTLEY, MD
Resident Physician, Department of Family Medicine, John Peter Smith Hospital, Fort Worth, Texas

ANITA C. JAYNES, CNM
Certified Nurse-Midwives and Clinical Instructors, Department of Obstetrics and Gynecology, University of Nebraska Medical Center, Omaha, Nebraska

AARON D. LANIK, MD
Thayer County Health Services, Hebron, Nebraska

LAWRENCE LEEMAN, MD, MPH
Associate Professor, Department of Family and Community Medicine; Associate Professor, Department of Obstetrics and Gynecology, University of New Mexico School of Medicine, Albuquerque, New Mexico

ANNE MARIE LOZEAU, MD
Associate Professor of Family Medicine, University of Wisconsin School of Medicine and Public Health; Northeast Family Medical Center, Madison, Wisconsin

A. ILDIKO MARTONFFY, MD
Assistant Professor of Family Medicine, University of Wisconsin School of Medicine and Public Health; Access-Wingra Family Medical Center, Madison, Wisconsin

EMILY NEWFIELD, MD, MS
Attending Physician, Department of Obstetrics and Gynecology, Contra Costa Regional Medical Center, Martinez, California

BETH POTTER, MD
Associate Professor of Family Medicine, University of Wisconsin School of Medicine and Public Health; Access-Wingra Family Medical Center, Madison, Wisconsin

KIRSTEN RINDFLEISCH, MD
Assistant Professor of Family Medicine, University of Wisconsin School of Medicine and Public Health; Access-Wingra Family Medical Center, Madison, Wisconsin

ROBERT L. RINGLER Jr, MD, FAAFP
Assistant Professor, Department of Family and Community Medicine, Eastern Virginia Medical School, Norfolk; Medical Director and Director of Family Medicine Obstetrics, Portsmouth Family Medicine, Department of Family and Community Medicine, Portsmouth, Virginia

JOHN R.M. RODNEY, MD
Maternal Child Health Fellow, Department of Family Medicine, John Peter Smith Hospital, Fort Worth, Texas

WM MACMILLAN RODNEY, MD
Professor and Chair, Medicos para la Familia, Memphis, Tennessee

KATHLEEN E. SCOTT, CNM
Certified Nurse-Midwives and Clinical Instructors, Department of Obstetrics and Gynecology, University of Nebraska Medical Center, Omaha, Nebraska

ZACHARY B. SELF, MD
Fellow, Surgical Family Medicine Obstetrics, Medicos para la Familia, Memphis, Tennessee

CINDY W. SU, MD
Department of Obstetrics and Gynecology, Contra Costa Regional Medical Center, Martinez, California

Contents

Electronic fetal monitoring assesses fetal health during the prenatal and intrapartum process. Intermittent auscultation does not detect key elements of fetal risk, such as beat-to-beat variability. Family medicine obstetric fellowships have contributed new knowledge to this process by articulating a method of analysis that builds on evidence-based recommendations from the American College of Obstetrics and Gynecology as well as the National Institute of Child Health and Development. This article summarizes the development, interpretation, and management of electronic fetal heart rate patterns and tracings.

This article reviews one of the less common but most dreaded complications of labor and delivery, shoulder dystocia, an infrequent but potentially devastating event that results from impaction of the fetal shoulders in the maternal pelvis. Shoulder dystocia occurs most commonly in patients without identified risk factors, and can result in both maternal and fetal morbidity. Because the vast majority of cases of shoulder dystocia are unpredictable, obstetric care providers must be prepared to recognize dystocia and respond appropriately in every delivery. Detailed documentation is essential after any delivery complicated by shoulder dystocia.

Cesarean delivery rates rose from 20 to 33% of births in the United States from 2006-2009 without an accompanying improvement in neonatal outcomes. The cesarean rate may be safely decreased by increasing vaginal birth after cesarean, encouraging external cephalic version for breech presentation, maintaining operative vaginal delivery skills, and applying stricter criteria for operative intervention in labor dystocia. A variety of cesarean operative techniques are supported by randomized controlled trials. Optimal maternity care outcomes depend on sound medical decision-making, appropriate operative technique and skills, and effective communication between maternity care team members.

Postpartum hemorrhage (PPH) is a very common obstetric emergency with high morbidity and mortality rates worldwide. Understanding its etiology is fundamental to effectively managing PPH in an acute setting. Active management of the third stage of labor is also a key component in its prevention. Management strategies include conservative measures (medications, uterine tamponade, and arterial embolization) as well as surgical interventions (arterial ligations, compression sutures, and hysterectomy). Creating a standardized PPH protocol and running simulation-based drills with a multidisciplinary team may also help decrease maternal morbidity and improve perinatal outcomes, although further studies are needed.

> Midwifery offers concepts and techniques for intrapartum care that could be integrated into the practice of a family physician. Normal birth has virtually been replaced by a medicalized model of maternity care in the American health care system, despite research indicating that many interventions are not necessary and even harmful. A low-tech, high-touch approach to low-risk women in labor is evidence based and results in improved perinatal outcomes as well as higher patient satisfaction with the birth experience.

VISIT THE CLINICS ONLINE!

Access your subscription at:
www.theclinics.com

Foreword
The Art of Prenatal Care

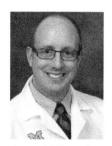

Joel J. Heidelbaugh, MD
Consulting Editor

The landscape of maternal care in the United States has evolved substantially over the last decades. Medical school used to turn out mostly male physicians years ago; recent decades have created a nearly 50:50 split of male and female graduates in most institutions, yet more obstetrical resident graduates in current day are female. The dramatic rise in nurse midwives has also shaped the workforce to create a more accessible choice for women to create their ideal prenatal care and childbirth experience. From community to academic practices, today's marketplace affords pregnant women with the best of all worlds in choosing the parameters of their pregnancy experience.

Each successive decade of medicine has seen a vast development of guidelines and evidence-based medicine. While I fully endorse the concept of evidence-based medicine (and my students and residents often pray for a break from my didactic lecturing of such practices!), what tends to get lost in day-to-day practice is the ability for clinicians to promote a practice based upon experience and their own expertise. Granted, there are very few "top-shelf" evidence-based practices in maternal care, which by definition would be based upon randomized controlled double-blinded trials, and in most cases aren't practical in obstetrical and prenatal care.

The bond that an expectant mother and her caregiver share often goes underappreciated, derided by the technical aspects of medical care and the fears of underlying pathology gone undetected or a split-second emergency during labor. The "art" of prenatal care characterized by Dr David Harnisch in his preface epitomizes what we strive for in patient care—a humanistic approach to the most germane and sensitive of life experiences. The articles that comprise this volume create the framework upon which a primary care clinician's practice builds its foundation in maternal care. From prenatal to intrapartum care, from genetic screening to management of commonly encountered obstetrical complications, the content herein outlines the construct of optimal maternal care.

Prim Care Clin Office Pract 39 (2012) xiii–xiv
doi:10.1016/j.pop.2011.11.012
0095-4543/12/$ – see front matter © 2012 Elsevier Inc. All rights reserved.

primarycare.theclinics.com

I sincerely thank Dr Harnisch and his authors for compiling a truly unique set of articles aimed at providing clinicians with the best current knowledge to care for our pregnant patients. This volume is extraordinary in that national experts have infused their own geographic practice standards, coupled with the best guideline recommendations for the salient conditions in prenatal care. It is my hope that our readers will use this edition of *Primary Care: Clinics in Office Practice* to re-infuse the art of maternal care into their practices.

Joel J. Heidelbaugh, MD
Ypsilanti Health Center
200 Arnet Street, Suite 200
Ypsilanti, MI 48198, USA

E-mail address:
jheidel@umich.edu

Preface

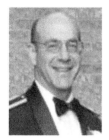

David R. Harnisch Sr, MD
Guest Editor

In the late 1970s when I was beginning my medical journey, I was struck by the "magic" of Obstetrics. By "magic" I refer to the answers I received to my questions about "why" and "how" things were done, receiving often the answer "that's just the way we do things here." Clearly the patterns established around my early training grounds were effective at getting babies delivered safely and moms through their pregnancies without inordinate difficulties; however, the "why" and the "how" seemed to be lacking. The "art" of this branch of medicine was strong.

Since my initiation and now about 30 years into the trip, I marvel at how far things have come. Through two residencies, practicing in eight states and the District of Columbia, at 16 different clinics, community hospitals, and medical centers, and serving on four residency program faculties, the development of the science of Obstetrics has been impressive. While answers are still being found and appropriately so, it seems to me that the science has caught up with the art of being an accoucheur.

As we know, pendulums swing both ways. Now the "art" is being forgotten and childbirth has been "medicalized." Somewhere in between lies the answer. While certainly there are times for intensive intervention and manipulation, at other times the best thing is to "let nature take its course." The urban medical centers seem to dominate (at least in the scientific literature), while the rural practitioners may be looked down on from the Ivory Towers. The obstetric intensivists (Maternal Fetal Medicine fellowship trained individuals) function on a different plane than the midwife—yet each has the same goal—a safe, happy, and healthy birth experience for mother and child.

In seeking to bring some balance to the debate, as guest editor of this volume from Elsevier, I have worked hard to find both ends of the spectrum in terms of practice style, geographical location, subspecialty, health care profession affiliation, and population center demographics. Represented in the articles that follow, I have been aided by practitioners who advocate birthing centers versus typical labor and delivery suites to incorporating perinatal intensive care units aided by high-risk pregnancy consultants; providers from both coasts and the great midlands of the

Prim Care Clin Office Pract 39 (2012) xv–xvi
doi:10.1016/j.pop.2011.11.008
0095-4543/12/$ – see front matter © 2012 Elsevier Inc. All rights reserved.

primarycare.theclinics.com

United States; obstetricians, family physicians, midwives, and dietitians; from large cities based at University quaternary care centers to the rural practitioner at a small community hospital. On top of this I have asked each of the authors to review the work and content of each others' articles and to comment on it from their unique perspective while always maintaining their local, regional, or national standards of care. Incorporated also into the authors' works are their perspectives from their ethical backgrounds.

What has resulted is this small work of 12 articles covering some of the significant topics of our day presented from a variety of perspectives seeking to balance the art and science of obstetrics for you. We, the authors, feel this work provides a cutting-edge review for you and will help to provide you with solid footing as well as necessary review for your practice.

David R. Harnisch Sr, MD
Clarkson Family Medicine
42nd and Douglas Streets
Omaha, NE 68046, USA

E-mail address:
dharnisch@nebraskamed.com

Preconception Counseling

Aaron D. Lanik, MD

KEYWORDS

- Preconception counseling • Medical history
- Reproductive history • Pregnancy

The preconception counseling visit is an ideal time to evaluate the patient and her future expectations regarding pregnancy. In fact at every patient encounter, whether for acute or chronic care, consideration should be given to any woman who, although not pregnant, may become pregnant, and what effect each ordered procedure, laboratory examination, or medication prescription might have on her or her fetus. Even providers who do not render prenatal services need to consider this in the course of their clinical practices; the preconception care they provide may in time become just as important as the prenatal care, as it lays the groundwork for the prenatal period and because they will be resuming care after delivery. If, however, the primary reason for the visit is preconception counseling, there are a few specific components that should be discussed besides a complete history and physical examination.

MEDICAL HISTORY

A complete medical history is the logical place to begin. Many patients are now postponing pregnancies until later in their reproductive lives, and there are many more women with long-standing medical problems who fall into this category. It therefore becomes essential to help patients optimize the medical management of these chronic medical problems to help ensure optimal outcomes during their future pregnancies. This section discusses some of the more common problems encountered in any busy primary care practice. However, a complete list of medical problems that a primary care provider may see in women who plan on becoming pregnant in the future is not provided.

Obesity

Based on the most recent data, approximately one-third of women in the United States are obese.[1] Despite the increased awareness of nutrition and obesity in general, this number has not decreased but rather has remained steady over the 8-year period from 1999–2000 to 2007–2008, from which the most recent data have

Thayer County Health Services, 120 Park Avenue, Hebron, NE 68370, USA
E-mail address: alanikmd@hotmail.com

Prim Care Clin Office Pract 39 (2012) 1–16
doi:10.1016/j.pop.2011.11.001

been taken.[2] Maternal obesity in pregnancy is associated with higher rates of gestational diabetes, hypertensive disorders, fetal macrosomia (with subsequent increased rates of cesarean delivery and shoulder dystocias), intrauterine fetal demise, antepartum venous thromboembolism, and congenital anomalies. These anomalies are headlined by neural tube defects but also include spina bifida, cardiovascular abnormalities, septal anomalies, cleft palate, cleft lip, anorectal atresia, hydrocephaly, and limb abnormalities. Children born to obese mothers are at an increased risk themselves of developing childhood obesity.[3]

Because of all these risks, the role of preconception counseling with regard to a patient's weight is important. The provider should discuss these risks with the patient with time enough before conception to make the necessary changes. The discussion from the provider should include diet (and many involve consultation with a dietitian), exercise, and weight loss, with the goal of returning to or nearing a normal healthy weight. As many pregnancies are also unplanned, it may also be beneficial to start folic acid supplementation (0.4–1.0 mg daily), if without contraindications, before a woman is planning on becoming pregnant to help decrease the risk of neural tube defects should the patient become pregnant before the success of weight loss strategies.[4] Specific nutrition guidelines during pregnancy are discussed in an article elsewhere in this issue.

Hypertension

Alongside the large percentage of people with clinical obesity and the number of women becoming pregnant at a later age, there has been a concomitant increase in the number of women with underlying essential hypertension. The Seventh Report of the Joint National Committee on Prevention, Detection, Evaluation, and Treatment of High Blood Pressure (JNC 7) defines hypertension in 2 stages. Stage 1 hypertension is defined as systolic blood pressure (sBP) between 140 and 159 mm Hg and/or diastolic blood pressure (dBP) between 90 and 99 mm Hg. Stage 2 hypertension is further defined as sBP 160 mm Hg or higher and/or dBP 100 mm Hg or higher. JNC 7 also further recommends that initial treatment of uncomplicated hypertension include thiazide diuretics and, if certain high risks are present, β-blockers or angiotensin-converting enzyme (ACE) inhibitors/angiotensin receptor blockers (ARBs).[5]

Some of these medicines are known teratogens and may have other nonteratogenic adverse effects on fetal growth and development. The ACE inhibitors have been associated with underdeveloped calvarial bone, renal failure, oligohydramnios, anuria, renal dysgenesis, pulmonary hypoplasia, intrauterine growth restriction (IUGR), and fetal/neonatal demise, and are contraindicated in pregnancy or in women who might become pregnant. There are fewer data on the ARB class of medication, but these agents are associated with adverse fetal and neonatal outcomes similar to those for the ACE inhibitors. β-Blockers in general, and in particular atenolol, have been associated with infants who are small for gestational age (SGA), and may cause IUGR. As diuretics can prevent normal expansion of the blood volume, there is a concern for an increased risk of uteroplacental perfusion and the development of IUGR.[6] Based on these concerns, it would be best to recommend discontinuation of these medications before becoming pregnant. Calcium-channel blockers are not associated with a major teratogenic risk and thus could play a role in the treatment of hypertension during pregnancy.[7]

The National High Blood Pressure Education Program Working Group on High Blood Pressure in Pregnancy defines chronic hypertension parameters slightly differently to JNC 7. Mild hypertension is defined as greater than 140/90 mm Hg and severe hypertension as greater than 180/110 mm Hg.[8] Both the National High Blood Pressure

Education Program Working Group on High Blood Pressure in Pregnancy and the American College of Obstetricians and Gynecologists (ACOG) state that women who are pregnant and have mild hypertension generally do well during pregnancy and do not necessarily require treatment with antihypertensive medications.[6,8] It may be reasonable to discontinue treatment in patients with mild hypertension and follow them expectantly. These groups do recommend treating women with severe hypertension or end-organ damage.[6,8] The specific treatment guidelines are discussed elsewhere in this issue. The ACOG also recommends obtaining baseline laboratory tests before or at the beginning of pregnancy to help determine whether there are any changes in the future that could correspond with superimposed preeclampsia, and these are listed in **Box 1**.[8]

Diabetes Mellitus

With the increase in the incidence of obesity, as also seen with hypertension, there has been an increase in the number of patients with diabetes. Uncontrolled diabetes has been associated with major congenital anomalies (including complex cardiac defects, central nervous system anomalies such as anencephaly and spina bifida, and skeletal malformations including sacral agenesis) occurring at rates as high as 6% to 10%.[9] Pregestational diabetes is also associated with an increased risk of miscarriage, spontaneous preterm labor, and preeclampsia.[10] Therefore, it is recommended that adequate glucose control be initiated before conception to allow enough time to evaluate the medical status of the patient and to normalize or maximize glycemic control to give the patent the best chance of reducing the risks of a pregnancy complicated by diabetes.[9,10] The American Diabetes Association (ADA) has created a list of 4 key elements of preconception care of patients with diabetes (**Box 2**).[11] Specific details of the control of diabetes during pregnancy are discussed elsewhere in this issue.

Depression

According to data from the National Health and Nutrition Examination Survey 2005-2006, approximately 6.7% of women in the United States suffer from depression[12] Approximately 64% of these women receive treatment for the depression, of whom 82% receive some sort of pharmacotherapy including selective serotonin reuptake inhibitors (SSRIs), tricyclic antidepressants (TCAs), and newer antidepressants such as venlafaxine, duloxetine, mirtazapine, and bupropion. With disease prevalence this high, many women contemplating pregnancy may present with or be undergoing treatment for depression.[13]

Untreated depression in pregnancy may be associated with miscarriage, low birth weight (<2500 g), SGA (birth weight <10% of age-adjusted weight), and preterm delivery. Infants born to mothers with a depressive disorder are also at an increased risk for irritability, decreased activity and attentiveness, and decreased facial expressiveness compared with offspring born to mothers without depression.[14]

Box 1
Laboratory tests to consider in patients with hypertension who are planning pregnancy

- Renal function tests (serum creatinine and blood urea nitrogen)
- 24-hour urine evaluation for total protein and creatinine clearance
- Liver function tests (aspartate aminotransferase, alanine aminotransferase, alkaline phosphatase)
- Hemoglobin/hematocrit and platelet level

Box 2
Key elements of preconception care of patients with diabetes mellitus

1. Patient education about the interaction of diabetes in pregnancy

2. Diabetes self-management education

3. Physician-directed medical care and laboratory testing

4. Counseling by a mental health professional when indicated to reduce stress and increase treatment plan adherence

---

Antidepressant use in pregnancy, including SSRIs, can have adverse effects on the pregnancy. Such effects can include low birth weight and SGA (when controlled for possible confounders including undertreated depression) and preterm birth (especially in patients with longer-term exposures to antidepressants). TCA usage in pregnancy is not associated with structural malformations. In general, SSRIs are also not considered to be teratogenic with the exception of paroxetine, especially with exposure early in pregnancy associated with an increased risk of cardiac defects. Based on the current limited data on the newer antidepressants, an increased risk of congenital malformations has not been observed, but the risk of preterm delivery is similar to that for SSRIs. Antidepressants including TCAs, SSRIs, and the newer antidepressants are also associated with poor neonatal adaptation after delivery, including tachypnea, hypoglycemia, temperature instability, irritability, weak or absent cry, and seizures. This disease spectrum is thought to reflect some sort of withdrawal or discontinuation syndrome. There has been an association made between the exposure of infants to SSRIs late in pregnancy and an increased risk of persistent pulmonary hypertension.[14]

According to the American Psychiatric Association and the ACOG, the preconception provider should first determine the severity of the symptoms. If the patient has mild or no symptoms for 6 months or longer on treatment, she may be considered a candidate for a medication taper or discontinuation prior to conception. If the patient has moderate to severe symptoms, it is recommended that, when possible, treatment be continued until a period of stability or euthymia has been achieved (often defined as 6–12 months) before conception is planned. In patients with a history of severe, recurrent major depressive disorders that require pharmacotherapy or a history of suicide attempts, discontinuation of the medication may not be an option. In these patients, it is recommended that other aspects of obstetric care be optimized to help decrease the risk of the pregnancy for patients on antidepressant therapy (such as psychotherapy, quitting smoking, and weight loss, among others).[14] It is imperative that the clinician providing preconception counseling discusses not only the risks and benefits of treatment but also the different treatment options, and document such discussions to aid in providing the best care for the patient.

Hypothyroidism

Hypothyroidism is a common condition affecting up to 1% to 2% of women in the United States, and complicates 0.3% of pregnancies.[15] It is associated with premature birth, preeclampsia, placental abruption, low birth weight, postpartum hemorrhage, and impaired neuropsychological development in childhood.[16]

Pregnancy alters the thyroid hormone levels as the increased estrogen levels present in the pregnant state result in a 2-fold to 3-fold increase in the thyroxine-binding globulin, which lowers the free thyroid hormone and thus stimulates the increased production of thyroid-stimulating hormone (TSH) through the hypothalamic-pituitary-thyroid axis. As a result of this action early in the pregnancy, some providers recommend empirically increasing the dose of thyroid hormone replacement by 30% as soon as a patient becomes pregnant. Preconception counseling is important to educate the patient, optimize her treatment, and, if needed, adjust the dose of levothyroxine.[15] Once stable, the TSH can be rechecked once every trimester.[17]

There is some controversy about screening for hypothyroidism in asymptomatic patients. The ACOG and the United States Preventative Services Task Force (USPSTF) do not recommend routine screening, whereas the American Association of Clinical Endocrinologists (AACE) does.[15,17] The routine screening of asymptomatic patients has also led to an increase in the diagnosis of subclinical hypothyroidism (increased level of TSH with a normal level of free T4). There have been a few case-control studies and observational studies indicating that the treatment of subclinical hypothyroidism in pregnancy leads to better neurocognitive outcomes in infants in the early development years. The endocrine community has used these studies to facilitate the recommendation by the AACE that subclinical hypothyroidism should be diagnosed and treated in pregnancy. The obstetric community has cautioned that more research is needed, and the ACOG recommends against routine screening for and treating subclinical hypothyroidism.[15,17,18] More research is necessary regarding these recommendations.

REPRODUCTIVE HISTORY

The discussion of a patient's reproductive history is the next important component of a preconception counseling visit. Taking this history allows the provider to evaluate the previous pregnancy or pregnancies, including complications and expectations. The following are a few components that may be elucidated and that may affect further management of the patient's future pregnancies.

Preterm Birth

In 2007, the rate of preterm delivery in the United States was 12.7%.[19] Women with a history of a previous preterm delivery have a 2.5-fold increase in the risk of preterm delivery with the subsequent pregnancy.[20] Overall, the earlier the preterm birth occurs (<32 weeks' gestation vs 32–36 weeks' gestation), the higher the risk of the second and subsequent pregnancies being complicated by preterm delivery.[21]

Research is ongoing to seek ways to prevent preterm delivery. Based on the most recent data, both the Cochrane database and the ACOG have identified and recommended the use of 17-hydroxyprogesterone for women with a history of spontaneous preterm birth.[22,23] Meta-analysis of the data used by the Cochrane database showed that women treated with progesterone were significantly less likely to have a preterm birth at less than 34 weeks as well as at less than 37 weeks, and a decrease in the risk of an infant with birth weight less than 2500 g. Pooled data in the Cochrane analysis, however, showed no statistical difference in secondary outcomes such as perinatal death, intrauterine fetal death, neonatal death, respiratory distress syndrome, intraventricular hemorrhage, retinopathy of prematurity, neonatal sepsis, and patent ductus arteriosus, whereas other studies have shown a difference in many of the complications associated with preterm birth.[22,24] There were also no documented differences in growth or developmental outcomes between those infants exposed in utero to progesterone and those exposed to placebo.[22]

Based on these data, the ACOG recommends offering progesterone supplementation to women with a history of preterm delivery and starting supplementation between 16 and 20 weeks' gestation. Studies on the route of administration (intra-vaginal vs intramuscular) and the dosage are currently under way.[23] Indentifying women with a history of preterm delivery before conception can allow the provider to discuss the importance of identifying the pregnancy early so that correct dates can be established and treatment started in the established time period, thus helping to decrease the risk of the subsequent pregnancy.

Preeclampsia

Women with a history of preeclampsia increase their risk of preeclampsia in a subse-quent pregnancy to around 15% from 1% without a history of preeclampsia, and this increases to around 30% if they have had the disease with 2 previous pregnancies.[25] To help women decrease the risk, the provider should identify and control, when possible, any other risk factors for preeclampsia. These factors include, but are not limited to, chronic hypertension, renal disease, diabetes mellitus, active con-nective tissue disease (such as lupus or rheumatoid arthritis), thrombophilias, and obesity.[26]

Recent evidence has shown that low-dose aspirin (50–150 mg daily) when started before 16 weeks' gestation is associated with a significant decrease in the incidence of preeclampsia in a subsequent pregnancy. The evidence also shows that the earlier in pregnancy the dose is started, the greater the benefits. When started after 16 weeks, there was no statistical benefit in decreasing the rate of preeclampsia.[27] The current guideline from the ACOG is that low-dose aspirin has shown no benefit in preventing preeclampsia in women who are low risk, therefore its use is not recom-mended in this group.[28] Further recommendations for women who are at high risk are still needed.

Previous Cesarean Delivery

In 2007, the rate of cesarean delivery in the United States was at an all-time high of 31.8%, which is an increase of 2% from the previous year and a more than 50% increase from 1996.[19] As many primary care providers may not be trained in cesarean delivery, it may be necessary to discuss with these patients the transfer of future preg-nancy care to a provider who does cesarean deliveries, or to manage the pregnancy and provide cesarean delivery services as a backup. A discussion should take place regarding the risk of trial of labor after cesarean delivery (TOLAC) versus the risk of repeat cesarean delivery. As many rural hospitals do not offer TOLAC because of coverage constraints, it may be necessary to discuss transfer of care to hospitals or providers that have this capability. Further discussion of operative deliveries and TOLAC can be found elsewhere in this issue.

Recurrent Miscarriages

Recurrent miscarriage or recurrent pregnancy loss is defined as 3 or more consecutive spontaneous abortions.[29] Although evaluation is typically completed by a fertility specialist, it is often the primary care provider to whom the patient may present initially. Therefore, primary care providers may be asked to initiate such an evaluation, which can include many factors: genetics, endocrine, immunologic, anatomic, throm-bophilic, and iatrogenic (such as medications, tobacco, alcohol, or caffeine use, among others). **Box 3** shows some of the tests that could be considered at the start of the evaluation process.[30,31] Although a complete evaluation is beyond the scope of this article, many of these tests can be ordered and evaluated by the primary care provider to provide part of the initial evaluation.

Box 3
Laboratory tests to consider in the initial evaluation of recurrent pregnancy loss

- Genetic
  - Genetic counseling
  - Cytogenetic analysis of the partners
- Endocrine
  - Hemoglobin A_{1c} or fasting glucose (trying to identify insulin resistance as seen with diabetes or polycystic ovarian syndrome)
  - TSH (thyroid dysfunction)
  - Prolactin level (hyperprolactinemia)
- Anatomic
  - Hysteroscopy or hysterosalpingogram
- Immunologic
  - Serum lupus anticoagulant and anticardiolipin antibodies (antiphospholipid antibody syndrome)
- Thrombophilic
  - Factor V Leiden
  - Prothrombin gene mutations
  - Fasting homocysteine
  - Antithrombin activity
  - Protein C and S levels

Infertility

Infertility is defined as the failure to achieve a successful pregnancy after 12 months of regular intercourse.[32] Although a fertility specialist may need to be consulted, a primary care provider may be the first person approached by a couple experiencing problems with infertility. Therefore, primary care providers should feel comfortable initiating an evaluation. A complete history and a physical examination are necessary with the focus on the medical, surgical, sexual, menstrual (in women), reproductive, social, and family histories of the couple. A common finding of physical examination in men with infertility problems is a varicocele. **Box 4** describes the laboratory tests that can be considered in the initial evaluation of infertility. **Box 5** describes a secondary laboratory evaluation for women if the initial tests are normal. If the secondary tests are positive, the primary care provider may initiate treatment of polycystic ovarian syndrome and/or initiate induction of ovulation with clomiphene if the partners are comfortable with this. Further tests and management options are beyond the scope of this text and may include a referral to a fertility specialist; however, in many circumstances the primary care provider may need to initiate the evaluation.[33]

SOCIAL HISTORY

Assessing for situations that not only place a patient's health at risk but may also affect the pregnancy is an important component of the preconception counseling session. By assessing risk before the patient becomes pregnant, the provider may be able to help initiate change in any behaviors that could negatively affect the future pregnancy. This section discusses a few items that should be assessed and addressed.

Box 4
Laboratory tests considered in the initial evaluation of infertility

- Males
  - Semen analysis
  - Testosterone levels
- Females
  - Complete blood count
  - Urinalysis
  - Sexually transmitted disease screen
  - Confirmation of varicella and rubella immunity
  - Pap smear
  - Follicle-stimulating hormone (FSH), luteinizing hormone
  - Prolactin level
  - TSH

Tobacco Use

The most recent figures estimate that 20.6% of adults in the United States (46.6 million) were current cigarette smokers; 17.9% of women are smokers.[34] Tobacco use in pregnancy has been associated with an increase in the risk for infertility, ectopic pregnancy, miscarriage, placental abruption, placenta previa, IUGR, preterm delivery, congenital defects such as cleft lip and cleft palate, and sudden infant death syndrome.[35] The USPSTF and ACOG recommend that clinicians ask all adults about tobacco use and provide tobacco cessation interventions for those who currently use tobacco products. Both groups recommend the use of the 5-A approach (**Box 6**).[36,37]

Alcohol Use

It is estimated that 53.9% of women in the United States have used alcohol in the last 30 days and that 23.3% have used it at binge-drinking levels (≥5 drinks on the same occasion).[38] Alcohol use in pregnancy can lead to birth defects and developmental disabilities, in particular fetal alcohol syndrome (FAS). FAS is characterized by a pattern of facial anomalies (including a smooth philtrum, thin upper lip, upturned nose, flat nasal bridge and midface, epicanthal folds, small palpebral fissures, and a small head circumference), prenatal and postnatal growth retardation, and functional or structural central nervous system abnormalities.[39] The prevalence of FAS is estimated to be between 0.5 and 2.0 per 1000 live births.[40] Although the incidence of FAS is linearly associated with higher levels of alcohol consumption, there have

---

Box 5
Secondary laboratory tests considered in women if the initial tests are normal

- FSH and estradiol level on day 3 of the menstrual cycle
- Hysterosalpingogram or hysteroscopy
- Testing for hyperandrogenism and insulin resistance (to help rule out polycystic ovarian syndrome)

Box 6
The 5-A approach to tobacco cessation
• Ask about tobacco use
• Advise to quit through a clear personalized message
• Assess willingness to quit
• Assist to quit
• Arrange follow-up and support

been studies linking fetal brain cell loss to as little as a single episode of drinking 2 alcoholic drinks (1 drink equals 12 oz [355 mL] of beer, 5 oz [148 mL] of wine, and 1.5 oz [45 mL] of liquor). Therefore, patients considering pregnancy should be advised to avoid alcohol from the time of conception throughout the pregnancy.[39]

Illicit Drug Use

According to the 2009 National Survey Drug Use and Health, it was estimated that 8.7% of the population in the United States used illicit drugs in the last 30 days. Some of the more commonly used illicit drugs were marijuana (6.6%), cocaine (0.7%), hallucinogens (0.5%), and methamphetamine (0.2%).[41] Use of illicit drugs during pregnancy is associated with an increased risk of maternal complications and adverse outcomes for the infant. Specifically, marijuana has been associated with a decrease in intellectual development, and cocaine with increased risks for low birth weight, prematurity, perinatal death, and placental abruption. It is recommended that patients be assessed for illicit drug use and, if discovered, the risks should be discussed and a recommendation made for the discontinuation of these substances.[42]

Sexually Transmitted Infection Risk

According to the most recent data provided by the Centers for Disease Control and Prevention (CDC), there are an estimated 19 million new cases of sexually transmitted infections in the United States annually. Rates of infection in 2009 varied among the 3 most common infections: chlamydia at 409.2 per 100,000 people, gonorrhea at 99.1 per 100,000, and syphilis at 4.6 per 100,000.[43] The estimated rate of diagnosis of human immunodeficiency virus (HIV) was estimated to be 17.4 per 100,000.[44] **Box 7** lists the prenatal effects of these infections.[45–47]

As the treatment of these diseases can decrease the risk for the newborn, the USPSTF recommends screening pregnant women for chlamydia and gonorrhea if they are younger than 25 years or engage in high-risk sexual behavior such as having multiple current sexual partners, having a new partner, inconsistent use of condoms, having sex under the influence of alcohol or drugs, or having sex in exchange for money or drugs. The USPSTF recommends screening all pregnant women for hepatitis B, HIV, and syphilis.[48] Therefore, it is imperative for the primary care provider to discuss sexual behavior with the patient during the preconception counseling visit, and it may be necessary to order these screening tests before pregnancy to ensure adequate treatment before the patient becomes pregnant and subsequently decrease the risk of infection during pregnancy, including the risks of fetal infection.

Box 7
Pregnancy and prenatal effects of sexually transmitted infections

- Chlamydia and gonorrhea
  - Risk factor for the development of pelvic inflammatory disease, which is a risk factor in the development of fertility issues
  - Risk of ophthalmologic disease, pulmonary disease, or sepsis if transmitted to the newborn at delivery
- Syphilis
  - Increased risk of miscarriage
  - Increased risk of stillbirth
  - Nonimmune hydrops
  - IUGR
  - Congenital syphilis
- HIV
  - Treatment during pregnancy reduces the risk of vertical transmission from mother to infant to approximately 1%–2%

Intimate Partner Violence Risk

Recent evidence has placed the rate of intimate partner violence (IPV) in the United States to be 5.3% before and 3.6% during pregnancy. Women at risk include women proximate to their divorce or separation, having a partner who has expressed that he does not want a pregnancy, and being close to someone with an alcohol or drug problem.[49] Adolescents are also at higher risk than adults.[50] Women affected by IPV are at risk for mental health disorders such as depression or anxiety, as well as for developing a substance abuse disorder, all of which are associated with an increased risk of poor pregnancy outcomes as noted earlier. Pregnant women affected by IPV are at higher risk for developing high blood pressure, severe nausea/vomiting associated with dehydration, and urinary tract infections or pyelonephritis. IPV is also associated with an increased risk for low birth weight, preterm labor, and perinatal death.[51]

Although IPV is common, the USPSTF does not recommend for or against universal screening, because of the lack of evidence concerning the effectiveness of universal screening.[52] Despite the lack of evidence of effectiveness, some professional groups (including the ACOG, the American Academy of Family Physicians, the American Academy of Pediatrics, and the American Medical Association) still recommend screening because the prevalence is so high.[53–56] Ongoing research is being undertaken not only to study the prevalence but also to help determine the best way to screen for IPV, and to help providers identify ways to best help women who are affected by IPV. It is important that the primary care provider knows of any local or state services equipped to help patients who screen positive for IPV.[51]

FAMILY HISTORY

The examination of the patient's family history including race, creed, ethnicity, and asking specifically about a family history of congenital defects or syndromes can help identify certain diseases that can be transferred from patient to child, such as congenital disease or metabolic syndromes. It is important to be aware of the patients' preferences or needs. The risks of transmission and the use of genetic screening is a complex issue, discussed in detail in an article elsewhere in this issue.

MEDICATION USE

As medications have the potential to affect the developing fetus, an examination of the patient's current use of medications (prescription, over-the-counter, and complementary and alternative medicines) should be reviewed. The US Food and Drug Administration (FDA) created a classification system that may be used with regard to the risk to the fetus during pregnancy. **Box 8** describes this system in detail.[57] The preconception counselor needs to conduct a review of the list and discuss the risks and benefits of each individual medication. Decisions should be made to continue or discontinue medications on an individual basis.

With the increase in availability and use of herbal supplements in the United States, the use of such agents should also be reviewed. In 1994, with the passage of the Dietary Supplement Health and Education Act of 1994 (DSHEA), dietary supplements (vitamins, minerals, herbals or other botanicals, and amino acids) were taken away from the jurisdiction of the FDA. It is now up to the manufacturer to determine the safety of such agents. The FDA is only allowed to evaluate products after they are sold on the market and if problems are reported. Therefore, products may not have undergone the strict studies that are required by prescription drugs before being placed on the market. Most of these products do not have any pregnancy safety

---

Box 8
FDA classification systems of medications in pregnancy

- Category A
  - Controlled studies show no fetal risk
  - Considered safe to use in pregnancy
- Category B
  - No evidence of risk in pregnancy
  - Considered safe to use in pregnancy
- Category C
  - Risk cannot be ruled out
  - Largest classification
  - Medications in this class used mainly on a risk versus benefit strategy
- Category D
  - Positive evidence of risk
  - There is documented risk as noted in human studies, but in some cases it still might be acceptable to use in certain individual situations and needs to be discussed with the patient on an individual basis
- Category X
  - Contraindicated in pregnancy
  - Medications show documented fetal abnormalities or death, and should be avoided in women who are pregnant or who may become pregnant

data; this should be discussed with the patient and the decision to continue using such supplements made on an individual basis.[58] Information can be found through the FDA (http://www.fda.gov) or the National Center for Complementary and Alternative Medicine, a division of the National Institutes of Health (http://nccam.nih.gov).

The final component of the medication history is the recommendation for a prenatal multivitamin or folic acid supplement. The ACOG recommends the use of folic acid to help decrease the risk of development of neural tube defects. The recommendation is for 0.4 mg of folic acid in low-risk women and 4 mg in women who are at high risk of neural tube defects (such as women on certain anticonvulsants) or women who have had a previous pregnancy complicated by a neural tube defect.[59]

VACCINATION HISTORY

Assessing a patient's immunization status is an important component when approaching a preconception counseling visit. Not only are there specific recommendations about which vaccines can be given during pregnancy, there are also recommendations about the time period during which a patient should avoid pregnancy after being administered a live attenuated vaccine.

The following are common vaccines that should be given or considered to be given around the time of pregnancy, based on the most current recommendations of the Advisory Committee on Immunization Practices (ACIP) at the time of writing. A complete listing of all recommendations and updates can be found on the CDC Web site at http://www.cdc.gov/vaccines.

Influenza

In 2010, the ACIP updated its current recommendations for influenza to include all people older than 6 months, including all women who are pregnant or may become pregnant during the influenza season (generally October 1 to March 31). The ACIP recommends using the trivalent inactivated influenza vaccine for this population.[60]

Tetanus/Pertussis

In 2010, because of an increase in the prevalence of pertussis in the United States over the last several years, the ACIP updated its current recommendations for the use of tetanus and acellular pertussis vaccine (Tdap). The ACIP states that adolescents aged 11 to 18 years who have completed the recommended childhood diphtheria and tetanus toxoids and pertussis (DTP) or diphtheria and tetanus toxoids and acellular pertussis (DTaP) vaccination series should receive a single dose of Tdap regardless of the length of time since previous vaccination. It also states that adults aged 19 to 64 years should receive a single dose of this vaccine regardless of the length of time since previous tetanus vaccination. If a Tdap booster has been given already, tetanus toxoid (Td) can be resumed on the previous schedule of every 5 to 10 years. Although Td has generally been considered safe to be given during pregnancy, no such safety data are available for the Tdap vaccine. When the indication for the use of Tdap rather than Td is present, this vaccine should be used and given either before planning on becoming pregnant (although this is not a live attenuated vaccine, no specific recommendation about the timing of the vaccine before pregnancy has been elucidated) or, if pregnant, after delivery and before discharge from the hospital.[61]

Hepatitis B

The ACIP recommends testing all pregnant women or women planning on becoming pregnant for the hepatitis B surface antigen (HBsAg) regardless of previous testing or vaccination status. This test is done to help ensure that all infants born to HBsAg-positive women receive the appropriate vaccination and prophylaxis regimen. The vaccine is not a live attenuated vaccine, and therefore may be given during pregnancy. If possible, the vaccine series should be given in its 3-dose regimen before pregnancy, as the data on its safety are still limited. If the patient is already pregnant, then only those women deemed at high risk of developing an acute hepatitis B infection during pregnancy should be vaccinated. Risk factors could include, but are not limited to, having more than 1 sex partner during the previous 6 months, having been evaluated or treated for a sexually transmitted infection, recent or current injected drug use, or having had an HBsAg-positive sex partner.[62]

Rubella

The ACIP recommends that all women who are pregnant or who may become pregnant be tested for rubella immunity. For the patient who is not immune to rubella, the measles-mumps-rubella (MMR) vaccine should be given. As this is a live attenuated vaccine, the patient should be counseled to wait at least 4 weeks after immunization before becoming pregnant. If pregnancy is planned sooner or if the patient is already pregnant, she should receive the MMR vaccine postpartum, before discharge from the hospital.[63]

Varicella

The ACIP recommends that all women who are pregnant or who may become pregnant be tested for varicella immunity to help prevent as much as possible a nosocomial infection and/or congenital varicella syndrome. For the patient who is not immune to varicella, the varicella (VZV) 2-dose vaccination series should be given 4 to 8 weeks apart. As this is another live attenuated vaccine, the patient should be counseled to wait at least 4 weeks after the second dose before becoming pregnant. If pregnancy is planned sooner or if the patient is already pregnant, she should receive the first dose of the VZV after delivery before discharge from the hospital, and the second dose 4 to 8 weeks later, which usually corresponds well with the timing of the postpartum visit.[64]

REFERENCES

1. Ogden CL, Carroll MD, Curtin LR, et al. Prevalence of overweight and obesity in the United States, 1999-2004. JAMA 2006;295(13):1549–55.
2. Flegal KM, Carroll MD, Ogden CL, et al. Prevalence and trends in obesity among United States adults, 1999-2008. JAMA 2010;303(3):235–41.
3. Davis E, Olson C. Obesity in pregnancy. Prim Care Clin Office Pract 2009;36(2): 341–56.
4. Lee CY, Koren G. Maternal obesity: effects on pregnancy and the role of preconception counseling. J Obstet Gynecol 2010;30(2):101–6.
5. Chobanian AV, Bakris GL, Black HR, et al. Seventh report of the Joint National Committee on Prevention, Detection, Evaluation, and Treatment of High Blood Pressure. Hypertension 2003;42(6):1206–52.
6. ACOG Committee on Practice Bulletins. ACOG practice bulletin. Chronic hypertension in pregnancy. Obstet Gynecol 2001;98(Suppl 1):177–85.
7. Magee LA, Schick B, Donnenfeld AE, et al. The safety of calcium channel blockers in human pregnancy: a prospective, multicenter cohort study. Am J Obstet Gynecol 1996;174(3):823–8.
8. Report of the National High Blood Pressure Education Program Working Group on High Blood Pressure in Pregnancy. Am J Obstet Gynecol 2000;183:S1–22.

9. Reece EA, Homko CJ. Prepregnancy care and the prevention of fetal malformation in the pregnancy complicated by diabetes. Clin Obstet Gynecol 2007;50(4): 990–7.
10. ACOG Committee on Practice Bulletins. ACOG practice bulletin. Pregestational diabetes mellitus. Obstet Gynecol 2005;105(3):675–85.
11. American Diabetes Association. Preconception care of women with diabetes. Diabetes Care 2005;27(Suppl 1):S76–8.
12. Pratt LA, Brody DJ. Depression in the United States household population, 2005-2006. NCHS Data Brief 2008;(7):1–8.
13. Marcus SC, Olfson M. National trends in the treatment for depression from 1998 to 2007. Arch Gen Psychiatry 2010;67(12):1265–73.
14. Yonkers KA, Wisner KL, Stewart DE, et al. The management of depression during pregnancy: a report from the American Psychiatric Association and the American College of Obstetricians and Gynecologists. Obstet Gynecol 2009;114(3):703–13.
15. Fitzpatrick DL, Russell MA. Diagnosis and management of thyroid disease in pregnancy. Obstet Gynecol Clin N Am 2010;37(2):173–93.
16. Davis LE, Leveno KJ, Cunningham FG. Hypothyroidism complicating pregnancy. Obstet Gynecol 1988;72(1):108–12.
17. ACOG Committee on Practice Bulletins. ACOG practice bulletin. Thyroid disease in pregnancy. Obstet Gynecol 2002;100(2):387–96.
18. Gyamfi C, Wapner RJ, D'Alton ME. Thyroid dysfunction in pregnancy. Obstet Gynecol 2009;133(3):702–7.
19. Martin JA, Hamilton BE, Sutton PD, et al. Births: final data for 2007. Natl Vital Stat Rep 2010;58(27):1–85.
20. Mercer MM, Goldenberg RL, Moawad AH, et al. The preterm prediction study: effect of gestational age and cause of preterm birth on subsequent obstetric outcome. National Child Health and Human Development Maternal-Fetal Medicine Units Network. Am J Obstet Gynecol 1999;185(5):1216–21.
21. Adams MM, Elam-Evans LD, Wilson HG, et al. Rates of and factors associated with recurrence of preterm delivery. JAMA 2000;283(12):1591–6.
22. Dodd JM, Flenady V, Cincotta R, et al. Prenatal administration of progesterone for preventing preterm birth in women considered to be at risk of preterm birth. Cochrane Database Syst Rev 2006;1:CD004947. DOI:10.1002/14651858. CD004947.pub2.
23. American College of Obstetricians and Gynecologists. Use of progesterone to reduce preterm birth, ACOG Committee Opinion No. 419, October 2008 (replaces No. 291, November 2003). Obstet Gynecol 2008;112(4):963–5.
24. Meis PJ, Klebanoff M, Thom E, et al. Prevention of recurrent preterm delivery by 17 alpha-hydroxyprogesterone caproate. National Institute of Child Health and Human Development Maternal-Fetal Medicine Units Network [published erratum appears in N Engl J Med 2003;349:1299]. N Engl J Med 2003;348:2379–85.
25. Hernandez-Diaz S, Toh S, Cnattingius S. Risk of pre-eclampsia In first and subsequent pregnancies: prospective cohort study. BMJ 2009;338:b2255.
26. Barton JR, Sibai BM. Prediction and prevention of recurrent preeclampsia. Obstet Gynecol 2008;112(2):359–72.
27. Gujold E, Roberge S, Lacasse Y, et al. Prevention of preeclampsia and intrauterine growth restriction with aspirin started in early pregnancy: a meta-analysis. Obstet Gynecol 2010;116(2):402–14.
28. ACOG Committee on Practice Bulletins. ACOG practice bulletin. Diagnosis and management of preeclampsia and eclampsia, number 33, January 2002. Obstet Gynecol 2002;99(1):159–67.

29. Stirrat GM. Recurrent miscarriage I: definition and epidemiology. Lancet 1990; 336:673–5.
30. Stephenson M, Kutteh W. Evaluation and management of recurrent early pregnancy loss. Clin Obstet Gynecol 2007;50(1):132–45.
31. ACOG Committee on Practice Bulletins. ACOG practice bulletin. Management of recurrent pregnancy loss, number 24, February 2001 (replaces technical bulletin number 212, September 1995). Int J Gynaecol Obstet 2002;78(2):179–90.
32. American Society of Reproductive Medicine Practice Committee. Definitions of infertility and recurrent pregnancy loss. Fertil Steril 2008;90(Suppl 5):S60.
33. Frey KA, Patel KS. Initial evaluation and management of infertility by the primary care physician. Mayo Clin Proc 2004;79(11):1439–43.
34. Centers for Disease Control and Prevention. Vital signs: current cigarette smoking among adults aged ≥18 years—United States, 2009. MMWR Morb Mortal Wkly Rep 2010;59(35):1135–40.
35. Einarson A, Riordan S. Smoking in pregnancy and lactation: a review of risks and cessation strategies. Eur J Clin Pharmacol 2009;65:325–30.
36. United States Preventive Services Task Force. Counseling and interventions to prevent tobacco use and tobacco caused disease in adults and pregnant women: United States Preventive Services Task Force Reaffirmation Recommendation Statement. Ann Intern Med 2009;150:551–5.
37. American College of Obstetricians and Gynecologists. Smoking cessation during pregnancy, ACOG Committee Opinion No. 316. Obstet Gynecol 2005;106(4): 883–8.
38. Muhuri PK, Gfroerer JC. Substance use among women: associations with pregnancy, parenting, and race/ethnicity. Matern Child Health J 2009;13:376–85.
39. Wattendorf DJ, Muenke M. Fetal alcohol spectrum disorders. Am Fam Physician 2005;72(2):279–82.
40. May PA, Gossage JP. Estimating the prevalence of fetal alcohol syndrome. Alcohol Res Health 2001;25(3):159–67.
41. Substance Abuse and Mental Health Services Administration. Results from the 2009 National Survey on Drug Use and Health: Volume I. Summary of national findings (Office of Applied Studies, NSDUH Series H-38A, HHS Publication No. SMA 10-4586 Findings). Rockville (MD): Substance Abuse and Mental Health Services Administration; 2010.
42. Floyd RL, Jack BW, Cefalo R, et al. The clinical content of preconception care: alcohol, tobacco, and illicit drug exposures. Am J Obstet Gynecol 2008; 199(6 Suppl 2):S333–9.
43. Centers for Disease Control and Prevention. Sexually transmitted disease surveillance 2009. Atlanta (GA): US Department of Health and Human Services; 2010.
44. Centers for Disease Control and Prevention. HIV surveillance report, 2009; vol. 21. Available at: http://www.cdc.gov/hiv/topics/surveillance/resources/reports/. Published February 2011. Accessed March 15, 2011.
45. Majeroni BA, Ukkadam S. Screening and treatment for sexually transmitted infections in pregnancy. Am Fam Physician 2007;76(2):265–70.
46. Genc M, Ledger WJ. Syphilis in pregnancy. Sex Transm Infect 2000;76:73–9.
47. Volmink J, Siegfried NL, van der Merwe L, et al. Antiretrovirals for reducing the risk of mother-to-child transmission of HIV infection. Cochrane Database Syst Rev 2007;1:CD003510.
48. Meyers D, Wolff T, Gregory K, et al. USPSTF recommendations for STI screening. Am Fam Physician 2008;77(6):819–24.

49. Chu SY, Goodwin MM, D'Angelo DV. Physical violence against U.S. women around the time of pregnancy, 2004-2007. Am J Prev Med 2010;38(3):317–22.
50. Chambliss LR. Intimate partner violence and its implication for pregnancy. Clin Obstet Gynecol 2008;81(2):385–97.
51. Sarkar NN. The impact of intimate partner violence on women's reproductive health and pregnancy outcome. J Obstet Gynecol 2008;28(3):266–71.
52. United States Preventative Services Task Force. Screening for family and intimate partner violence: recommendation statement. Ann Fam Med 2004;2(2):156–60.
53. American College of Obstetricians and Gynecologists. Psychosocial risk factors: perinatal screening and intervention, ACOG Committee Opinion No. 343. Obstet Gynecol 2006;108(2):469–77.
54. American Academy of Family Physicians. Policy on family and intimate partner violence and abuse. Available at: www.aafp.org/online/en/home/policy/policies/f/familyandintimatepartner-violenceandabuse.html. Accessed March 12, 2011.
55. American Academy of Pediatrics, Committee on Child Abuse and Neglect. The role of the pediatrician in recognizing and intervening on behalf of abused women. Pediatrics 1998;101:1091–2.
56. American Medical Association. Diagnostic and treatment guidelines on domestic violence. Arch Fam Med 1992;1(1):39–47.
57. Mehta N, Larson L. Pharmacotherapy in pregnancy and lactation. Clin Chest Med 2011;32(1):43–52.
58. US Food and Drug Administration. Dietary supplements. Available at: http://www.fda.gov/Food/DietarySupplements/default.htm. Accessed March 15, 2011.
59. ACOG Committee on Practice Bulletins. ACOG practice bulletin. Neural tube defects, number 44, July 2003. Obstet Gynecol 2003;102(1):203–13.
60. Centers for Disease Control and Prevention. Prevention and control of influenza with vaccines: recommendations of the Advisory Committee on Immunization Practices (ACIP), 2010. MMWR 2010;59(No. RR-8):32–7.
61. Centers for Disease Control and Prevention. Updated recommendations for use of tetanus toxoid, reduced diphtheria toxoid and acellular pertussis (Tdap) vaccine from the Advisory Committee on Immunization Practices, 2010. MMWR 2011;60(No. RR-1):13–5.
62. Centers for Disease Control and Prevention. A comprehensive immunization strategy to eliminate transmission of hepatitis B virus infection in the United States: recommendations of the Advisory Committee on Immunization Practices (ACIP) part 1: immunization of infants, children, and adolescents. MMWR 2005;54(No. RR-16):12–4.
63. Centers for Disease Control and Prevention. Measles, mumps, and rubella—vaccine use and strategies for elimination of measles, rubella, and congenital rubella syndrome and control of mumps: recommendations of the Advisory Committee on Immunization Practices (ACIP). MMWR 1998;47(No. RR-8):32–3.
64. Centers for Disease Control and Prevention. Prevention of varicella: recommendations of the Advisory Committee on Immunization Practices (ACIP). MMWR Recomm Rep 2007;56(No. RR-4):16–7, 24–6.

Prenatal Care: Touching the Future

Erin Kate Dooley, MD, MPH[a],*, Robert L. Ringler Jr, MD[b,c]

KEYWORDS

- Antenatal • Prenatal • Pregnancy • Preconception
- Testing and screening • Patient education

The provision of preconception and prenatal care is a critical and time-honored role for family physicians. It could even be termed the first preventive care a human being receives. It has been suggested by some studies that, because of the continuity of care that is considered a cornerstone of family practice, family physicians provide prenatal care that may improve birth outcome.[1,2] Although prenatal care is acknowledged as important for a healthy pregnancy and delivery, there is debate regarding the true efficacy of prenatal care. This debate leads one to question, "Is prenatal care really important? If so, why and what components make it so?"

PRENATAL CARE: A BRIEF HISTORY

In 1985, the Institute of Medicine issued a report promoting a national policy goal of enrolling all pregnant women into a system of prenatal care to reduce the risk of delivering a low birth weight infant.[3] This report resulted in changes and legislative initiatives passed by the US Congress, expanding Medicaid eligibility to low-income pregnant women and children independent of their welfare status.[3] Since that time, great expense and effort have been expended to clarify barriers to timely prenatal care and subsequently to increase enrollment and participation in prenatal care programs with some success. Prenatal care is now one of the most frequently used health services in the United States and, after general medical examination, prenatal care is the most frequently cited preventive health service.[4] Although still slightly less than the Healthy People 2000 and Healthy People 2010 objectives of 90% initiation of prenatal care within the first trimester, participation has increased to more than 83% of women.[5]

The authors have nothing to disclose.
[a] Médicos Para La Familia, Department of Surgical Family Medicine, 3030 Covington Pike, Memphis, TN 38128, USA
[b] Department of Family and Community Medicine, Eastern Virginia Medical School, PO Box 1980, Norfolk, VA 23501, USA
[c] Portsmouth Family Medicine, Department of Family and Community Medicine, 600 Crawford Street, Suite 300, Portsmouth, VA 23704, USA
* Corresponding author.
E-mail address: erinkatedooley@gmail.com

Prim Care Clin Office Pract 39 (2012) 17–37
doi:10.1016/j.pop.2011.11.002   primarycare.theclinics.com
0095-4543/12/$ – see front matter © 2012 Elsevier Inc. All rights reserved.

Despite these strides, there are still large disparities in adequate use between teenagers and adults. Higher-risk women are less likely to begin care as early as low-risk women.[4,6] Although the gap has narrowed, African American women and women with less education lag behind in their use of timely prenatal care.[5–7] Several variables have been identified in the literature as barriers to timely care (**Box 1**).[8–12]

Efforts to target these different barriers are under way through a variety of different programs and practices. Yet the questions remain: are these efforts appropriate and effective? Is prenatal care really a good investment?

The Institute of Medicine estimated that for every dollar spent on prenatal care for women at high risk, $3.38 is saved in medical care costs for low birth weight infants.[13] However, a comprehensive literature review by Fiscella in 1995 found that "studies of the cost effectiveness of prenatal care...overestimated the impact of prenatal care on birth outcomes." Alexander and Kotelchuck[3] came to a similar conclusion, stating that "our current prenatal care approaches are not particularly effective and cannot be given a wholehearted endorsement" as being effective in preventing preterm births. Preterm bias, which refers to the fact that premature delivery results in fewer prenatal visits, is a confounding factor that may have overestimated the impact of prenatal care on reducing premature delivery and low birth weights (often a concurrent circumstance). When controlled for preterm bias, prenatal care has not proved to improve birth outcomes, reduce rates of preterm delivery, or reduce low birth weight to a statistically significant degree.[2,3,13]

Nevertheless, many believe that prenatal care is effective, but research has focused in the wrong area. Some caution that cost-effectiveness and live birth outcomes should not be the only measure of effectiveness. In his 1995 article, Fiscella points out that prenatal care serves as a gateway to ongoing, continuous health care for women.[13] Similarly, prenatal care may have benefits for reducing maternal morbidity and mortality that go unaccounted when research focuses purely on live infant birth outcomes.[3] In addition, studies failed to note the impact of prenatal care on fetal mortality. Early detection of fetal problems or distress may enable earlier therapeutic intervention or interruption of pregnancy to reduce the risk of fetal morbidity and mortality.[3] Thus, although the baby may still potentially be born prematurely with a lower birth weight (thus prenatal care is deemed ineffective by these measures), consistent prenatal care was possibly able to avoid the death or injury of the child. Perhaps most importantly, prenatal care also offers an opportunity for health education and has been cited as a means of reducing ethnic variations in adverse pregnancy

---

Box 1
Barriers to timely prenatal care

- Sociodemographic characteristics
  - Educational attainment
  - Mental status
  - Language difficulties
- Varying attitudes and beliefs regarding importance of prenatal care
- Stressful life events/circumstances
- Logistic barriers
  - Transportation
  - Difficulty getting appointments

outcomes.[8] Counseling, education, and communication can have a long-lasting impact on morbidity and overall health of the mother and the baby through early interventions on risk factors such as smoking, alcohol and drug use, education regarding proper dietary precautions and balance, and detection and management of sexually transmitted diseases (STDs).[7,14,15]

Prenatal care may not be able to reliably change the timeline or progression of labor to prevent preterm births and the concomitant low birth weights; prenatal care is a critical health service that cannot be abandoned or minimized because of the opportunity it affords to offer health education in the course of a patient's life. Perhaps the key to the preventive aspects of prenatal care arises from education and counseling. If this is true, clear and open communication is the key to quality prenatal care. This idea is supported by the findings of Bennett and colleagues in their 2006 study[7] of prenatal care among African American women of low and high literacy. In this study, Bennett and colleagues found that "women described poor-quality clinicians as unable to provide health information in a clear, accessible form. Some women reported that they did not tell the clinician when they did not understand. Some stated a belief that their clinicians knew that they did not understand and still did nothing to help them." Although this was a small study, women who experienced good communication generally had better prenatal care use, which also corresponded with better outcomes in some measures.

Studies such as this highlight the importance of the communication and educational components of care. Nevertheless, it must be acknowledged that these are surrogate measures lacking randomized trials based on outcomes.

PRECONCEPTION

The preconception visit is an opportunity to initiate preventive care and open discussion for counseling. Please refer to the article elsewhere in this issue for more on this subject. According to the Institute for Clinical Systems Improvement, a preconception visit is defined as a health maintenance visit, within the 12 months preceding a pregnancy, in which topics and guidance specifically related to pregnancy and maternal health are discussed. This process can easily be incorporated in to the annual well woman examination for any woman of child-bearing age who is trying to conceive or simply not taking pregnancy preventive measures with reliable contraception. During these visits, patients should be counseled regarding prevention and risk reduction measures and healthy lifestyle choices to optimize health in preparation for a pregnancy. Among important topics to discuss are maintenance of a healthy weight (or weight loss or gain as needed), physical activity, substance use, appropriate vaccinations and immunity (especially distancing live-virus immunizations from time of conception), and environmental safety, including intimate partner violence screening and counseling.[15–25] In addition, all women should be counseled on preconception folic acid supplementation to prevent neural tube defects.[15,26,27]

Women with preexisting conditions or a history of other conditions complicating pregnancy (eg, gestational diabetes, pregnancy-induced hypertension) may require further screening and counseling. Medications and herbal supplements should be reviewed and assessed for safety in early pregnancy. Teratogenic medications such as angiotensin-converting enzyme inhibitors, statins, and anticonvulsants should be changed to an agent that is known to be safe in pregnancy. Women with risk factors for gestational diabetes or a history of gestational diabetes should undergo annual diabetic screening.[17,28–30] In addition, abnormal blood pressures in the preconception period should be assessed and managed appropriately with a special focus on healthy lifestyle changes to optimize therapy.

TIMING VISITS

In 1989, the American College of Obstetrics and Gynecology produced a set of guidelines from the Public Health Services Expert Panel that laid out recommendations on the timing and content of prenatal care visits. This schedule reduced the total number of visits from previously adopted models and emphasized educational components at different stages of pregnancy.[31–35] During weeks 4 to 28 of gestational age, routine visits are suggested every 4 weeks. The recommended frequency increases to every 2 to 3 weeks between 28 and 36 weeks' gestation followed by weekly visits thereafter until delivery.[36] This timeline has not been universally adopted and varies widely among nations.

FIRST VISIT

Because education and counseling have been shown to be an important and effective component of prenatal care, the first visit takes on greater importance. In addition, because of the quantity of information that must be exchanged during this visit, it may be useful to divide the visit into 2 closely spaced visits to facilitate thoroughness on the part of the physician and improved absorption and understanding on the part of the patient.[37]

The initial prenatal visit requires a thorough patient history to include past medical history (including chronic conditions and current medications), obstetric and gynecologic history, sexual history, past surgeries (including cervical procedures), family history (focusing on inherited or congenital health issues), and a social history. This information helps the physician to determine which screenings and follow-up counseling are appropriate. In addition, the history opens the door for educational topics, including nutrition and weight gain, prenatal vitamins and supplementation, domestic violence, alcohol and drug use, genetic screening, and occupational conditions that affect pregnancy.

Along with a complete history and physical examination, several important screening laboratory tests are indicated early in pregnancy and help determine appropriate treatment or interventions as the pregnancy progresses. These tests include:

- Complete blood count (CBC)
- Blood typing and antibody screen
- Urinalysis and culture
- Cervical cytology
- Syphilis screening
- Gonorrhea and chlamydia testing
- Human immunodeficiency virus (HIV) testing
- Hepatitis B surface antigen testing
- Rubella and varicella immunity verification
- Hemoglobin electrophoresis, tuberculosis, toxoplasmosis, and hepatitis C testing in special populations.

CBC, Blood Typing, Antibody Screen, and Hemoglobinopathies

The CBC is used to identify anemia early in pregnancy. The World Health Organization defines anemia in pregnancy as a hemoglobin value less than 11 g/dL. Iron deficiency is the most common cause of anemia in pregnancy worldwide.[38] There is a physiologic anemia seen in pregnancy secondary to the relatively greater expansion of plasma volume compared with the increase in red blood cell mass, resulting in a decrease in the concentration of hemoglobin in the blood. This process serves the function of decreasing the viscosity of the blood and, thus, in theory, enhances placental perfusion.[39] For this reason, treatment of anemia and the hemoglobin level at which to initiate therapy are controversial. There are known risks of complications, with blood loss during the delivery and an increased risk for cardiac heart failure with hemoglobin levels less than 7 g/dL. Several studies suggest that hemoglobin levels between 7 and 10 g/dL are also a risk factor for fetal death, prematurity, low birth weight, and other adverse outcomes. Therefore, it is generally accepted that treatment is indicated for hemoglobin levels less than 10 g/dL.[40–42] However, it may be acceptable and even beneficial to mother and fetus to monitor but refrain from iron therapy treatment of mild anemia (Hb 10–11 g/dL).[38,39,42]

Blood typing and antibody screening indicate the need to test and prophylactically treat ABO and Rh incompatibility. Women who are Rh(D) negative and may be pregnant with an Rh(D)-positive fetus require prophylaxis with RhoGAM whenever there is a potential exposure to fetal blood in the maternal circulation (ie, trauma, abortion, amniocentesis, chorionic villus sampling [CVS], or external cephalic version). Because the Rh(D) status of the fetus is unknown until delivery, these precautions are generally taken with all Rh(D)-negative women. This therapy is also indicated at 28 weeks' gestational age (and post partum if the baby tests positive for Rh+ blood type) for Rh(D)-negative women.

Some populations require special screening for various forms of hemoglobinopathies. Individuals of African descent may be screened for sickle cell anemia with a CBC and electrophoresis.[43–45] Similarly, individuals at known risk for thalassemia may be screened initially with CBC and electrophoresis. A CBC and red blood count index are usually sufficient for patients who are not of African descent. However, if results show anemia with a reduced mean corpuscular volume and normal iron studies, an electrophoresis should also be obtained in addition to this screen because this may represent risk of thalassemia or other hemoglobinopathy.[14] This topic is not without dissenting opinion, and 1 author has never seen a management-changing result from such screening because patients with known sickle cell crisis are referred to maternal-fetal medicine management.

Urinalysis and Culture

In the United States, urinalysis and culture are recommended for all women at the initial visit to identify asymptomatic bacteriuria (ASB). The prevalence of ASB in pregnancy is approximately 2.5% to 11%. ASB becomes a risk factor for more serious infection, with 20% to 40% of untreated women developing pyelonephritis during pregnancy.[46–48] However, this situation is rare; at Médicos Para La Familia in Memphis, Tennessee, 1 in 500 patients per year have ASB and there have been no linked cases of pylonephritis in 20 years of practice.

Sexually Transmitted Infection Screening

Because of the significant complications that can be posed by sexually transmitted infection (STI) during pregnancy, the Center for Disease Control recommends comprehensive STI screening for all women early in pregnancy and again near delivery (if indicated based on personal risk factors or regional prevalence data). Because of the relative risk bias that drives this screening, other countries disagree and opt to save precious medical funding by not participating in this type of screening. Women with an STI are at higher risk for premature labor, premature rupture of membranes, and postpartum endometritis.[49,50] In addition, risks to the fetus include stillbirth, low birth weight, pneumonia, conjunctivitis, neonatal sepsis, neurologic damage, blindness, deafness, and liver damage or disease.[51–53] These outcomes are largely preventable with appropriate treatment, thus emphasizing the necessity of early screening.

Immunity Verification

Because of the potentially devastating effects of maternal infection with rubella and varicella, screening for immunity is a common component of early prenatal care. Immunization for both of these conditions during pregnancy is not possible but awareness of the lack of immunity should raise the patient's precautionary measures around any others that may have active infection. Immunization should be offered after delivery,[53] typically with measles, mumps, rubella vaccine rather than rubella vaccine alone (for cost reasons).

FIRST-TRIMESTER COUNSELING

Informed and educated families are critical to healthy pregnancies for mother and baby. The first trimester and the first few visits can involve sharing a large amount of information. Weaving this education into patient history-taking may make the information more relevant to the patient. Clear and simple handouts with appropriate reading level text and pictures can be helpful to the patient.

Nutrition, Vitamins and Supplements, and Weight Gain

Women should eat a well-balanced diet throughout pregnancy, with a diet geared toward appropriate weight gain based on prepregnancy weight. In addition, supplementation with a daily prenatal multivitamin is commonly recommended. Calcium supplementation to attain a daily recommended intake of 1000 to 1300 mg is recommended to decrease blood pressure and preeclampsia.[54,55] Folic acid supplementation from 4 to 12 weeks' gestational age is recommended to prevent neural tube defects (0.4–0.8 mg for primary prevention, 4 mg/d in a pregnant woman with a history of a fetus with a neural tube defect).[15,56] There is mixed evidence on recommendations for iron and vitamin D supplementation, and this should be considered on a case-by-case basis.

Women whose prepregnancy body mass index (BMI, calculated as weight in kilograms divided by the square of height in meters) is less than 18.5 (under weight) are encouraged to increase their caloric intake more than those with a BMI in the normal (18.5–24.9), overweight (25–29.9), or obese (>30) categories. According to the Institute of Medicine guidelines (which are summarized in **Table 1**), total weight gain and rate of weight gain in the second and third trimester for an overweight patient are half that recommended for an underweight patient. This point is particularly important on both ends of the spectrum in reducing risks for preterm birth (for the underweight patient)[57,58] or gestational diabetes, preeclampsia, induction of labor or primary

| Table 1 | | |
| Institute of Medicine guidelines for weight gain in pregnancy | | |
Prepregnancy BMI	Total Target Weight Gain (lbs)	Weight Gain Target Rate (lbs/wk)
Underweight (<18.5)	28–40 (12.7–18.2)	1–1.3 (0.45–0.59)
Normal (18.5–24.9)	25–35 (11.4–15.9)	0.8–1 (0.36–0.45)
Overweight (25–29.9)	15–25 (6.8–11.4)	0.5–0.7 (0.23–0.32)
Obese (>30)	11–20 (5–9.1)	0.4–0.6 (0.18–0.27)

cesarean section, shoulder dystocia, and postsurgical complication (for the over-weight patient).[57–64] Please see the article elsewhere in this issue for more information on this subject.

Drug and Alcohol Use

There is strong evidence on the catastrophic effects of alcohol, tobacco, and illicit drug use during pregnancy. Fetal alcohol spectrum disorder is the most common preventable cause of mental disability[25,65,66]; tobacco use increases the risk of low birth weight infants[37,67–70]; and illicit drugs have various deleterious effects from increased risk of placental abruption to an association with other high-risk behaviors.[71–79] Consistent screening and counseling have been shown to be effective in reducing exposure to these substances.[25,65,70,80]

Intimate Partner Violence

Screening for intimate partner violence is recommended both during preconception counseling and during prenatal care, especially because some studies suggest pregnancy as a risk factor in and of itself. Up to 46% of pregnant women reported a history of abuse at some point in the past, with 7% to 18% of women reporting physical abuse during their current pregnancy.[81–84] Counseling and intervention have not been shown to statistically significantly improve morbidity or mortality for mother or baby; however, at least 1 study reported that safety behaviors during and after pregnancy improved in those women offered intervention or resources.[85]

Genetic Screening

Antepartum genetic screening is an important modality for helping to identify and address some factors that might make a pregnancy high risk. Screening can be tailored based on patient demographics or predisposing factors and should consider both maternal and paternal factors, including age, race, family history, history of previous pregnancy loss, substance abuse, and serious health conditions of the mother. With any screening that is undertaken, it is important that the patient and family understand the test itself, the sensitivity and specificity, and the decisions or options that may need to be considered based on the results of the test. This discussion should happen before testing is undertaken and may even affect the decision to screen or not to screen for certain conditions. In Latin cultures, this type of screening is rare.

Occupational Issues in Pregnancy

Most employment is not a risk factor for suboptimal outcomes in pregnancy. However, specific characteristics such as heavy lifting, prolonged standing (>4 hours per shift), noisy or cold environments, mental stress, or excessive work hours (>36 hours per week or 10 hours per day) have all been shown to place affected women at higher risk for preterm labor, low birth weight, or pregnancy-induced hypertension.[86–89] In addition, occupations that expose patients to anesthetic agents, radiation, solvents, inhaled agents, or pesticides are also associated with increased risk of miscarriage, malformations, and other poor outcomes. Patients should be advised of these risks, and assisted with work-related documentation that may be required to reduce or eliminate these risks.

ROUTINE VISITS

There is mixed evidence as to the usefulness of different components traditionally used in a routine visit. Numerous studies have been conducted on every procedure from fundal height measurement and maternal weight gain tracking to routine urinalysis and fetal heart tone measurements.[47,59,90,91] Generally, the following components are included in routine assessment:

- Fundal height
- Maternal weight
- Maternal blood pressure
- Fetal heart auscultation
- Urine testing for protein and glucose[a]
- Fetal movement monitoring (FMM).

[a]This is the most controversial component and is not universally performed on a routine basis.

VISITS 4 TO 12

Components of the initial antepartum visit have already been detailed. During the period between 10 and 12 weeks' gestational age, fetal heart tones should be identifiable and this test can be incorporated into the routine visit.

For women with uncertain or atypical (onset, duration, amount of flow) last menstrual dates, early ultrasonography is essential. Because gestational age drives the timing of all other screening tests, as well as interventions late in pregnancy, it is critical that accurate dating be established as early as possible. Early dating ultrasonography is usually preformed between estimated weeks 6 and 12 of gestation for best accuracy.

Although not a required standard, early ultrasonography also permits measurement of nuchal translucency between weeks 10 and 14 of gestational age as part of a first-trimester genetic screening program (not recommended at 14 or greater weeks of gestation), at which time maternal serum screening tests are also drawn (described in greater detail later). If these results show increased risk, confirmatory testing with CVS between 10 and 12 weeks' gestational age may also be offered. Alternatively, these results may also be held until tetra screen results are drawn at 15 to 21 weeks' gestation.[92,93] The first-trimester nuchal skin fold or nuchal translucency measuring requires specialized ultrasonography training and may not be available at all treatment facilities.

In addition, some populations may benefit from early glucola screening (at the first prenatal visit) to identify gestational diabetes (or even preexisting but undiagnosed nongestational diabetes mellitus). At-risk women should be screened as early as possible to facilitate intervention and treatment.[94–99] According to American Diabetes Association recommendations, women diagnosed with a positive 1-hour glucose tolerance test in the first trimester or at first presentation should be diagnosed with nongestational diabetes mellitus in pregnancy rather than gestational diabetes.

Regional Highlight: Deep South

According to the US Centers for Disease Control (CDC), the Deep South region has one of the highest rates of obesity and diabetes in the United States and has been dubbed the Diabetes Belt. More than 75% of counties in the region have 27% or more of the entire population fitting the diagnosis of obese and 11.3% or more of the population diagnosed with diabetes. It is also estimated that 25% of those who would meet the diagnostic criteria for diabetes have not yet been diagnosed. This finding emphasizes the importance of early gestational diabetes screening for at-risk patients in this region who may have the condition before pregnancy but have not sought care or have not been diagnosed.

WEEKS 12 TO 28

During this period of pregnancy, the gravid condition becomes a more obvious reality to the patient and the family, with quickening taking place around 20 weeks' gestational age for nulliparous and 18 to 20 weeks for multiparous women. Educational topics usually begin to turn to more concrete topics of pregnancy, labor, and delivery. Several additional screening procedures also take place during this phase.

Between weeks 15 and 19 of gestation, all pregnant women may be offered serum marker screening for trisomies 21 and 18 and open neural tube defects.[14,37] As mentioned earlier, these screening tests are ideally discussed in the visits before the window in which the markers are drawn for greatest accuracy. This strategy allows patients to consider their options and make informed and personal decisions regarding screening. This screening test usually consists of midtrimester triple (human chorionic gonadotropin, unconjugated estradiol, and α-fetoprotein) or quad or tetra (triple plus inhibin-A) maternal serum screening. Some facilities have the ability to add fetal nuchal translucency by ultrasound screening. If the serum screening examination is positive, women should be offered confirmatory testing with amniocentesis. Amniocentesis may be performed after 15 weeks' gestation.[100–102] Discussing positive reasons for the testing, such as early diagnosis of conditions that may change the location and intensity of care provided to the patient and her infant at delivery, rather than for purposes of detecting a defect for which termination may be considered, may make all the difference in the patient's desiring or rejecting this testing.

Ultrasound assessment for morphology, ideally scheduled between weeks 18 and 20 of gestation, has also become a standard part of prenatal care. Although there is no evidence that ultrasonography improves overall outcomes, there has been nothing to show that ultrasound imaging poses any risks. Furthermore, the ease of access and high-quality imaging available to parents makes it a popular option. The Routine Antenatal Diagnostic Imaging with Ultrasound Study (RADIUS) found that 85% of patients had recognized indications for ultrasonography, and thus it is an insurance-covered service for most patients with such coverage.[14,103,104]

Screening for gestational diabetes is ideally performed between weeks 24 and 28 of gestation.[105–110] Initial screening usually consists of a 1-hour glucola screening test, which involves blood glucose testing 1 hour after a 50-g oral glucose load. The definition of positive screening results varies between greater than 130 mg/dL and greater than 140 mg/dL. A positive screening test should be followed up with a diagnostic 3-hour glucose tolerance test. A positive fasting value, or 2 values more than the normal levels at any point during the test, are considered diagnostic for gestational diabetes.[94,111–115] Again, there are 2 diagnostic standards, both detailed in **Table 2**.

Even although treatment has been shown to benefit mother and baby by reducing delivery complications and serious perinatal outcomes without increasing the rate of

Table 2		
Diagnostic criteria for 100-g oral glucose tolerance test		
	Blood Glucose Reading (mg/dL) (Carpenter-Coustan Scale)	Blood Glucose Reading (mg/dL) (National Diabetes Data Group Scale)
Fasting	95	105
1 h	180	190
2 h	155	165
3 h	140	145

cesarean sections,[116] screening has not been shown to be beneficial (see the article on gestational diabetes mellitus elsewhere in this issue).

As discussed earlier, women with Rh(D)-negative blood types should receive Rho-GAM to prevent isoimmunization and its feared complication of erythroblastosis fetalis. Several trials in the late 1980s proved that administration of immunoglobulin D at 28 weeks' gestational age for unsensitized women successfully reduces antenatal isoimmunization to less than 2% overall.[117]

SECOND-TRIMESTER COUNSELING AND EDUCATION

As mentioned earlier, topics for education in the second trimester tend to address the emerging and preeminent issues of the developing pregnancy. Among the many important topics to discuss in this trimester are pain and discomforts of middle pregnancy, sexuality, breastfeeding decisions, signs and symptoms of preterm labor, and anesthesia in labor. Many of these discussions can allow the patient time to consider choices that must be made, as well as having a greater sense of control during the process of pregnancy.

Pain and Discomfort During Pregnancy

Discomfort or pain is a common complaint in pregnancy, especially as it advances closer to term. According to a 2008 Cochrane review, more than two-thirds of American women reported experiencing lower back pain in pregnancy and approximately 20% of pregnant women reported pelvic pain.[118] For decades, both physicians and caring supporters have offered a plethora of suggestions for managing and reducing this discomfort using everything from special exercises, frequent rest, hot and cold compresses, supportive belts, massage, acupuncture and chiropractic treatments to aromatherapy, relaxation, herbs, yoga, and Reiki.[118] This same review found that few quality studies have been performed to assess the efficacy of most of these methods, and those studies that were performed tended to be small, have significant bias, and showed small effect size. These limited studies focused on exercise, acupuncture, and a specific form of supportive pillow, all of which showed some positive effect but, as mentioned, the studies were flawed. Nevertheless, this is a major issue in pregnancy and one that is important to address with women. The provider needs to help to set appropriate expectations of what is normal or expected in pregnancy as well as what is beyond that range. In addition, although there may be little scientific evidence that some of the time-honored suggestions are effective, there is also little evidence of harm, and therefore, as long as the patient understands this lack of evidence, it may be beneficial to suggest various methods so that each patient may find her best means of reducing discomfort.

Sexuality During Pregnancy

Sexuality is often an unspoken and unaddressed issue in pregnancy. Numerous studies spanning several decades have reported a fairly consistent pattern of behavior for women during pregnancy that, although it certainly does not dictate limitations or appropriate behavior to any individual patient, may be a helpful tool to reassure and validate patients' experiences as normal. Often, the frequency of sexual intercourse declines slightly in the first trimester. This finding has been attributed to unpleasant symptoms in early pregnancy such as nausea, breast pain, and fatigue.[119] However, as these symptoms improve in the second trimester, sexual activity often increases and women report higher energy levels and libido, which increases enjoyment. However, by the third trimester, surveys report a sharp decline in sexual activity, because it becomes physically more difficult and sometimes uncomfortable to engage in intercourse.[119,120] Although not borne out in medical literature, there may also be a perception among some patients (or their partners) that intercourse during pregnancy or during specific periods during pregnancy is not safe or poses increased risk of preterm labor or harm to the fetus. Appropriate reassurance can be critical in putting the patient and her partner at ease.

Breastfeeding

Breastfeeding has been shown to have benefits for both mother and infant. Benefits ranging from reduced risk of childhood obesity, diabetes, hypercholesterolemia, otitis media infections, necrotizing enterocolitis, asthma, and improved cognitive development in infants have all been studied. In addition, mothers benefit with improved postpartum weight loss and reduced risk of breast and ovarian cancer. Nevertheless, the decision to breastfeed is not necessarily an easy or convenient choice, and mothers may need significant encouragement and support to successfully undertake that task. For some women, breastfeeding may be contraindicated, and discussion of this issue is also important. Early discussion provides women with time and room to discuss the benefits, challenges, and adjustments that may be required to facilitate their decision.[121–126]

Signs and Symptoms of Labor

The second trimester is a good time to begin discussing the signs of labor and the labor process. This discussion is particularly important for first-time mothers, for whom these changes and sensations are new. Distinguishing false labor or Braxton Hicks contractions from active labor, recognizing rupture of membranes, and knowing when to seek medical attention by coming to the labor and delivery department are all critical topics not only at term but also to help patients recognize preterm labor. Further guidance on how to manage contractions and effectively reduce discomfort can help patients reduce unnecessary visits to the labor and delivery department. In addition, beginning education on the stages of labor and the typical timeline of labor helps establish realistic expectations and plans for labor.

Anesthesia

Intrapartum analgesia/anesthesia administered through an epidural catheter has become an increasingly popular option over the last 30 years, with more than half of all deliveries now using this form of pain control.[127] Nevertheless, there are strong cultural and personal factors that contribute to patients' desire for or refusal of epidural analgesia/anesthesia. As patients approach their due dates, it is important that they understand the options for intrapartum pain control, the risks and benefits, timing of initiating therapy, and circumstances that may modify or even preclude the use of an epidural.

Regional Highlight: Far North (Alaska)

Because of extremely remote conditions in most areas of rural Alaska, special accommodations are made by some Alaska native health systems to bring women into the hospital to board at 35 weeks' gestational age. This strategy provides immediate access to labor and delivery services when labor begins and complies with American College of Obstetricians and Gynecologists (ACOG) travel recommendations against air travel in the last 4 weeks of gestation.[1]

WEEKS 28 TO 40

Testing tapers down in the third trimester, and visits increasingly focus on patient education and monitoring of fetal growth and well-being by simple office and home techniques such as measurement of fundal height, fetal heart rate auscultation, maternal blood pressure, and FFM or kick counting. ACOG recommends rescreening at-risk patients for STDs including HIV,[128] syphilis,[129] hepatitis B, gonorrhea, and chlamydia in the third trimester.[49,50,53,130]

Universal screening for vaginal group B streptococcus (GBS) colonization at 35 to 37 weeks' gestation is recommended to determine the need for intrapartum antibiotic prophylaxis. In addition, the CDC recommends antibiotic chemoprophylaxis for all women with GBS bacteriuria during the current pregnancy or with a history of previous delivery of a GBS-infected infant. This prophylaxis can be undertaken without additional screening. If the result of GBS culture is not known at the onset of labor, intrapartum chemoprophylaxis should be administered to women with any of the following risk factors: gestation less than 37 weeks, duration of membrane rupture 18 hours or greater, or a temperature of 100.4°F or greater (**Fig. 1**).[131]

THIRD-TRIMESTER COUNSELING AND EDUCATION

Third-trimester counseling continues to build on some of the themes that were initiated in the previous trimester, but the emphasis begins to turn toward looking beyond pregnancy and encompassing the postpartum period. Early discussions promote educated decision-making on the part of the patient. Topics to consider include FFM, options and plans for the birthing experience, preparations for newborn care, male circumcision, and postpartum depression.

FFM

FFM is a basic and simple method used as an indicator of fetal well-being that encourages the patient to perform a daily count of the fetal movements she feels as the assessment tool.[132] There are various methods and techniques with differing

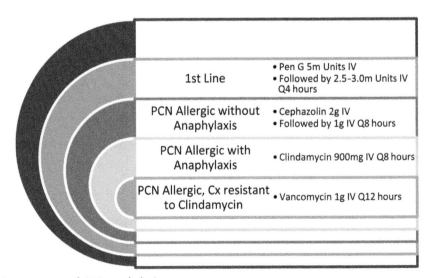

Fig. 1. Agents of GBS prophylaxis.

parameters of normal. Studies show markedly higher patient compliance with the Cardiff count method, which involves once-daily counts (rather than multiple periods) up to 10 movements and compares the relative time it takes to achieve 10 movements, where a significantly longer period may indicate fetal distress and trigger more advanced monitoring.[132]

Birthing Experience/Options

Counseling on the labor process that started in the second trimester continues into the third trimester as the event comes ever closer. Patients should be encouraged to work with their delivering provider to develop a mutually agreeable and appropriate plan for birth. Some hospital facilities offer a variety of birthing options from tubs to birthing balls to birthing chairs. Practitioners may discuss these options and inform the patient of what they feel comfortable in using as a provider. In addition, patients should be informed how the guests and visitors policy of the hospital is applied and how many supporters can be present during delivery so that patients may discuss and decide what their own preferences are within the policy.

Preparing for Baby, Choosing a Doctor, and Childhood Vaccinations

Late pregnancy is a good time to begin discussion and education about newborn care and preparation. Car-seat acquisition before hospital discharge, cosleeping and sleep safety, and infant soothing techniques are topics that are of immediate necessity and may require some preparation. In addition, one of the first decisions that needs to be made by the new parent(s) is choice of family doctor or pediatrician for the newborn; this decision may determine hospital nursery care and destination for newborn screening results. The new parent is also asked to make the decision regarding the first childhood vaccine (hepatitis B) while still in the hospital. Opening the discussion about childhood vaccinations during late pregnancy allows parents to ask questions and feel reassured about the strong medical evidence behind this preventive measure.

Circumcision

Parent(s) expecting a male infant face an additional decision regarding circumcision. This procedure is common and usually performed within the first 2 days of life. The decision to circumcise a male infant is usually deeply personal and largely based on religious or cultural factors.[133] Parents who are not predisposed to 1 decision or another may enquire about health benefits and risks and desire to discuss the issue before making the decision.

Postpartum Blues and Depression

Postpartum depression is the most common condition complicating the postpartum period, affecting approximately 13% of all postpartum women.[134] For this reason, it is important that lines of communication be opened early and patients informed that this condition is a high risk. Having this discussion before the emergence of symptoms may help reduce any sense of guilt, inadequacy, or shame that the new mother struggling with this condition may feel. Postpartum blues is even more common, but less debilitating and more transient. Helping women understand the causes behind postpartum blues and equipping them to recognize warning signs of the more serious depression may facilitate earlier use of support and treatment.[135,136] The Edinburgh Postnatal Depression Scale is a validated and commonly used tool for assessing postpartum depression at follow-up visits after delivery.

GROUP PRENATAL VISITS

Looking toward the future, providing prenatal care in groups is a model that is increasingly being piloted and used in different practices across the country. This model usually involves a cohort of 10 to 15 women with similar due dates and a multidisciplinary provider team and is conducive to patient education.

SUMMARY

Prenatal care offers a unique opportunity for in-depth, continuous, and frequent patient education and the unrivaled opportunity to deepen the physician-patient relationship, potentially providing the foundation for a lifetime of preventive care for the entire family.

REFERENCES

1. ACOG Committee on Obstetric Practice. Committee opinion: number 264, December 2001. Air travel during pregnancy. Obstet Gynecol 2001;98(6):1187–8.
2. Boss DJ, Timbrook RE. Clinical obstetric outcomes related to continuity in prenatal care. J Am Board Fam Pract 2001;14(6):418–23.
3. Alexander GR, Kotelchuck M. Assessing the role and effectiveness of prenatal care: history, challenges, and directions for future research. Public Health Rep 2001;116(4):306–16.
4. Kogan MD, Martin JA, Alexander GR, et al. The changing pattern of prenatal care utilization in the United States, 1981-1995, using different prenatal care indices. JAMA 1998;279(20):1623–8.
5. Alexander GR, Kogan MD, Nabukera S. Racial differences in prenatal care use in the United States: are disparities decreasing? Am J Public Health 2002; 92(12):1970–5.
6. Markovitz BP, Cook R, Flick LH, et al. Socioeconomic factors and adolescent pregnancy outcomes: distinctions between neonatal and post-neonatal deaths? BMC Public Health 2005;5:79.
7. Bennett I, Switzer J, Aguirre A, et al. 'Breaking it down': patient-clinician communication and prenatal care among African American women of low and higher literacy. Ann Fam Med 2006;4(4):334–40.
8. Yu SM, Alexander GR, Schwalberg R, et al. Prenatal care use among selected Asian American groups. Am J Public Health 2001;91(11):1865–8.
9. Braveman P, Marchi K, Egerter S, et al. Barriers to timely prenatal care among women with insurance: the importance of prepregnancy factors. Obstet Gynecol 2000;95(6 Pt 1):874–80.
10. Goldenberg RL, Patterson ET, Freese MP. Maternal demographic, situational and psychosocial factors and their relationship to enrollment in prenatal care: a review of the literature. Women Health 1992;19(2–3):133–51.
11. Lia-Hoagberg B, Rode P, Skovholt CJ, et al. Barriers and motivators to prenatal care among low-income women. Soc Sci Med 1990;30(4):487–95.
12. Poland ML, Ager JW, Olson JM. Barriers to receiving adequate prenatal care. Am J Obstet Gynecol 1987;157(2):297–303.
13. Fiscella K. Does prenatal care improve birth outcomes? A critical review. Obstet Gynecol 1995;85(3):468–79.
14. Health Care Guideline: Routine Prenatal Care. Institute for Clinical Systems Improvement; 2010. Fourteenth. Available at: http://www.icsi.org/prenatal_care_4/prenatal_care__routine__full_version__2.html. Accessed April 14, 2011.

15. Kirkham C, Harris S, Grzybowski S. Evidence-based prenatal care: Part I. General prenatal care and counseling issues. Am Fam Physician 2005;71(7): 1307–16.
16. Bronstein JM, Felix HC, Bursac Z, et al. Providing general and preconception health care to low income women in family planning settings: perception of providers and clients. Matern Child Health J 2011. Availale at: http://www. springerlink.com/content/g4173m6653464754/. Accessed November 2, 2011.
17. Brennan M. Pre-pregnancy care for diabetes. Pract Midwife 2010;13(11):16, 18–9.
18. Witters I, Bogaerts A, Fryns JP. Preconception care. Genet Couns 2010;21(2): 169–82.
19. Heavey E. Don't miss preconception care opportunities for adolescents. MCN Am J Matern Child Nurs 2010;35(4):213–9.
20. Das S, Rao V, Chaudhuri JD. Preconception counseling in the prevention of fetal alcohol syndrome: a unique window of opportunity. Clin Ter 2009;160(4): 315–22.
21. Carl J, Hill DA. Preconception counseling: make it part of the annual exam. J Fam Pract 2009;58(6):307–14.
22. Solomon BD, Jack BW, Feero WG. The clinical content of preconception care: genetics and genomics. Am J Obstet Gynecol 2008;199(6 Suppl 2):S340–4.
23. Elsinga J, de Jong-Potjer LC, van der Pal-de Bruin KM, et al. The effect of preconception counselling on lifestyle and other behaviour before and during pregnancy. Womens Health Issues 2008;18(Suppl 6):S117–25.
24. Hillemeier MM, Weisman CS, Chase GA, et al. Women's preconceptional health and use of health services: implications for preconception care. Health Serv Res 2008;43(1 Pt 1):54–75.
25. Tough SC, Clarke M, Clarren S. Preventing fetal alcohol spectrum disorders. Preconception counseling and diagnosis help. Can Fam Physician 2005;51: 1199–201.
26. Gardiner PM, Nelson L, Shellhaas CS, et al. The clinical content of preconception care: nutrition and dietary supplements. Am J Obstet Gynecol 2008; 199(6 Suppl 2):S345–56.
27. Wilson RD, Johnson JA, Wyatt P, et al. Pre-conceptional vitamin/folic acid supplementation 2007: the use of folic acid in combination with a multivitamin supplement for the prevention of neural tube defects and other congenital anomalies. J Obstet Gynaecol Can 2007;29(12):1003–26.
28. Lipscombe LL, McLaughlin HM, Wu W, et al. Pregnancy planning in women with pregestational diabetes. J Matern Fetal Neonatal Med 2011;24(9):1095–101.
29. Slocum J, Barcio L, Darany J, et al. Preconception to postpartum: management of pregnancy complicated by diabetes. Diabetes Educ 2004;30(5):740, 742–4, 747–53.
30. Crocker A, Farrell T. Pregnancy and pre-existing diabetes: key concerns. Hosp Med 2004;65(6):351–4.
31. American College of Obstetricians and Gynecologists, Committee on Professional Standards. Standards for obstetric-gynecologic hospital services. Standards for obstetric-gynecologic services. 6th edition. Washington, DC: American College of Obstetricians and Gynecologists; 1985.
32. Huntington J, Connell FA. For every dollar spent–the cost-savings argument for prenatal care. N Engl J Med 1994;331(19):1303–7.
33. Carroli G, Villar J, Piaggio G, et al. WHO systematic review of randomised controlled trials of routine antenatal care. Lancet 2001;357(9268):1565–70.

34. Clement S, Candy B, Sikorski J, et al. Does reducing the frequency of routine antenatal visits have long term effects? Follow up of participants in a randomised controlled trial. Br J Obstet Gynaecol 1999;106(4):367–70.

35. Villar J, Khan-Neelofur D. Patterns of routine antenatal care for low-risk pregnancy. Cochrane Database Syst Rev 2000;2:CD000934.

36. American Academy of Pediatrics, American College of Obstetricians and Gynecologists. March of Dimes Birth Defects Foundation. Guidelines for perinatal care. 6th edition. Elk Grove Village (IL), Washington, DC: American Academy of Pediatrics; American College of Obstetricians and Gynecologists; 2007. xiv, p. 450.

37. National Collaborating Centre for Women's and Children's Health. Antenatal care: routine care for the healthy pregnant woman, 2008. Availale at: http://www.nice.org.uk/nicemedia/live/11947/40145/40145.pdf. Accessed November 2, 2011.

38. McLean E, Cogswell M, Egli I, et al. Worldwide prevalence of anaemia, WHO Vitamin and Mineral Nutrition Information System, 1993-2005. Public Health Nutr 2009;12(4):444–54.

39. Lops VR, Hunter LP, Dixon LR. Anemia in pregnancy. Am Fam Physician 1995; 51(5):1189–97.

40. Msolla MJ, Kinabo JL. Prevalence of anaemia in pregnant women during the last trimester. Int J Food Sci Nutr 1997;48(4):265–70.

41. Bayoumeu F, Subiran-Buisset C, Baka NE, et al. Iron therapy in iron deficiency anemia in pregnancy: intravenous route versus oral route. Am J Obstet Gynecol 2002;186(3):518–22.

42. Reveiz L, Gyte GM, Cuervo LG. Treatments for iron-deficiency anaemia in pregnancy. Cochrane Database Syst Rev 2007;2:CD003094.

43. Tsianakas V, Calnan M, Atkin K, et al. Offering antenatal sickle cell and thalassaemia screening to pregnant women in primary care: a qualitative study of GPs' experiences. Br J Gen Pract 2010;60(580):822–8.

44. Dormandy E, Gulliford M, Bryan S, et al. Effectiveness of earlier antenatal screening for sickle cell disease and thalassaemia in primary care: cluster randomised trial. BMJ 2010;341:c5132.

45. Rogers DT, Molokie R. Sickle cell disease in pregnancy. Obstet Gynecol Clin North Am 2010;37(2):223–37.

46. Krcmery S, Hromec J, Demesova D. Treatment of lower urinary tract infection in pregnancy. Int J Antimicrob Agents 2001;17(4):279–82.

47. Murray N, Homer CS, Davis GK, et al. The clinical utility of routine urinalysis in pregnancy: a prospective study. Med J Aust 2002;177(9):477–80.

48. Rouse DJ, Andrews WW, Goldenberg RL, et al. Screening and treatment of asymptomatic bacteriuria of pregnancy to prevent pyelonephritis: a cost-effectiveness and cost-benefit analysis. Obstet Gynecol 1995;86(1):119–23.

49. Sexually transmitted diseases treatment guidelines 2002. Centers for Disease Control and Prevention. MMWR Recomm Rep 2002;51(RR-6):1–78.

50. Nelson HD, Helfand M. Screening for chlamydial infection. Am J Prev Med 2001; 20(Suppl 3):95–107.

51. Hong FC, Liu JB, Feng TJ, et al. Congenital syphilis: an economic evaluation of a prevention program in China. Sex Transm Dis 2010;37(1):26–31.

52. Johnson HL, Ghanem KG, Zenilman JM, et al. Sexually transmitted infections and adverse pregnancy outcomes among women attending inner city public sexually transmitted diseases clinics. Sex Transm Dis 2011;38(3):167–71.

53. Kirkham C, Harris S, Grzybowski S. Evidence-based prenatal care: part II. Third-trimester care and prevention of infectious diseases. Am Fam Physician 2005; 71(8):1555–60.

54. Hofmeyr GJ, Lawrie TA, Atallah AN, et al. Calcium supplementation during pregnancy for preventing hypertensive disorders and related problems. Cochrane Database Syst Rev 2010;8:CD001059.

55. Sibai BM. Calcium supplementation during pregnancy reduces risk of high blood pressure, pre-eclampsia and premature birth compared with placebo? Evid Based Med 2011;16(2):40–1.

56. Anwar A, Salih A, Masson E, et al. The effect of pre-pregnancy counselling for women with pre-gestational diabetes on maternal health status. Eur J Obstet Gynecol Reprod Biol 2011;155(2):137–9.

57. Spinillo A, Capuzzo E, Piazzi G, et al. Risk for spontaneous preterm delivery by combined body mass index and gestational weight gain patterns. Acta Obstet Gynecol Scand 1998;77(1):32–6.

58. Rasmussen T, Stene LC, Samuelsen SO, et al. Maternal BMI before pregnancy, maternal weight gain during pregnancy, and risk of persistent positivity for multiple diabetes-associated autoantibodies in children with the high-risk HLA genotype: the MIDIA study. Diabetes Care 2009;32(10):1904–6.

59. Saftlas A, Wang W, Risch H, et al. Prepregnancy body mass index and gestational weight gain as risk factors for preeclampsia and transient hypertension. Ann Epidemiol 2000;10(7):475.

60. Langer O, Yogev Y, Xenakis EM, et al. Overweight and obese in gestational diabetes: the impact on pregnancy outcome. Am J Obstet Gynecol 2005;192(6): 1768–76.

61. Robinson HE, O'Connell CM, Joseph KS, et al. Maternal outcomes in pregnancies complicated by obesity. Obstet Gynecol 2005;106(6):1357–64.

62. Ju H, Rumbold AR, Willson KJ, et al. Borderline gestational diabetes mellitus and pregnancy outcomes. BMC Pregnancy Childbirth 2008;8:31.

63. Ouzounian JG, Hernandez GD, Korst LM, et al. Pre-pregnancy weight and excess weight gain are risk factors for macrosomia in women with gestational diabetes. J Perinatol 2011;31(11):717–21.

64. Heude B, Thiebaugeorges O, Goua V, et al. Pre-pregnancy body mass index and weight gain during pregnancy: relations with gestational diabetes and hypertension, and birth outcomes. Matern Child Health J 2011. Available at: http://www.mendeley.com/research/prepregnancy-body-mass-index-weight-gain-during-pregnancy-relations-gestational-diabetes-hypertension-birth-outcomes/. Accessed November 2, 2011.

65. Chang G, McNamara TK, Orav EJ, et al. Brief intervention for prenatal alcohol use: a randomized trial. Obstet Gynecol 2005;105(5 Pt 1):991–8.

66. O'Connor MJ, Whaley SE. Brief intervention for alcohol use by pregnant women. Am J Public Health 2007;97(2):252–8.

67. Lu MC, Tache V, Alexander GR, et al. Preventing low birth weight: is prenatal care the answer? J Matern Fetal Neonatal Med 2003;13(6):362–80.

68. Khoury JC, Miodovnik M, Buncher CR, et al. Consequences of smoking and caffeine consumption during pregnancy in women with type 1 diabetes. J Matern Fetal Neonatal Med 2004;15(1):44–50.

69. ACOG Committee on Health Care for Underserved Women, ACOG Committee on Obstetric Practice. ACOG committee opinion. Number 316, October 2005. Smoking cessation during pregnancy. Obstet Gynecol 2005;106(4):883–8.

70. Rosenthal AC, Melvin CL, Barker DC. Treatment of tobacco use in preconception care. Matern Child Health J 2006;10(Suppl 5):S147–8.

71. Little BB, Snell LM, Van Beveren TT, et al. Treatment of substance abuse during pregnancy and infant outcome. Am J Perinatol 2003;20(5):255–62.

72. Ebrahim SH, Gfroerer J. Pregnancy-related substance use in the United States during 1996-1998. Obstet Gynecol 2003;101(2):374–9.
73. Miles DR, Lanni S, Jansson L, et al. Smoking and illicit drug use during pregnancy: impact on neonatal outcome. J Reprod Med 2006;51(7):567–72.
74. Ludlow J, Christmas T, Paech MJ, et al. Drug abuse and dependency during pregnancy: anaesthetic issues. Anaesth Intensive Care 2007;35(6):881–93.
75. Kuczkowski KM. The effects of drug abuse on pregnancy. Curr Opin Obstet Gynecol 2007;19(6):578–85.
76. Domenici C, Cuttano A, Nardini V, et al. Drug addiction during pregnancy: correlations between the placental health and the newborn's outcome–elaboration of a predictive score. Gynecol Endocrinol 2009;25(12):786–92.
77. Keegan J, Parva M, Finnegan M, et al. Addiction in pregnancy. J Addict Dis 2010;29(2):175–91.
78. Moore DG, Turner JD, Parrott AC, et al. During pregnancy, recreational drug-using women stop taking ecstasy (3,4-methylenedioxy-N-methylamphetamine) and reduce alcohol consumption, but continue to smoke tobacco and cannabis: initial findings from the Development and Infancy Study. J Psychopharmacol 2010;24(9):1403–10.
79. de Moraes Barros MC, Guinsburg R, de Araujo Peres C, et al. Exposure to marijuana during pregnancy alters neurobehavior in the early neonatal period. J Pediatr 2006;149(6):781–7.
80. Dawes MG, Grudzinskas JG. Repeated measurement of maternal weight during pregnancy. Is this a useful practice? Br J Obstet Gynaecol 1991; 98(2):189–94.
81. Brown HL. Trauma in pregnancy. Obstet Gynecol 2009;114(1):147–60.
82. O'Reilly R, Beale B, Gillies D. Screening and intervention for domestic violence during pregnancy care: a systematic review. Trauma Violence Abuse 2010; 11(4):190–201.
83. Renker PR, Tonkin P. Women's views of prenatal violence screening: acceptability and confidentiality issues. Obstet Gynecol 2006;107(2 Pt 1):348–54.
84. Shah PS, Shah J. Maternal exposure to domestic violence and pregnancy and birth outcomes: a systematic review and meta-analyses. J Womens Health (Larchmt) 2010;19(11):2017–31.
85. Gielen AC, Faden RR, O'Campo P, et al. Women's protective sexual behaviors: a test of the health belief model. AIDS Educ Prev 1994;6(1):1–11.
86. Klebanoff MA, Shiono PH, Carey JC. The effect of physical activity during pregnancy on preterm delivery and birth weight. Am J Obstet Gynecol 1990;163(5 Pt 1):1450–6.
87. Berkowitz GS. Employment-related physical activity and pregnancy outcome. J Am Med Womens Assoc 1995;50(5):167–9, 174.
88. Luke B, Mamelle N, Keith L, et al. The association between occupational factors and preterm birth: a United States nurses' study. Research Committee of the Association of Women's Health, Obstetric, and Neonatal Nurses. Am J Obstet Gynecol 1995;173(3 Pt 1):849–62.
89. Peoples-Sheps MD, Siegel E, Suchindran CM, et al. Characteristics of maternal employment during pregnancy: effects on low birthweight. Am J Public Health 1991;81(8):1007–12.
90. Neilson JP. Symphysis-fundal height measurement in pregnancy. Cochrane Database Syst Rev 2000;2:CD000944.
91. Gribble RK, Fee SC, Berg RL. The value of routine urine dipstick screening for protein at each prenatal visit. Am J Obstet Gynecol 1995;173(1):214–7.

92. Comstock CH, Malone FD, Ball RH, et al. Is there a nuchal translucency millimeter measurement above which there is no added benefit from first trimester serum screening? Am J Obstet Gynecol 2006;195(3):843–7.

93. Taslimi MM, Acosta R, Chueh J, et al. Detection of sonographic markers of fetal aneuploidy depends on maternal and fetal characteristics. J Ultrasound Med 2005;24(6):811–5.

94. Agarwal MM, Dhatt GS, Shah SM. Gestational diabetes mellitus: simplifying the international association of diabetes and pregnancy diagnostic algorithm using fasting plasma glucose. Diabetes Care 2010;33(9):2018–20.

95. Bhattacharya SM. Fasting or two-hour postprandial plasma glucose levels in early months of pregnancy as screening tools for gestational diabetes mellitus developing in later months of pregnancy. J Obstet Gynaecol Res 2004;30(4):333–6.

96. Bito T, Nyari T, Kovacs L, et al. Oral glucose tolerance testing at gestational weeks < or =16 could predict or exclude subsequent gestational diabetes mellitus during the current pregnancy in high risk group. Eur J Obstet Gynecol Reprod Biol 2005;121(1):51–5.

97. Chatzi L, Plana E, Pappas A, et al. The metabolic syndrome in early pregnancy and risk of gestational diabetes mellitus. Diabetes Metab 2009;35(6):490–4.

98. Nahum GG, Wilson SB, Stanislaw H. Early-pregnancy glucose screening for gestational diabetes mellitus. J Reprod Med 2002;47(8):656–62.

99. Seshiah V, Cynthia A, Balaji V, et al. Detection and care of women with gestational diabetes mellitus from early weeks of pregnancy results in birth weight of newborn babies appropriate for gestational age. Diabetes Res Clin Pract 2008;80(2):199–202.

100. American College of Obstetricians and Gynecologists. ACOG Practice Bulletin No. 88, December 2007. Invasive prenatal testing for aneuploidy. Obstet Gynecol 2007;110(6):1459–67.

101. Bornstein E, Lenchner E, Donnenfeld A, et al. Complete trisomy 21 vs translocation Down syndrome: a comparison of modes of ascertainment. Am J Obstet Gynecol 2010;203(4):391 e391–5.

102. South ST, Chen Z, Brothman AR. Genomic medicine in prenatal diagnosis. Clin Obstet Gynecol 2008;51(1):62–73.

103. Crane JP, LeFevre ML, Winborn RC, et al. A randomized trial of prenatal ultrasonographic screening: impact on the detection, management, and outcome of anomalous fetuses. The RADIUS Study Group. Am J Obstet Gynecol 1994;171(2):392–9.

104. Whitworth M, Bricker L, Neilson JP, et al. Ultrasound for fetal assessment in early pregnancy. Cochrane Database Syst Rev 2010;4:CD007058.

105. Summaries for patients. Screening for gestational diabetes during pregnancy: recommendation from the U.S. Preventive Services Task Force. Ann Intern Med 2008;148(10):I60.

106. U.S. Preventive Services Task Force. Screening for gestational diabetes mellitus: U.S. Preventive Services Task Force recommendation statement. Ann Intern Med 2008;148(10):759–65.

107. Blatt AJ, Nakamoto JM, Kaufman HW. Gaps in diabetes screening during pregnancy and postpartum. Obstet Gynecol 2011;117(1):61–8.

108. Carr CA. Evidence-based diabetes screening during pregnancy. J Midwifery Womens Health 2001;46(3):152–8.

109. Lu GC, Luchesse A, Chapman V, et al. Screening for gestational diabetes mellitus in the subsequent pregnancy: is it worthwhile? Am J Obstet Gynecol 2002;187(4):918–21.

110. Maegawa Y, Sugiyama T, Kusaka H, et al. Screening tests for gestational diabetes in Japan in the 1st and 2nd trimester of pregnancy. Diabetes Res Clin Pract 2003;62(1):47–53.
111. American Diabetes Association. Diagnosis and classification of diabetes mellitus. Diabetes Care 2010;33(Suppl 1):S62–9.
112. Dashora U, Dashora V, Kennedy L. Two-hour 75-g oral glucose tolerance test early in pregnancy detects most cases of gestational diabetes. Diabetes Care 2002;25(4):803 [author reply: 804].
113. de Sereday MS, Damiano MM, Gonzalez CD, et al. Diagnostic criteria for gestational diabetes in relation to pregnancy outcome. J Diabetes Complications 2003;17(3):115–9.
114. Hadar E, Hod M. Establishing consensus criteria for the diagnosis of diabetes in pregnancy following the HAPO study. Ann N Y Acad Sci 2010;1205:88–93.
115. Serlin DC, Lash RW. Diagnosis and management of gestational diabetes mellitus. Am Fam Physician 2009;80(1):57–62.
116. Crowther CA, Hiller JE, Moss JR, et al. Effect of treatment of gestational diabetes mellitus on pregnancy outcomes. N Engl J Med 2005;352(24): 2477–86.
117. Trolle B. Prenatal Rh-immune prophylaxis with 300 micrograms immune globulin anti-D in the 28th week of pregnancy. Acta Obstet Gynecol Scand 1989;68(1): 45–7.
118. Young G, Jewell D. Interventions for preventing and treating pelvic and back pain in pregnancy. Cochrane Database Syst Rev 2002;1:CD001139.
119. Murtagh J. Female sexual function, dysfunction, and pregnancy: implications for practice. J Midwifery Womens Health 2010;55(5):438–46.
120. Katz A. Sexually speaking: sexual changes during and after pregnancy. Am J Nurs 2010;110(8):50–2.
121. Crume TL, Ogden L, Maligie M, et al. Long-term impact of neonatal breastfeeding on childhood adiposity and fat distribution among children exposed to diabetes in utero. Diabetes Care 2011;34(3):641–5.
122. Khresheh R, Suhaimat A, Jalamdeh F, et al. The effect of a postnatal education and support program on breastfeeding among primiparous women: a randomized controlled trial. Int J Nurs Stud 2011;48(9):1058–65.
123. Monica KC, du Plessis RA. Discussion of the health benefits of breastfeeding within small groups. Community Pract 2011;84(1):31–4.
124. Murtagh L, Moulton AD. Working mothers, breastfeeding, and the law. Am J Public Health 2011;101(2):217–23.
125. Oddy WH, Li J, Whitehouse AJ, et al. Breastfeeding duration and academic achievement at 10 years. Pediatrics 2011;127(1):e137–45.
126. Hoddinott P, Tappin D, Wright C. Breast feeding. BMJ 2008;336(7649):881–7.
127. Vincent RD Jr, Chestnut DH. Epidural analgesia during labor. Am Fam Physician 1998;58(8):1785–92.
128. Centers for Disease Control and Prevention. Revised recommendations for HIV screening of pregnant women. MMWR Recomm Rep 2001;50(RR-19):63–85 [quiz: CE61-19a62–CE66-19a62].
129. U.S. Preventive Services Task Force. Screening for syphilis infection in pregnancy: U.S. Preventive Services Task Force reaffirmation recommendation statement. Ann Intern Med 2009;150(10):705–9.
130. Centers for Disease Control and Prevention (CDC). Chlamydia screening among sexually active young female enrollees of health plans–United States, 2000-2007. MMWR Morb Mortal Wkly Rep 2009;58(14):362–5.

131. Verani JR, McGee L, Schrag SJ, et al. Prevention of perinatal group B streptococcal disease: revised guidelines from CDC, 2010. Atlanta (GA): Dept. of Health and Human Services, Centers for Disease Control and Prevention; 2010.
132. Mangesi L, Hofmeyr GJ. Fetal movement counting for assessment of fetal wellbeing. Cochrane Database Syst Rev 2007;1:CD004909.
133. Circumcision policy statement. American Academy of Pediatrics. Task Force on Circumcision. Pediatrics 1999;103(3):686–93.
134. Wisner KL, Parry BL, Piontek CM. Clinical practice. Postpartum depression. N Engl J Med 2002;347(3):194–9.
135. Chandra PS, Sudhir P. Post-partum depression. Br J Psychiatry 2006;188:84 [author reply: 84–5].
136. Hannah P, Adams D, Lee A, et al. Links between early post-partum mood and post-natal depression. Br J Psychiatry 1992;160:777–80.

Family Medicine Obstetrics: Pregnancy and Nutrition

Jean M. Harnisch, BS, RD[a], Patricia H. Harnisch, BS, MEd, RD[b],
David R. Harnisch Sr, MD[c],*

KEYWORDS

- Prenatal care • Nutrition • Antepartum care • Postpartum care
- BMI • Vitamins • Minerals • Lactation

THE PREPREGNANCY TIME FRAME: PRECONCEPTION NUTRITION

Without reprinting here mountains of tables and charts, it seems that 2 assumptions are made by most providers of obstetric care: (1) a woman with a normal body mass index (BMI) is a healthier woman (nutritionally and in many other ways) and (2) prenatal vitamins with iron and calcium supplementation make up for a general lack of the basic nutrients, vitamins, or minerals needed to keep patients as nutritionally healthy as possible. These 2 simplistic statements can help guide the health care team in the care of their patients in most cases.

BMI

The patient's BMI should be considered another vital sign along with pulse, temperature, and respirations. Simply stated, BMI is a measure of body fat based on height and weight. By calculating this and using it as a vital sign, it is possible to determine if a patient is underweight, normal weight, overweight, or obese.

The formulas for calculating BMI are as follows:

1. BMI (metric) = weight (kg)/height (meters squared)
2. BMI (English) = 703 (weight [lb]/height [inches squared]).

There are also numerous tables available for quick conversion as well as BMI calculators on the Internet. Clinic staff can be trained to calculate and record this for physicians as another vital sign to follow.

Using the metric scale, the BMI is interpreted as in **Table 1**.

This work received no grant funding.

[a] Central Alabama Veterans Health Care System, Montgomery, AL, USA

[b] Papillion, NE, USA

[c] Clarkson Family Medicine Residency, The Nebraska Medical Center, 42nd and Douglas Streets, Omaha, NE 68046, USA

* Corresponding author.

E-mail address: dharnisch@nebraskamed.com

Prim Care Clin Office Pract 39 (2012) 39–54

doi:10.1016/j.pop.2011.11.003   primarycare.theclinics.com

Table 1 The BMI scale[1]	
	BMI
Underweight	<18.5
Normal	18.5–24.9
Overweight	25.0–29.9
Obese	≥30

This is the scale as used by the Centers for Disease Control and Prevention[1] and the Institute of Medicine.[2,3] There are several tables and calculators with other breakdowns of the BMI categories available online, but this will suffice.

We care about our patient's BMI before pregnancy because there are significant risks to underweight and obese patients and, probably by logical extension, to overweight patients as well.[4,5]

A woman with a BMI in the obese range is subject to the following complications during pregnancy (and this is not an exhaustive list): increased risk of cesarean delivery, increased risk of preterm delivery, increased birth weight of fetus, fetal macrosomia, pregnancy-induced hypertension, postterm pregnancies, shoulder dystocia, maternal weight retention (with the lifelong consequences of obesity such as increased risks of osteoarthritis, diabetes, hypertension, urinary tract infections, obstructive sleep apnea, coronary artery disease, cerebrovascular accidents, and endometrial cancer), increased perinatal mortality, increased rates of congenital malformations, gestational and nongestational diabetes, venous thromboembolic disease, and an increased rate of twinning with all its attendant fetal and maternal risks. The woman is also at risk of increased complications from cesarean delivery if she were to undergo this procedure, and these risks include, but are not limited to, infection, hemorrhage, poor wound healing, and wound breakdown. The fetus would be at increased risks from the preterm delivery of all the complications of prematurity, including death, retinopathy of prematurity, necrotizing enterocolitis, and neurologic damage, as well as all the risks from shoulder dystocia should that occur, particularly the brachial plexus injuries.[6,7]

A woman who is underweight or has a BMI less than 18.5 is also at risk for complications of pregnancy (as well as the complications of anorexia or bulimia in general), and these include an increased risk of preterm delivery, low birth weight of the neonate, small-for-gestational-age fetus, intrauterine growth restriction, and stillbirth.[5]

The BMI is an excellent tool to help in the management of the entire duration of pregnancy, and a treatment team including the primary care obstetric provider and a clinical dietitian is useful at each prenatal visit. Patients approached in a nonjudgmental manner through a team approach tend to respond better with improved BMIs. Other consultants (including maternal fetal medicine, mental health, physical therapy, cardiology, gastroenterology, and so forth) may be involved as needed. If cesarean delivery is anticipated, an anesthesiology consult is advised in morbidly obese patients. Consideration of place of delivery is also an issue, particularly if cesarean delivery is likely. Extra medical assistance may be needed in the operating room, a neonatal intensive care unit may be needed, and a special operating room table may be needed for the patients whose BMI is extremely high.

The Diet History

A general medical history, including assessment of medications and complementary and alternative medications, is very important and discussed in further depth in article by Aaron Lanik elsewhere in this issue. For example, a patient on antiepileptic medications may have special dietary needs.

Aside from BMI, 4 other special nutrition concerns may be evident or discovered prenatally and should be addressed by the treatment team.

First, a general dietary history can determine any glaring nutrient deficiencies or diet disorders that might cause a deficiency. This information can then be addressed by the treatment team.

Second, a diet history will provide information on whether a patient is a vegetarian (and there are different degrees of being a vegetarian mostly centering on egg, cheese, or milk ingestion.) Vegetarianism may lead to a deficiency of proteins or certain other nutrients, and the dietitian can help guide efforts to supplementation or diet augmentation as needed.[8]

Third, some patients and some regions of the country are subject to pica, which is an eating disorder typically defined as the persistent ingestion of nonnutritive substances for a period of at least 1 month at an age at which this behavior is developmentally inappropriate and can include the ingestion of starch, ice, clay, dirt, and other substances. This behavior may be associated with iron deficiency.[9]

Fourth, obesity itself may impair the patient's ability to conceive. Increased BMI is associated with subfertility (possibly because of association with polycystic ovarian syndrome). Obesity is also a risk factor for spontaneous abortion, and the pregestational effect of obesity on glucose metabolism has profound effects on the human body up to and including such feared complications as retinopathy, neuropathy, and nephropathy.[10–15]

There are 2 final points to consider regarding information that is obtained in a general medical history. First, if provider concerns are aroused regarding deficiencies or excesses of calories, vitamins, minerals, or other substances, then a general laboratory screen could be helpful to detect potential deficiencies. For instance, a microcytic hypochromic anemia could potentially signify iron deficiency. A general laboratory screen could include determination of B12 or folate levels, serum protein levels, serum albumin levels, and serum prealbumin levels or complete blood cell count with indices and a peripheral smear, all of which may indicate a disorder of nutrition. Second, we would be remiss if we did not give special attention to folic acid supplementation. Folic acid deficiency is now well known to be associated with neural tube and cardiac defects. It is now recommended that all pregnant women ingest at least 400 μg (0.4 mg) of folic acid daily, and, if a woman has a history of a neural tube defect in a previous pregnancy, it is recommended that she be supplemented with at least 4000 μg (4 mg) of folic acid daily. If a woman is thinking of conceiving or, in the opinion of the health care provider, might conceive, then preconception supplementation of folic acid is highly recommended.

THE PREGNANCY TIME FRAME: ANTEPARTUM

If our patients take our prepregnancy counseling to heart, it often makes for much smoother sailing during pregnancy. In this section of the article, we discuss the pregnant female and the implications of weight gain for her in regard to her prepregnancy BMI, necessary levels of certain vitamins and minerals, complications of deficiencies or excesses of nutrients, and certain dietary restrictions.

BMI and Weight Gain

The subject of the exact amount of weight to gain during pregnancy comes up frequently. As we work to dispel the "you are eating for 2" and "eat all you want, you are pregnant" myths, it is clear that for many women their pregnancies are times when they put on pounds that remain with them forever and that this is a sequential phenomenon, that is, the excess weight from each pregnancy remains oftentimes for the rest of the patient's life.

Observing BMI tables and leaning on the work of the Institute of Medicine as well as recommendations put forth by numerous investigators, the American College of Obstetricians Gynecologists, and the World Heath Organization, the recommendations in **Table 2** has been suggested as a guide. **Table 3** provides information on weight gained on average in a healthy patient.

This leads to a gain of 20.5 to 21.5 lb (9.3–9.8 kg) on average. About 6 to 8 more pounds of fat stores are gained in preparation for lactation and for energy for use during the pregnancy.

One other easy to use rule of thumb for weight gain is 1 lb in the first trimester, half pound per week in the second trimester (6 lb total), and 1 lb/wk in the third trimester (13 lb) for a total of 20 lb.

As outlined in the first section of the article, the dangers of obesity are pervasive in a pregnancy and absolutely need to be avoided. Aside from the previously mentioned complications of obesity in pregnancy, there are other risks included in pregnancy, such as increased lengths of labor with increasing BMI, increased rates of induction of labor, decreased chance of trial of labor after cesarean success, decreased chance of external cephalic version success, increased rates of cesarean delivery, and increased rates of shoulder dystocia. Other negative effects in women who are obese (and even overweight) include gestational diabetes, preeclampsia, emergency cesarean delivery, pelvic infection, and stillbirth.[7]

Perhaps one of the most significant factors of obesity is that children born to obese women often become obese as adults. There is a direct association with maternal preconception obesity and childhood obesity. This leads to a cycle of obesity and a drain on medical and financial resources.[11–13]

As mentioned previously, the BMI is a type of vital sign, and most clinics performing prenatal care at least check their patient's weights at each visit to check for adequacy and an acceptable rate of gain. Women who are obese at the start of their pregnancy should have a first trimester glucose tolerance test (GTT) in addition to the traditional 24- to 28-week GTT. Women who are gaining excess weight should be evaluated to rule out multiple gestations, preeclampsia (with water retention), or simple overeating with resulting weight gain.[16–23]

Table 2
New recommendations for total and rate of weight gain during pregnancy by prepregnancy BMI[2,3]

Prepregnancy BMI	BMI (kg/m²) (World Health Organization)	Total Weight Gain Range (lb)	Rates of Weight Gain[a] During Second and Third Trimester (Mean Range in lb/wk)
Underweight	<18.5	28–40	1 (1–1.3)
Normal weight	18.5–24.9	25–35	1 (0.8–1)
Overweight	25.0–29.9	15–25	0.6 (0.5–0.7)
Obese (includes all classes)	≥30.0	11–20	0.5 (0.4–0.6)

[a] Calculations assume a 0.5–2 kg (1.1–4.4 lbs) weight gain in the first trimester.
(based on Siega-Riz et al., 1994; Abrams et al., 1995; Carmichael et al., 1997).

Table 3		
Weight gained on average in a healthy population[18]		
	Weight Gained (lb)	**Weight Gained (kg)**
The placenta	1.5	0.7
Uterus	2.0	0.9
Amniotic fluid	2.0	0.9
Fetus	7.0–8.0	3.2–3.6
Blood		
Cellular components	3.0–4.0	1.4–1.8
Plasma	2.0–3.0	0.9–1.4

Gaining too little weight during a pregnancy is a problem because even women who are extremely obese (BMI>40) are still encouraged to gain a minimum of 15 lb or so.[2,3]

Too little weight gain is also potentially a problem because starting out with a low BMI can be a risk factor for preterm delivery and stillbirth as mentioned in the first section. There are signs that should be watched for that might serve as red flags for future problems. Some of these signs include hyperemesis gravidarum, no or poor weight gain, a known history of an eating disorder, hyperkalemia, poor dentition, and a fetus with intrauterine growth restriction. Any of these signs that are noted during the course of a pregnancy would be grounds for further evaluation, with special consideration given for protein and calorie malnutrition.

Vitamins and Minerals

The issue of supplementing the diet of pregnant women has long received significant interest in obstetric care. The nutritional requirements of many substances have been reviewed, and there have been many tables published listing these values. It seems, however, that a normally nourished women or, put differently, a woman consuming a nutritionally complete diet will not have any nutritional deficiencies, and iron and vitamin deficiencies might not be found in many of these women in this population on performing a laboratory screen.

A table containing these recommendations as published at the Web site Perinatology.com and reviewed by investigators is attached (**Table 4**).[24]

A counter proposal to the management of this issue is the prenatal vitamin. Rather than performing expensive tests for deficiencies, there have been standard general recommendations that all pregnant women, all lactating women, and even women thinking about conceiving ought to be taking a prenatal vitamin to ensure that their iron and vitamin "tanks" are topped off and thus the fetus will have no void of raw materials. What about some of the specifics.

In the first section of this article, folic acid supplementation (0.4 and 4.0 mg) was reviewed. Similarly, iron plays a key role in pregnancy and childbirth. All pregnancies end with a "hemorrhage" (500 mL is the average blood loss in pregnancy), and it is known that although there is a physiologic anemia in pregnancy, there is an overall increase in plasma and red cell mass to help compensate for the bleeding during delivery.

The blood volume of a normal pregnant woman is 40% to 45% greater than that of a nonpregnant woman, with the plasma volume increasing more than the red cell volume (but red cell volume does go up.) About 1000 mg of iron is required for pregnancy, with 300 mg of it going to the fetus and placenta, 200 mg lost to either nonabsorption or excretion or routine red cell death, and 500 mg of it going to help increase the red cell volume by around 450 mL.

Table 4
Daily dietary reference intakes[a] during pregnancy[24]

Nutrient (Units)	Age≤18 y	Age, 19–50 y	Some Natural Sources
Water (L)	3	3	Tap or bottled water, juices, carbonated beverages, tea, milk, soup, iceberg lettuce, cucumber, papaya, watermelon
Carbohydrate (g)	175	175	Canned condensed milk, pie crust, barley, white rice, tapioca, couscous, dates, raisins, cornmeal, wheat flour, bulgur, chocolate
Protein (g)	71	71	Duck, chicken, fish, turkey, lamb, beef, soybeans, ricotta and cottage cheese, pork
Total fiber (g)	28	28	Barley, bulgur, beans, peas, lentils, wheat fiber, oat bran, artichokes, dates, chickpeas
Linoleic acid (g)	13	13	Safflower oil, sunflower seeds, corn oil, soybean oil, pine nuts, pecans, sesame oil, chicken fat
α-Linolenic acid (g)	1.4	1.4	Flaxseed oil, walnuts, canola oil soybean oil, fatty fish
Vitamin A (µg RAE[b] [IU as preformed vitamin A])	750 (2500); UL = 2800 (9240)	770 (2565); UL = 3000 (10,000)	Turkey and chicken giblets, carrots, pumpkin, sweet potato, spinach, collards, kale, cantaloupe, turnip greens, beet greens, winter squash
Vitamin E (mg)	15; UL = 800	15; UL = 1000	Ready-to-eat cereals, tomato, sunflower seeds, nuts, spinach, safflower oil, turnip greens
Vitamin K (µg)	75; UL = ND	90; UL = ND	Kale, collards, spinach, turnip greens, beet greens, dandelion greens, mustard greens, Brussels sprouts, broccoli
Vitamin C (mg)	80; UL = 1800	85; UL = 2000	Oranges, grapefruit, sweet red peppers, papaya, cranberries, strawberries, broccoli, Brussels sprouts
Vitamin B1 (thiamine) (mg)	1.4; UL = ND	1.4; UL = ND	Ready-to-eat cereals, enriched white rice, wheat flour, oat bran, pork loin, enriched cornmeal
Vitamin B2 (riboflavin) (mg)	1.4; UL = ND	1.4; UL = ND	Turkey giblets, milk, ready-to-eat cereals, duck, yogurt, soybeans, spinach
Niacin (mg)	18; UL = 30	18; UL = 35	Chicken, fish, duck, wheat flour, barley, ready-to-eat cereals, tomatoes, turkey, enriched white rice, buckwheat flour, yellow cornmeal, pork loin, ham, bulgur, beef, couscous, lamb, peanuts

Nutrient			Food sources
Vitamin B6 (pyridoxine) (mg)	1.9; UL = 80	1.9; UL = 100	Ready-to-eat cereals, chickpeas, fish, beef, turkey, enriched white rice, potatoes, chestnuts, buckwheat flour, chicken breast and giblets, pork loin, prune juice, duck, bananas, plantains
Folate (µg)	600; UL = 800 ACOG recommends that women who have had a pregnancy affected by a neural tube defect (eg, spina bifida or anencephaly) and are planning a pregnancy should receive 4 mg of folic acid supplementation per day for 1 mo before conception through the first 3 mo of pregnancy[8,9]	600; UL = 1000	Enriched white rice, ready-to-eat cereals, cornmeal, turkey giblets, wheat flour, lentils, cowpeas (black-eyed peas), beans, chickpeas (garbanzo beans), okra, spinach, asparagus, beef
Vitamin B12 (cyanocobalamin) (µg)	2.6; UL = ND	2.6; UL = ND	Cooked clams, turkey giblets, cooked oysters, cooked crab, fish, ready-to-eat cereals, beef, lamb
Iron (mg)	27; UL = 45	27; UL = 45	Beef, turkey, duck, cooked clams, chicken, soybeans, fortified cereals, lentils, spinach, lima beans, refried beans, chickpeas, tomatoes, and prune juice
Iodine (µg)	220; UL = 900	220; UL = 1100	Cheese, bread, milk, salt, cooked seafood
Vitamin D (cholecalciferol) (µg [IU])	5 (200); UL = 50 (2000)	5 (200); UL = 50 (2000)	Salmon, rockfish, tuna, milk with added vitamin D, ready-to-eat cereals, skin exposure to sunlight
Biotin (µg)	30; UL = ND	30; UL = ND	Cooked egg, cheddar cheese, whole-wheat bread, cooked salmon, pork, avocado
Choline (mg)	450; UL = 3000	450; UL = 3500	Egg, salmon, turkey, beef, pork lion, lamb, soybeans, baked beans, ham, chickpeas (garbanzo beans), kidney beans
Pantothenic acid (mg)	6; UL = ND	6; UL = ND	Ready-to-eat cereals, beef, mushrooms, chicken, turkey, duck, canned, condensed, or evaporated milk, sunflower seeds, couscous, rice, bulgur, yogurt, corn, peas
Calcium (mg)	1300; UL = 2500	1000; UL = 2500	Ready-to-eat cereals, milk, cheese, cornmeal, yogurt, wheat flour, collards, rhubarb, sardines, spinach, soybeans, turnip greens
Phosphorous (mg)	1250; UL = 3500	700; UL = 3500	Cornmeal; canned, condensed, or evaporated milk, raw oat bran, fish, ricotta cheese, duck, barley, clam chowder, soybeans, bulgur

(continued on next page)

Table 4
(continued)

Nutrient (Units)	Age≤18 y	Age, 19–50 y	Some Natural Sources
Magnesium (mg)	400; UL = 350 (from pharmacologic agent)	360; UL = 350 (from pharmacologic agent)	Buckwheat flour, bulgur, oat bran raw, semisweet chocolate, fish, wheat flour, spinach, barley, pumpkin seeds, cornmeal, soybeans, white beans
Copper (µg)	1000; UL = 8000	1000; UL = 10,000	Beef, cooked oysters, cooked crab, mushrooms, chocolate, tomato products, nuts, mature soybeans, sunflower seeds, chili con carne, cooked clams
Zinc (mg)	12; UL = 34	11; UL = 40	Cooked oyster, ready-to-eat cereals, baked beans, turkey, beef, cooked crab, chicken, duck, lamb, pork, kidney beans
Chromium (µg)	29; UL = ND	30; UL = ND	Broccoli, grape juice, orange juice, English muffin, waffle, potatoes, garlic, basil, beef, turkey breast
Manganese (mg)	2; UL = 9	2; UL = 11	Raw oat bran, wheat, bulgur, pineapple, barley, nuts, ready-to-eat cereals, white rice, spaghetti, okra, brown rice, chickpeas, spinach, raspberries, lima beans
Molybdenum (µg)	50; UL = 1700	50; UL = 2000	Beans, lentils, peas, nuts, cereals, peas spinach, broccoli
Selenium (µg)	60; UL = 400	60; UL = 400	Nuts, chicken or turkey giblets, fish, cooked oysters, turkey, duck, wheat flour, enriched white rice, oat bran, pork, ricotta cheese
Fluoride (mg)	3; UL = 10	3; UL = 10	Fluoridated drinking water, cooked seafood, tea

Abbreviations: ACOG American Congress of Obstetricians and Gynecologists; ND, not determinable; UL, the maximum level of daily nutrient intake that is likely to pose no risk of adverse effects.

[a] Recommended dietary allowances and adequate intakes.

[b] RAE, retinol activity equivalents; 3.33-IU vitamin A, 1-µg RAE; 6.66-IU β-carotene from supplement, 1-µg RAE.

Data from Institute of Medicine, Food and Nutrition Board, Committee on Nutritional Status During Pregnancy, part I: nutritional status and weight gain. Washington, DC: National Academy Press; 2000; and Available at: www.iom.edu/CMS/3788/4819I/68004/68230.aspx. Accessed August 8, 2011.

To provide this 1000 mg of iron, it has been estimated that 27 to 30 mg of iron per day by mouth should be sufficient. Most prenatal vitamins with iron compounded in them meet this level of supplementation. There are several potential problems with iron supplements: (1) they make the color of stools darker, (2) they can cause gastric irritation, and (3) they can cause constipation. The color change is easy enough, but, to a woman queasy from morning sickness, the prenatal vitamin's taste and iron content may be enough to move the patient from nausea to emesis and will oftentimes be eliminated from the patient's medicine cabinet unless the patient is counseled about these potentialities. The constipation resulting in a woman who is already bound up from the high progesterone state will also discourage iron's further use. Standard recommendations are to hold the iron till the second trimester or to give the iron with a stool softener to help avoid the constipation. Preemptive counseling will help empower the patient in this regard.[25–28]

A lot of these issues can be forestalled by having patients meet with a dietitian to talk about their basic nutritional needs and also to answer questions regarding iron and vitamins and to help dispel myths about these substances.

Some other basic facts about the generic patient's diet are that a pregnant woman only needs 100 to 300 cal (average of 250 cal) extra per day. Her protein intake needs go up to about 5 to 6 g/d.[29]

Calcium supplementation merits a special comment. There have been efforts to encourage even greater replacement of calcium in the mother's diet to help in fetal skeleton construction and to help prevent theft of the mother's skeletal calcium resulting in osteopenia or osteoporosis. There has also been mention about preventing preeclampsia via calcium supplementation; however, this has not been proven to be accurate.[29]

In general, a generic prenatal vitamin with 27 to 30 mg of iron and a stool softener included in its compounding ought to suffice for most patients to meet their requirements for iron, vitamins, and minerals.

A word of caution regarding the fat-soluble (A, D, E, and K) vitamins. It is certainly not physiologic or desirable to supersupplement with these vitamins, particularly vitamin A which is a known teratogen. Occasionally patients may need specific counseling with specific regard to this issue.

There has been significant interest in attempting to prevent preeclampsia through dietary means if possible. A recent study suggested that vitamin E and vitamin C might be of benefit in prevention, but other similar studies have not corroborated this. Calcium supplementation (acting through the renin-angiotensin system) has been studied and has been found to help reduce hypertension and reduce preeclampsia (apparently in women at high risk to develop preeclampsia), but there have been no significant differences in randomized controlled studies between supplemented or nonsupplemented populations, and, at this time, the benefit of calcium supplements in pregnancy to prevent preeclampsia is uncertain.[30–44]

Dietary Advice and Restrictions

Pregnant women should eat a variety of foods from all the food groups as outlined in the MyPyramid[45] program or in the newer MyPlate program.[45] Women should seek to achieve a normal BMI before pregnancy and follow the weight gain guidelines during pregnancy. Consuming a prenatal vitamin helps ensure that any minimal to mild deficiencies will be remedied. Women should avoid alcohol during pregnancy to avoid any chance of fetal alcohol syndrome. About 100 to 300 cal extra per day are all that is required.[46] Folic acid supplementation and iron supplements were discussed previously. Calcium consumption should be about 1000 mg/d before, during, and after pregnancy to ensure strong maternal bones, healthy fetal skeleton, and adequate calcium for lactation postpartum.

What about foods to avoid? In general, according to the Food and Drug Administration, there are 4 areas for concern in the food market that pertain especially to pregnant women and their fetuses (aside from alcohol as mentioned earlier).

The first substance is methylmercury from consumption of top-end fish predators. The ocean-going food chain results in the meat from top-end predators (king mackerel, swordfish, tilefish, and shark) containing high levels of methylmercury. Methylmercury poisoning (extreme example is Minamata disease in Japan) can result in microcephaly, cerebral palsy, developmental delay and/or mental retardation, blindness, muscle weakness, and seizures. In general, however, consumption of cold-water fish provides valuable sources of protein and omega-3 fatty acids. "The FDA suggests that pregnant patients may safely eat 12 ounces a week (340 g, or two average meals) of most types of cooked fish including store bought small ocean fish (salmon, Pollock, catfish), shellfish (king crab, shrimp), or canned fish (including light tuna) Fish sticks and fast-food fish are likely made from fish with lower levels of methylmercury."[47]

Toxoplasmosis is an often discussed food contaminant; however, it seems that in pregnant patients, the main source of toxoplasmosis is exposure to cat feces.[48–53] That being said, it is important to thoroughly cook foods (eg, pork or bear) that might be contaminated with the cysts of toxoplasmosis so that they may be killed and new infection prevented. (Also, although this is not a nutritional topic, someone else should change the litter box for the pregnant patient, or, if the woman must do the changing, she should thoroughly clean her hands with hot soapy water afterward; pregnant women should wear gloves when gardening or handling sand from a sandbox and should not get themselves any new pet cats while pregnant.) Toxoplasmosis is relevant in pregnancy because it can cause infection of the fetal central nervous system or ocular system with significant long-term damage.[49]

Listeria is a bacterium that can grow even at refrigerated temperatures and can be found in luncheon meats. The rules for handling these foods and preventing disease transmission are as follows: (1) do not eat hot dogs or luncheon meats unless they are reheated steaming hot, (2) avoid soft cheeses unless they are made with pasteurized milk (and avoid other milk or milk-containing foods with unpasteurized milk in them), (3) avoid refrigerated meat spreads, and (4) do not eat refrigerated smoked seafood unless it is in a cooked dish. Although listeria is usually not harmful to pregnant mothers, it can cause stillbirth, miscarriage, premature delivery, or a life-threatening neonatal infection.

All pregnant women should be aware of the dangers of excess caffeine use. Recently studies have shown that ingestion of large amounts of caffeine may lead to miscarriage. The exact "dose" of caffeine necessary to cause miscarriage is unknown, but there is at least a 1.9-fold increase with caffeine ingestion more than 300 to 500 mg daily. The confounder is that the dosing of caffeine in caffeine-containing beverages is extremely variable depending on brewing times and formulations. In general, moderation is wise in this regard.[54]

THE PREGNANCY TIMEFRAME: POSTPARTUM NUTRITION

The pregnancy is over now. Everyone can relax and go home, right? Well not quite. Pregnancy is only a 9-month window in someone's life. It is a time when women seem very receptive to provider counseling. How many times has a provider seen a woman quit tobacco or drugs or alcohol cold turkey after having her pregnancy test result turn positive? So now that the patients have quit these addictions, the health care team should continue their efforts to promote healthy lifestyles.

Lactation

As the messages continue to sink in, it is known without a shadow of a doubt that breast is best. There are many reasons why physicians should be encouraging their patients to breastfeed: it is recommended by the American Academies of Pediatrics[55] and Family Practice and by the American Dietetic Association[56]; reduction in breast,[57–62] endometrial,[63] and ovarian[64–66] cancers in lactating mothers; decreased cancers in children/adults[67–69] who were breastfeed; decreased asthma,[70] otitis media,[71,72] and diarrhea[73,74] in the neonates; increased intelligence quotient in breast-fed babies[75–79]; continued weight reduction in mothers who nurse[80–83]; decreased maternal blood loss postpartum; and many others that are being researched, including possible reductions in sudden infant death syndrome.[84–91]

Lactating women do have special nutritional needs. There is a need to consume an extra 500 to 1000 mL of fluid per day. Once lactation is established, the rate of production of breast milk is about 30 oz/d (this of course may vary). It would take roughly 800 kcal extra to produce this milk unless maternal energy (mostly fat) stores are used.[44] There is great potential for weight reduction in a properly counseled mother (again aiming for that normal BMI). Prenatal vitamins should be continued to account for the maternal need for extra phosphorus, magnesium, folate, and calcium. The key here could be that by coordinating counseling of the dietitian, health care provider, and the lactation counselor, a new mother could reduce extra weight simply by nursing and not replacing (or over replacing) her caloric expenditures. Statistically, most women experience a net gain of weight with each successive pregnancy. A well–thought-out lactation program helps to eliminate this trend.

The good habits that pregnant patients have picked up during their pregnancies should be lauded and the patients urged to continue with these positive practices. Lactation helps promote mother-baby closeness and strengthens family bonds. There is also a sense of accomplishment for lactating mothers when they see how they are able to provide for their children's needs.

Attention should also be paid to restoring the iron, vitamins, and minerals that may have been lost to the neonate and through the child-bearing process. If patients were able to optimize their nutritional health during pregnancy as described earlier, then they should have adequate stores; however, if they were, for instance, iron deficient, then they may need iron supplementation postpartum. Laboratory studies may need to be followed depending on the magnitude of the perceived deficiencies. With restoration also should come preparation for the next pregnancy. Some information is coming out now on the optimal spacing of children, and, it is conceivable that if children are born at too close an interval, especially in the light of suboptimal nutritional replacement of the body's building blocks, then the long-term health of the mother and potentially of future children could theoretically be harmed. Further studies are needed to test this theorem, but it certainly makes teleologic sense. There is information developing now regarding the skeletal health of postmenopausal women, and more and more evidence is piling up showing that a strong well-developed skeleton in a child will go further toward a strong skeleton in a woman who is postmenopausal than all the pharmacologic interventions started with her first hip fracture.[92]

SUMMARY

This article has discussed the approach to pregnancy and nutrition from a lifetime health perspective rather than from a momentary tick in time. There are some general principles listed that may be followed and punctuated with specific emphasis where most applicable. If these guidelines are followed, the patient and her fetus will benefit dramatically, and, with the help of the health care team including the dietitian, the lactation consultant, and the physician or nurse midwife, happier and healthier pregnancies, labors, deliveries, and lives can be ensured for mothers and their children (and their children's children.)

REFERENCES

1. Body mass index. Centers for Disease Control and Prevention. Available at: http://www.cdc.gov/healthyweight/assessing/bmi/. Accessed August 8, 2011.
2. Institute of Medicine. Food and Nutrition Board, Committee on Nutritional Status During Pregnancy, part I: nutritional status and weight gain. Washington, DC: National Academy Press; 2000.
3. Available at: www.iom.edu/CMS/3788/48191/68004/68230.aspx. Accessed August 8, 2011.
4. Nuthalapaty FS, Lockwood CJ, Rouse DJ, et al. The impact of obesity on fertility and pregnancy. UpToDate. Available at: http://www.uptodate.com/contents/the-impact-of-obesity-on-fertility-and-pregnancy?source=search_result&selectedTitle=1%7E150. Accessed August 8, 2011.
5. Lusskin SI, Yager J, Solomon D, et al. Eating disorders in pregnant women. UpToDate. Available at: http://www.uptodate.com/contents/eating-disorders-in-pregnant-women?source=search_result&selectedTitle=1%7E150. Accessed August 8, 2011.
6. ACOG Practice Bulletin. Bariatric surgery and pregnancy, June 2009, Number 105. Available at: http://www.acog.org/publications/educational_bulletins/pb105.cfm. Accessed August 8, 2011.
7. Cunningham, Leveno K, Bloom S, et al. Obesity and pregnancy complications. 23rd edition, Williams Obstetrics. The McGraw-Hill Companies; 2010. p. 201; 950ff.
8. American Dietetic Association. Position of the American Dietetic Association and Dietitians of Canada: vegetarian diets. Can J Diet Pract Res 2003;64(2):62–81.
9. Ellis CR. Eating disorder, pica. Available at: http://emedicine.medscape.com/article/914765-overview. Accessed August 8, 2011.
10. Fraser A, Tilling K, Macdonald-Wallis C, et al. Association of maternal weight gain in pregnancy with offspring obesity and metabolic and vascular traits in childhood. Circulation 2010;121:2557.
11. Singer JE, Westphal M, Niswander K. Relationship of weight gain during pregnancy to birth weight and infant growth and development in the first year of life. Obstet Gynecol 1968;31:417.
12. Mamun AA, O'Callaghan M, Callaway L, et al. Associations of gestation weight gain with offspring body mass index and blood pressure at 21 years of age: evidence from a birth cohort study. Circulation 2009;119:1720.
13. Van der Steeg JW, Steures P, Eljkemans MJ, et al. Obesity affects spontaneous pregnancy chances in subfertile, ovulatory women. Hum Reprod 2008;23:324.
14. Gesink Law DC, Maclehose RF, Longnecker MP. Obesity and time to pregnancy. Hum Reprod 2007;22:414.
15. Ramlau-Hansen CG, Thulstrup AM, Nohr EA, et al. Subfecundity in overweight and obese couples. Hum Reprod 2007;22:1634.

16. Weight gain during pregnancy: reexamining the guidelines, report brief. Institute of Medicine; 2009. Available at: http://www.iom.edu/Reports/2009/Weight-Gain-During-Pregnancy-Reexamining-the-Guidelines.aspx. Accessed August 8, 2011.

17. Weight gain during pregnancy: reexamining the guidelines, resource sheet. Institute of Medicine; 2009. Available at: http://www.iom.edu/Reports/2009/Weight-Gain-During-Pregnancy-Reexamining-the-Guidelines.aspx. Accessed August 8, 2011.

18. Tse, Macones G. Weight gain in pregnancy. UpToDate. Available at: http://www.uptodate.com/contents/weight-gain-in-pregnancy?view=print. Accessed August 8, 2011.

19. Committee on Maternal Nutrition/Food and Nutrition Board. Maternal nutrition and the course of pregnancy. Washington, DC: National Research Council; 1970.

20. Greene GW, Smiciklas-Wright H, School TO, et al. Postpartum weight change: how much of the weight gained in pregnancy will be lost after delivery? Obstet Gynecol 1988;71:701.

21. Viswanathan M, Siega-Riz AM, Moos MK, et al. Outcomes of maternal weight gain. Evid Rep Technol Assess (Full Rep) 2008;(168):1–223.

22. Norwitz ER. Prevention of spontaneous preterm birth. Up to Date. Available at: http://www.uptodate.com/contents/prevention-of-spontaneous-preterm-birth?source=search_result&selectedTitle=1%7E150. Accessed August 8, 2011.

23. Lockwood C, Magriples U. The initial prenatal assessment and routine prenatal care. UpToDate. Available at: http://www.uptodate.com/contents/the-initial-prenatal-assessment-and-routine-prenatal-care?source=search_result&selectedTitle=1%7E150. Accessed August 8, 2011.

24. Perinatolgy.com. Available at: http://www.perinatology.com/Reference/RDApregnancy.htm. Accessed August 8, 2011.

25. Pritchard JA, Adams RH. Erythrocyte production and destruction during pregnancy. Am J Obstet Gynecol 1960;79:750.

26. Pritchard JA, Mason RA. Iron stores of normal adults and their replenishment with oral iron therapy. JAMA 1964;190:897.

27. Pritchard JA, Scott DE. Iron demands during pregnancy. In: Vanotti A, editor. Iron deficiency pathogenesis: clinical aspects and therapy. London: Academic Press; 1970. p. 173.

28. Ueland K, Metcalfe J. Circulatory changes in pregnancy. Clin Obstet Gynecol 1975;18:41.

29. Gillen-Goldstein J, Funai EF, Roque H. Nutrition in pregnancy. UpToDate. Available at: http://www.uptodate.com/contents/nutrition-in-pregnancy?source=search_result&selectedTitle=1%7E150. Accessed August 8, 2011.

30. Sibai BM, Dekker G, Kupfermic M. Pre-eclampsia. Lancet 2005;365:785.

31. Sibai BM. Prevention of preeclampsia: a big disappointment. Am J Obstet Gynecol 1998;179:1275.

32. Hatton DC, McCarron DA. Dietary calcium and blood pressure in experimental models of hypertension: a review. Hypertension 1994;23:513.

33. Belizan JM, Villar J, Repke J. The relationship between calcium intake and pregnancy induced hypertension: up to date evidence. Am J Obstet Gynecol 1988;158:898.

34. Sanchez-Ramos L, Briones DK, Jaunitz AM, et al. Prevention of pregnancy-induced hypertension by calcium supplementation in angiotensin-II sensitive patients. Obstet Gynecol 1994;84:349.

35. Lopez-Jaramillo P, Narvaez M, Weigel RM, et al. Calcium supplementation reduces the risk of pregnancy-induced hypertension in an Andes population. Br J Obstet Gynaecol 1987;96:648.
36. Villar J, Repke JT. Calcium supplementation during pregnancy may reduce preterm delivery in high-risk populations. Am J Obstet Gynecol 1990;163:1124.
37. Belizan JM, Villar J, Gonzalez L, et al. Calcium supplementation to prevent hypertensive disorders of pregnancy. N Engl J Med 1991;325:1399.
38. Lopez-Jaramillo P, Narvaez M, Felix C, et al. Dietary calcium supplementation and prevention of pregnancy hypertension. Lancet 1990;335:293.
39. Lopez-Jaramillo P, Delgado F, Jacoine P, et al. Calcium supplementation and the risk of preeclampsia in Ecuadorian pregnant teenagers. Obstet Gynecol 1997;90:162.
40. Levine RJ, Jauth JC, Curet LB, et al. Trial of calcium to prevent preeclampsia. N Engl J Med 1997;337:69.
41. Herrera JA, Arevalo-Herrara M, Herrara S. Prevention of preeclampsia by linoleic acid and calcium supplementation: a randomized controlled trial. Obstet Gynecol 1998;91:585.
42. Crowther CA, Hiller JE, Pridmore B, et al. Calcium supplementation in nulliparous women for the prevention of pregnancy-induced hypertension, preeclampsia and preterm birth: an Australian randomized trial. Aust N Z J Obstet Gynaecol 1999;39:12.
43. Rogers MS, Fung HY, Hung CY. Calcium and low-dose aspirin prophylaxis in women at high risk of pregnancy-induced hypertension. Hypertens Pregnancy 1999;18:165.
44. Gabbe SG, Simpson JL, Niebyl JR, et al. Obstetrics—normal and problem pregnancies, 5th edition, Hypertension. Philadelphia (PA): Churchill Livingstone; 2007. p. 604, 871 ff.
45. MyPyramid and MyPlate programs, United States Department of Agriculture programs. Available at: http://www.choosemyplate.gov/. Accessed August 8, 2011.
46. Cunningham, Leveno K, Bloom S, et al. Recommended dietary allowances. 23rd edition, Williams Obstetrics. The McGraw-Hill Companies; 2010. p. 202.
47. Apply the Heat Campaign, US Food and Drug Administration Center for Food Safety and Applied Nutrition. Available at http://www.fda.gov/Food/ResourcesForYou/HealthEducators/ucm082539.htm. Accessed August 8, 2011.
48. Eat right during pregnancy. American Dietetic Association web-based resources; also mentioned in the American Dietetic Association's publication "Expect the Best: Your Guide to Healthy Eating Before, During, and After Pregnancy". Available at: http://www.eatright.org/search.aspx?search=eat+right+during+pregnancy&type=Site. Accessed August 8, 2011.
49. Food safety for moms to be. US Food and Drug Administration. Available at: http://www.fda.gov/Food/ResourcesForYou/HealthEducators/ucm081819.htm. Accessed August 8, 2011.
50. Methylmercury and pregnancy. Organization of Teratology Information Specialists. Available at: http://www.otispregnancy.org/files/methylmercury.pdf. Accessed August 8, 2011.
51. Consumption Advice: Joint Federal Advisory for mercury in fish. US Environmental Protection Agency. Available at: http://www.google.com/search?sourceid=navclient&ie=UTF-8&rlz=1T4SUNA_enUS292US293&q=consumption+advice%3a+joint+federal+advisory+for+mercury+in+fish. Accessed August 8, 2011.
52. What you need to know about mercury in fish and shellfish. US Environmental Protection Agency. Available at: http://www.epa.gov/mercury/advisories.htm. Accessed August 8, 2011.

53. Oken E. Risks and benefits of fish consumption and fish oil supplements during pregnancy. UpToDate. Available at: http://www.uptodate.com/contents/risks-and-benefits-of-fish-consumption-and-fish-oil-supplements-during-pregnancy?source=search_result&selectedTitle=1%7E150. Accessed August 8, 2011.
54. Weng X, Odouli R, Li D. Maternal caffeine consumption during pregnancy and the risk of miscarriage: a prospective cohort study. Am J Obstet Gynecol 2008; 198(3):279, e1–279.
55. AAP Breastfeeding Policy Statement. Breastfeeding and the use of human milk pediatrics. vol. 115, No. 2, February 2005. Available at: aappolicy.aappublications.org/cgi/content/full/pediatrics;115/2/496. Accessed August 8, 2011.
56. ADA Website. Available at: http://www.eatright.org/WorkArea/linkit.aspx?LinkIdentifier=id&ItenID=8425. Accessed August 8, 2011.
57. Jernstorm H, Lubinski J, Lynch H, et al. Breast-feeding and the risk of breast cancer in BRCA1 and BRCA2 mutation carriers. J Natl Cancer Inst 2004;96: 1094–8.
58. Lee SY, Kim M, Kim S, et al. Effect of lifetime lactation on breast cancer risk: a Korean women's cohort study. Int J Cancer 2003;105:390–3.
59. Collaborative Group on Hormonal Factors in Breast Cancer. Breast cancer and breastfeeding: collaborative reanalysis of individual data from 47 epidemiological studies in 30 countries, including 50,302 women with breast cancer and 96,973 women without the disease. Lancet 2002;360:187–95.
60. Zheng, Duan L, Zhang B, et al. Lactation reduces breast cancer risk in Shandong Province, China. Am J Epidemiol 2000;152(12):1129.
61. Newcomb PA, Storer BE, Longnecker MP, et al. Lactation and a reduced risk of premenopausal breast cancer. N Engl J Med 1994;330:81–7.
62. Eiger MS, Wendkos Olds S. The complete book of breastfeeding. New York: Workman Publishing Co., Inc; 1999.
63. Rosenblatt KA, Thomas DB. Prolonged lactation and endometrial cancer. Int J Epidemiol 1995;24:499–503.
64. Hartage, Whittemore AS, Itnyre J, et al. Rates and risks of ovarian cancer in subgroups of white women in the United States. Obstet Gynecol 1994;84(5): 760–4.
65. Rosenblatt KA, Thomas DB. Lactation and the risk of epithelial ovarian cancer. Int J Epidemiol 1993;22:192–7.
66. Gwinn ML. Pregnancy, breastfeeding and oral contraceptives and the risk of epithelial ovarian cancer. J Clin Epidemiol 1990;43:559–68.
67. Freudenheim J, Marshall JR, Graham S, et al. Exposure to breast milk in infancy and the risk of breast cancer. Epidemiology 1994;5:324–31.
68. Uvnas-Moberg K, Eriksson M. Breastfeeding: physiological, endocrine and behavioral adaptations caused by oxytocin and local neurogenic activity in the nipple and mammary gland. Acta Paediatr 1996;85(5):525–30.
69. Shu XO, Linet M, Steinbuch M, et al. Breastfeeding and the risk of childhood acute leukemia. J Natl Cancer Inst 1999;91:1765–72.
70. Oddy WH, Holt PG, Sly PD, et al. 'Association between breast feeding and asthma in 6 year old children: findings of a prospective birth cohort study'. British Medical Journal 1999;319:815–9.
71. Aniansson G, Alm B, Andersson B, et al. A prospective cohort study on breast-feeding and otitis media in Swedish infants. Pediatr Infect Dis J 1994; 13:183–8.
72. Duncan B, Ey J, Holberg C, et al. Exclusive breastfeeding for at least four months protects against otitis media. Pediatrics 1993;91:867–72.

73. Beaudry M, Dufour R, Marcoux S. Relation between infant feeding and infections during the first six months of life. J Pediatr 1995;126:191–7.
74. Howie PW, Forsyth JS, Ogstron SA, et al. Protective effect of breast feeding against infection. BMJ 1990;300:11–6.
75. Mortensen EL, Michaelsen K, Sanders S, et al. The association between duration of breastfeeding and adult intelligence. JAMA 2002;287:2365–71.
76. Anderson JW, Johnstone B, Remley D. Breastfeeding and cognitive development: a meta-analysis. Am J Clin Nutr 1999;70:525–35.
77. Horwood LJ, Fergusson DM. Breastfeeding and later cognitive and academic outcomes. Pediatrics 1998;101(1):E9.
78. Lucas A. Breast milk and subsequent intelligence quotient in children born preterm. Lancet 1992;339:261–2.
79. Wang YS, Wu SY. The effect of exclusive breastfeeding on development and incidence of infection in infants. J Hum Lact 1996;12:27–30.
80. Lovelady CA, Garner K, Moreno K, et al. The effect of weight loss in overweight lactating women on the growth of their infants. N Engl J Med 2000;342:449–53.
81. Kramer F. Breastfeeding reduces maternal lower body fat. J Am Diet Assoc 1993; 93(4):429–33.
82. Dewey KG, Heinig MJ, Nommwen LA. Maternal weight-loss patterns during prolonged lactation. Am J Clin Nutr 1993;58:162–6.
83. Chua S, Arulkumaran S, Lim I, et al. Influence of breastfeeding and nipple stimulation on postpartum uterine activity. Br J Obstet Gynaecol 1994;101:804–5.
84. Horn RS, Parslow P, Ferens D, et al. Comparison of evoked arousability in breast and formula fed infants. Arch Dis Child 2004;89(1):22–5.
85. Alm, Wennergren G, Norvenius S, et al. Breastfeeding and the sudden infant death syndrome in Scandinavia. Arch Dis Child 2002;86:400–2.
86. McVea KL, Turner P, Peppler D. The role of breastfeeding in sudden infant death syndrome. J Hum Lact 2000;16:13–20.
87. Fredrickson DD. Relationship between sudden infant death syndrome and breastfeeding intensity and duration. Am J Dis Child 1993;147:460.
88. Ford RP, Taylor BJ, Mitchell EA, et al. Breastfeeding and the risk of sudden infant death syndrome. Int J Epidemiol 1993;22(5):885–90.
89. Scragg LK, Mitchell EA, Tonkin SL, et al. Evaluation of the cot death prevention programme in South Auckland. N Z Med J 1993;106:8–10.
90. Betran, deOnis M, Laurer J, et al. Ecological study of effect of breastfeeding on infant mortality in Latin America. BMJ 2001;323:1–5.
91. Dewey KG, Heinig MJ, Nommsen-Rivers LA. Differences in morbidity between breast-fed and formula-fed infants. J Pediatr 1995;126:696–702.
92. Teegarden D, Proulx WR, Martin BR. Peak bone mass in young women. J Bone Miner Res 1995;10(5):711–5.

Genetic Screening and Counseling: Family Medicine Obstetrics

K.M. Rodney Arnold, MD[a],*, Zachary B. Self, MD[b]

KEYWORDS

- Genetic screening • Family medicine • Obstetrics
- Genetic counseling

Genetic screening and counseling have become a routinely offered part of prenatal care in the United States, involving invasive and noninvasive options for assessing fetal genetics. Methods of fetal genetic evaluation include the quadruple screen, nuchal skin fold testing, chorionic villus sampling (CVS), and amniocentesis. As DNA testing continues to expand proportionately to the increasing ability to detect hundreds of genetic variations, ethical and fiscal concerns are more relevant. The challenge of processing and incorporating this multiplying, complex information highlights the specialty of genetic counseling. Overall, balancing this burgeoning information and the emotional implications of the results generated can be exhausting and is a learned art, hopefully taught during medical training.

Approximately 3% of live-born infants have genetically linked congenital anomalies. More than 50% of first trimester spontaneous abortions may have chromosomal abnormalities. Furthermore, congenital abnormalities account for 20% to 25% of perinatal deaths.

Societal shifts, such as delayed childbearing and the associated genetic consequences, have made antenatal genetic screening more common. Societal trends, in part, also have generated improved and more available genetic screening for pregnant patients. Still, genetic screening may be confounded by inaccurate information, false-positives, socioeconomic barriers to testing, and cultural differences.

This article reviews and addresses these concerns and provides a summary and framework for training in family medicine obstetrics and other providers of obstetric care.

The authors have nothing to disclose.

[a] University of Tennessee College of Medicine Chattanooga, 1100 East, 3rd Street, Chattanooga, TN 37404, USA
[b] Surgical Family Medicine Obstetrics, Medicos para la Familia, 3030 Covington Pike, Suite 100, Memphis, TN 38128, USA
* Corresponding author.
E-mail address: krodneyarnold@gmail.com

GENETIC CATEGORIES

The field of medical genetics studies the origin, pathogenesis, and natural history of human disease related to mutations in the human genetic code. Phenotypic variation may be divided by origin into chromosomal abnormalities, single-gene (mendelian) disorders, polygenic and multifactorial disorders, and teratogenic disorders.

Chromosomal Abnormalities

The reported incidence of chromosomal abnormalities is 1 in 160 (**Table 1**). Chromosomal abnormalities increase with maternal age. The term *advanced maternal age*

Table 1 Chromosomal abnormalities in newborn infants	
Type of Abnormality	**Incidence**
Numeric aberrations	
Sex chromosomes	
47,XYY	1/1000 MB
47,XXY	1/1000 MB
Other (men)	1/1350 MB
47,X	1/10,000 FB
47,XXX	1/1000 FB
Other (females)	1/2700 FB
Autosomes	
Trisomies	
13–15 (D group)	1/20,000 LB
16–18 (E group)	1/8000 LB
21–22 (G group)	1/800 LB
Other	1/50,000 LB
Structural aberrations	
Balanced	
Robertsonian	
t(Dq; Dq)	1/1500 LB
t(Dq; Gq)	1/5000 LB
Reciprocal translocations and insertional inversions	1/7000 LB
Unbalanced	
Robertsonian	1/14,000 LB
Reciprocal translocations and insertional Inversions	1/8000 LB
Inversions	1/50,000 LB
Deletions	1/10,000 LB
Supernumeraries	1/5000 LB
Other	1/8000 LB
Total	1/160 LB

Abbreviations: FB, female births; LB, live births; MB, male births.

Data from Simpson JL, Holzgreve W. Genetic Counseling and Genetic Screening. In: Gabbe SG, Niebyl JR, Simpson JL, editors. Obstetrics: Normal and Problem Pregnancies. 5th edition. Philadelphia: Elsevier; 2007. p. 139.

denotes a woman 35 years of age or older (at the time of delivery) and reflects the age at which the risk of giving birth to a living child with any chromosomal abnormality (1/204) roughly equals the risk of a fetus dying from complications of genetic amniocentesis (roughly 1/200 or 0.5%). **Table 2** shows maternal age as it relates to the incidence of trisomy 21, Down syndrome, and other chromosomal abnormalities.

Single-Gene Disorders

Roughly 1% of live births are phenotypically abnormal secondary to a single-gene mutation. These mendelian disorders account for 40% of congenital defects noted

Table 2
Maternal age and chromosomal abnormalities (live births)

Maternal Age	Risk for Down Syndrome	Risk for Any Chromosome Abnormalities
20	1/1667	1/526
21	1/1667	1/526
22	1/1429	1/500
23	1/1429	1/500
24	1/1250	1/476
25	1/1250	1/476
26	1/1176	1/476
27	1/1111	1/455
28	1/1053	1/435
29	1/1100	1/417
30	1/952	1/384
31	1/909	1/385
32	1/769	1/322
33	1/625	1/317
34	1/500	1/260
35	1/385	1/204
36	1/294	1/164
37	1/227	1/130
38	1/175	1/103
39	1/137	1/82
40	1/106	1/65
41	1/82	1/51
42	1/64	1/40
43	1/50	1/32
44	1/38	1/25
45	1/30	1/20
46	1/23	1/15
47	1/18	1/12
48	1/14	1/10
49	1/11	1/7

Data from Simpson JL, Holzgreve W. Genetic counseling and genetic screening. In: Gabbe SG, Niebyl JR, Simpson JL, editors. Obstetrics: normal and problem pregnancies. 5th edition. Chapter 6. Philadelphia: Elsevier; 2007. p. 139.

in live-born infants, although each individual gene disorder is uncommon. For example, cystic fibrosis, the most common single-gene disorder in Caucasians, occurs in 1 in 2500 Caucasians of Ashkenazi Jewish or European origin.

Polygenic/Multifactorial Disorders

Approximately another 1% of abnormal newborns possess mutations at more than one genetic locus (ie, polygenetic/multifactorial disorders). These mutations are usually limited to a single organ system and affect between 1% and 5% of siblings of the proband (**Box 1**).

Teratogenic Disorders

The known contribution of teratogens to the development of anomalies is fairly small. Two well-known and well-researched teratogens include alcohol and antiepileptiform medications. Multiple medications, however, have either mild or poorly described teratogenic effects. For example, growing scrutiny borders the selective serotonin reuptake inhibitors (SSRIs), because 2% to 13% of all pregnant women are treated with antidepressants, representing a twofold to fourfold increase in exposure in Western populations during the past decade. An association exists between SSRIs and cardiac malformations, mainly septal defects. Persistent debate surrounds the validity of these data, and further study is ongoing. Because of the lack of evidence about the safety profile of pharmacologic treatments during gestation, the general consensus is to avoid unnecessary medication intake during pregnancy and to encourage the lowest dosage for the shortest time when benefits outweigh the risks.[1–3]

Box 1
Polygenic/multifactorial traits

Hydrocephaly (excepting some forms of aqueductal stenosis and Dandy-Walker syndrome)

Neural tube defects (anencephaly, spina bifida, encephalocele)

Cleft lift, with or without cleft plate

Cleft lip (alone)

Cardiac anomalies (most types)

Diaphragmatic hernia

Pyloric stenosis

Omphalocele

Renal agenesis (unilateral or bilateral)

Ureteral anomalies

Posterior urethral values

Hypospadias

Müllerian fusion effects

Müllerian aplasia

Limb reduction defects

Talipes equinovarus (clubfoot)

Data from Simpson JL, Holzgreve W. Genetic counseling and genetic screening. In: Gabbe SG, Niebyl JR, Simpson JL, editors. Obstetrics: normal and problem pregnancies. 5th edition. Chapter 6, 7. Philadelphia: Elsevier; 2007. p. 138–83.

GENETIC SCREENING

Genetic screening may be used to monitor for the presence (or absence) of a given condition in otherwise apparently normal individuals. The options for genetic screening are trimester-dependent, and include the preconceptual and postpartum periods. It is important for physicians to recognize current options for screening and to develop protocols for offering genetic counseling or diagnostic screening. These protocols may change as new information and technologies develop. For instance, the American College of Obstetricians and Gynecologists (ACOG) guidelines recommend that all women, regardless of age, be offered screening for Down syndrome, whereas previously, women were only automatically offered this counseling and diagnostic evaluation if they were of advanced maternal age.[4,5]

Although Down syndrome screening theoretically is offered to all pregnant women, multiple studies have shown that predictors of prenatal testing include insurance status, inclination to terminate pregnancy, language preference, and desire for minimal intervention.[6,7] Despite these models of predictability, it remains the physician's responsibility to educate and offer an equal choice to each patient.

Preconception Screening

Genetic history

A genetic history is the first step in preconception screening. This process begins with collecting data related to the family history of diseases and malformations, and connecting patterns consistent with modes of inheritance. The ultimate goal is to identify appropriate candidates for referral to a genetic counselor, whose role involves constructing a pedigree (**Fig. 1**).

The American Academy of Family Physicians (AAFP) developed the mnemonic "SCREEN" to provide focus for a potentially time-consuming history within the typical patient visit (**Box 2**).[8]

Adverse outcomes, such as repetitive spontaneous abortions, stillbirths, and anomalous live-born infants, should be listed clearly. These events may signal couples in need of chromosomal studies to exclude balanced translocations. Birth defects in second- or third-degree relatives typically do not confer substantially increased risk of that anomaly over what is seen in the general population.

Advanced paternal age, defined as age older than 50 years, confers a 1% increase for aneuploidy, with single genetic mutations being the most common.

The ACOG recommends screening for a limited number of autosomal recessive disorders that are amenable to prenatal diagnosis through selecting asymptomatic heterozygotes in families without affected progeny (**Table 3**).

The following three diseases portray heritable autosomal recessive disorders commonly explored during preconception counseling.

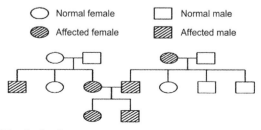

Fig. 1. Pedigree of Tay-Sachs disease.

Box 2
AAFP SCREEN mnemonic

- Some Concerns: Do you have any (some) concerns about diseases or conditions that seem to run in your family
- Reproductions: Have there been any problems with pregnancy, infertility or birth defects in your family?
- Early disease, death or disability: Have any members of your family been diagnosed with a chronic disease at an early age, or have members of your family died at an early age?
- Ethnicity: How would you describe your ethnicity? What country did your ancestors come from?
- Nongenetic conditions: Are you aware of any nonmedical conditions or risk factors, such as smoking or problem drinking, that are present in your family?

Tay-Sachs disease

Tay-Sachs disease involves deterioration of mental and physical health beginning at the age of 6 months, with progressive decline until death at approximately 4 years of age. Within the Ashkenazi Jewish population, the heterozygote frequency of this

---

Table 3
Genetic screening in various ethnic groups

Ethnic Group	Disorder	Screening Test
All ethnic groups	Cystic fibrosis	DNA analysis of selected panel of 23 CFTR mutations (alleles present in 0.1% of the general US population)
Black	Sickle cell anemia	MTV<80%, followed by hemoglobin electrophoresis
Ashkenazi Jewish	Tay-Sachs disease	Decreased serum hexosaminidase-A or DNA analysis for selected alleles
	Canavan disease	DNA analysis for selected alleles
	Familial dysautonomia	DNA analysis for selected alleles
Cajun	Tay-Sachs disease	DNA analysis for selected alleles
French Canadian	Tay-Sachs disease	DNA analysis for selected alleles
Mediterranean (Italian, Greek)	β-Thalassemia	MCV<80%, followed by hemoglobin electrophoresis if iron deficiency excluded
Southeast Asian (Filipino, Chinese, African, Vietnamese, Laotian, Cambodian, Filipino)	α-Thalassemia	MCV<80%, followed by hemoglobin electrophoresis if iron deficiency excluded

Abbreviation: CFTR, cystic fibrosis transmembrane conductance regulator; MCV, mean corpuscular volume.
Data from Simpson JL, Holzgreve W. Genetic counseling and genetic screening. In: Gabbe SG, Niebyl JR, Simpson JL, editors. Obstetrics: normal and problem pregnancies. 5th edition. Chapter 6. Philadelphia: Elsevier; 2007. p. 145.

disease is 1 in 30. Physicians are recommended to screen all Jewish couples and couples in which only one partner is Jewish.

Thalassemias

Thalassemia describes a group of genetic diseases affecting the synthesis of the α- or β-globin chains, leading to abnormal hemoglobin molecules. Abnormal hemoglobin production can lead to different cases of anemia, with the most severe causing death. Screening for β-thalassemia is recommended for individuals of Mediterranean descent and begins by measuring the mean corpuscular volume (**Table 4**).

Cystic fibrosis

Cystic fibrosis (CF) is a multisystem disease caused by a mutation in the gene for the protein cystic fibrosis transmembrane conductance regulator (CFTR), which affects the production of sweat, mucus, and digestive secretions. The most common mutation is ΔF508, reported to be responsible for approximately 70% of the cases worldwide and 90% of the mutations in the United States.

The ACOG recently revised a Committee Opinion regarding preconception and prenatal screening for CF. Prior recommendations included screening whites of non-Jewish descent and Ashkenazi Jews because of an increased proportion of heterozygotes in these populations. The 2011 guidelines recommend that CF screening be offered to all women of childbearing age, preferably preconceptually. Additionally, women who are CF carriers and their reproductive partners may need additional screening tests and referrals for genetic and reproductive counseling.[9]

First-Trimester Genetic Screening and Genetic Testing

First-trimester screening for trisomy 21 and other aneuploidies

Many obstetric providers prefer to screen for trisomy 21 in the first trimester at 11 to 14 weeks' gestational age. Screening can be invasive (CVS) or through analyte analysis separately or in combination with ultrasound-derived measures of nuchal translucency. For noninvasive first-trimester screening, plasma protein A (PAPP-A) and β human chorionic gonadotropin (β-hCG) are the most useful markers for detecting Down syndrome. Low PAPP-A levels and elevated free β-hCG levels reflect a positive screen. Combining PAPP-A and free β-hCG with the ultrasound measurement of fetal nuchal translucency increases detection rates (**Table 5**).

Nuchal translucency describes a fluid-filled space that can be observed at the posterior aspect of the fetal neck between 11 and 14 weeks' gestation, and an increased nuchal translucency measurement (>3.5 mm) is associated with Down syndrome and other aneuploidies (**Fig. 2**).

Table 4		
Hematologic indices of α-thalassemia and β-thalassemia in adults		
Test	**α-Thalassemia**	**β-Thalassemia**
MCV<80 mg/dL (beginning screen)	Low	Low
RDW	Normal	Normal; occasionally high
Ferritin	Normal	Normal
Hb electrophoresis	Normal	Increased HbA2, reduced HbA, and probably increased HbF

Abbreviations: Hb, hemoglobin; HbF, fetal hemoglobin; MCV, mean corpuscular volume; RDW, red blood cell distribution width.

Table 5
Down syndrome detection rates

	DR %[a]
Age, PAPP-A, free β-hCG	68
Age, PAPP-A, free β-hCG, NT	84

Abbreviations: DR, detection rate; NT, nuchal translucency.

[a] At a 5% false-positive rate.

Data from Palomaki GE, Knight GJ, Neveux LM, et al. Maternal serum invasive trophoblast antigen and first trimester Down syndrome screening. Clin Chem 2005;51:1499–504.

Increased NT itself is not a fetal abnormality, but rather a marker that confers increased risk. The ACOG recommends that patients with increased fetal nuchal translucency measurements be offered a targeted ultrasound, echocardiogram, or both. Studies have shown similar detection rates, at a constant false-positive rate, for

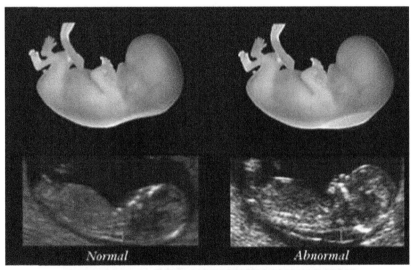

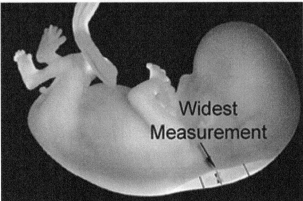

Fig. 2. Nuchal translucency. (*Reproduced from* DeVore GR. Nuchal translucency imaging. Fetal Diagnostic Centers Web site. Available at: http://www.fetal.com/NT%20Screening/02%20NT%20Imaging.html. Accessed June 15, 2011; with permission.)

first- and second-trimester screening tests. The ACOG considers first-trimester screening a reasonable option.[5]

Indications for prenatal genetic studies

Although every chromosomal disorder is potentially detectable in utero, performing invasive procedures in every pregnancy to find them is not appropriate. For many parents, the risk of an invasive procedure will outweigh the possible benefits of the test. Commonly cited indications for prenatal genetic studies include advanced maternal age, parental chromosome rearrangements, previous affected child, positive aneuploidy screening test, and abnormal ultrasound markers and/or ultrasound findings.

Advanced maternal age Historically, advanced maternal age has been the most common reason for women to pursue antenatal cytogenetic studies. In the United States, standard practice was to offer invasive chromosomal diagnosis to all women who at their expected delivery date would be at least 35 years of age. Currently, the ACOG recommends that fetal chromosomal screening be offered to all women, regardless of age, before 20 weeks' estimated gestational age.

Previous child with chromosomal abnormality After one offspring with autosomal trisomy is born, the likelihood that subsequent progeny will have autosomal trisomy is increased. Recurrence risk is approximately 1% for these trisomies, and exists even when parental chromosomal complements are normal. Referral to a genetic counselor for precise patient information and risk stratification should be discussed.

Ultrasound markers Abnormal ultrasound markers, such as a shortened femur, intracardiac hyperechogenic foci, choroid plexus cyst, renal pyelectasis, and hyperechogenic bowel, merit a detailed scan, including the possibility of a fetal echocardiogram.

Whether all obstetric patients should undergo ultrasound screening, and whether this screening improves pregnancy outcomes, is controversial. Some authors claim the that Eurofetus Trial, the largest study of routine ultrasonographic examination in an unselected population, shows that the most accurate sensitivity rates for ultrasound detection of all anomalies approaches approximately 50%.[10,11] Although detection rates of anomalies differ among trials and are dependent on operator experience, the Radius Trial, the first randomized trial of routine obstetric ultrasound screening in the United States, failed to show an improvement in perinatal outcomes under study.[12] The study design of this trial, however, raises debate.

Regardless, the ACOG states that the benefits and limitations of ultrasonography as a screening tool should be discussed with patients, and performance of the procedure is reasonable in patients who request it.[13]

First-Trimester Karyotype Analysis

CVS

CVS sampling is typically performed at 10 to 12 weeks' estimated gestation age. If the woman has an increased risk of fetal aneuploidy, genetic counseling and CVS, and second-trimester amniocentesis, can be offered to analyze fetal tissue for definitive diagnosis. CVS may be performed using either a transcervical or a transabdominal approach. Transcervical CVS is performed using a flexible polyethylene catheter that encircles a metal obturator and extends distal to the catheter tip. Using simultaneous ultrasound visualization, the catheter is introduced transcervically. The catheter is guided in the direction of the trophoblastic tissue surrounding the gestational sac, and 10 to 25 mg of villi are aspirated into a 20- or 30-mL syringe containing tissue culture media.

To perform transabdominal CVS (TA-CVS), an 18- or 20-gauge spinal needle is directed into the placenta under direct ultrasound guidance (**Fig. 3**). Villi are then aspirated into a 20-mL syringe containing tissue culture media. transabdominal CVS can be performed at any time during the course of pregnancy.

The risk of pregnancy loss after CVS is comparable to the risk associated with second-trimester amniocentesis. Studies state that the risk is up to 1% in experienced hands. Several variables have been identified as adversely influencing fetal loss rates in CVS. These factors include fundal location of the placenta, number of catheter passages, small sample size, and prior bleeding during the pregnancy.

Second-Trimester Genetic Screening and Genetic Testing

The quadruple screen

The quadruple screen is the leading test available for Down syndrome screening for women who present after 13 weeks of pregnancy. The test involves measurement of the serum markers maternal serum α-fetoprotein (AFP), unconjugated estriol, hCG, and inhibin A. Evaluation occurs ideally between 15 and 18 weeks' gestation and includes screening for open neural tube defects and trisomy 18 using the AFP component of the test (**Table 6**).

Selected cutoffs determine the test result; the screen is considered negative or positive based on preestablished levels of the serum analytes. Screen-negative women still carry a risk of having a child with Down syndrome; therefore, no test

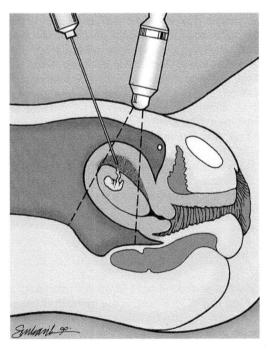

Fig. 3. Transabdominal chorionic villus sampling. (*From* Simpson JL, Holzgreve W. Genetic counseling and genetic screening. In: Gabbe SG, Niebyl JR, Simpson JL, editors. Obstetrics: normal and problem pregnancies. 5th edition. Philadelphia: Elsevier; 2007; with permission.)

Table 6
Quadruple screen interpretations

	MSAFP	hCG	uE3	Inhibin A
ONTD	Increased risk			
Down syndrome	Decreased risk	Increased risk	Decreased risk	Increased risk
Trisomy 18	Decreased risk	Decreased risk	Decreased risk	

Abbreviations: MSAFP, maternal serum α-fetoprotein; ONTD, open neural tube defect; uE3, unconjugated estriol.

should be described as "normal," because the fetus' karyotype remains unknown. Furthermore, screen-positive women should be informed that the test has a false-positive rate of at least 5% that is secondary to a variety of factors, including incorrect data entry, woman's age, woman's weight, gestational age information, and fetal number.[14]

Women with increased risk might then elect an invasive procedure (amniocentesis), whereas women with decreased risk may decide against testing. Either way, women may refuse all testing in acceptance of the natural course of the pregnancy.

Second-Trimester Karyotype Analysis

Amniocentesis

Amniocentesis is the most commonly used prenatal diagnostic invasive procedure. It is a procedure that is typically performed at between 15 and 17 weeks' gestation. Using ultrasound guidance, a 21- or 22-gauge spinal needle with stylet is inserted percutaneously, with care to avoid fetus, cord, and placenta. Normally, approximately 20 mL of amniotic fluid is aspirated, with the first 1 or 2 mL being discarded to avoid maternal cell contamination.

In experienced hands, the procedure-specific risk (of fetal loss) is 0.5% to 1%.[15] Other maternal risks include symptomatic amnionitis, which occurs at an approximate rate of 0.1%, and transient vaginal spotting or amniotic fluid leakage, which occurs in approximately 1% of cases and is usually self-limited. More significant complications may include intra-abdominal viscus injury or hemorrhage. The most serious of reported maternal complications is sepsis, with maternal mortality exceedingly rare.

Common Diagnostic Dilemmas in Prenatal Cytogenetic Diagnosis

Several technical issues may result in inaccurate or uninterpretable results. Cells may not grow at all or sufficiently for proper analysis. Maternal rather than fetal cells may be collected mistakenly. Chromosomal abnormalities detected in villi (placental tissue) or amniotic fluid may not accurately reflect the status of the fetus. For instance, chromosomal aberrations may arise in culture, or chromosomal aberrations may be confined to placental tissue. These complications should be discussed with the patient before procedure referral.

Despite the focus on determining chromosomal abnormalities in community medical practice, one-third of anomalies have been trivial (**Fig. 4**) and another third have been significant but not life-threatening (**Fig. 5**).

GENETIC COUNSELING

The National Society of Genetic Counselors defines genetic counseling as the process of helping people understand and adapt to the medical, psychological, and familial

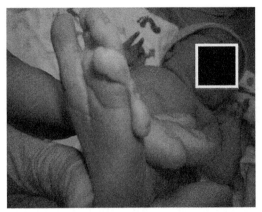

Fig. 4. Polydactly. (*Courtesy of* Wm. MacMillan Rodney, *Medicos para la Familia*; with permission.)

implications of genetic contributions to disease.[16] The family history obtained by a genetic specialist is more detailed and time-consuming than what is feasible in a routine patient care setting. The physician's role is to target patients who qualify for counseling, with the goal of improving the health and quality of life of the fetus and mother.

Ethics

Some patients have expressed uncertainty and concern about genetic discrimination as a result of genetic testing. To prevent patients from avoiding important health information out of fear, the physician should remind patients that legal protection exists through the Genetic Information Nondiscrimination Act (GINA). This act prohibits discrimination by health insurers and employers based on genetic information.[17]

Psychosocial Literacy

Although genetic counseling may require referral to a clinical geneticist, multiple barriers exist within daily patient care. Referrals are often guided by the economic,

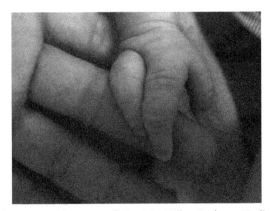

Fig. 5. Failure of formation. (*Courtesy of* Wm. MacMillan Rodney, *Medicos para la Familia*; with permission.)

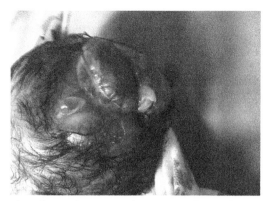

Fig. 6. Amniotic band syndrome. (*Courtesy of* Wm. MacMillan Rodney, *Medicos para la Familia*; with permission.)

social, and religious framework of the patient. Beyond these obstacles is the potential that patients who are not matched appropriately for this counseling might be further confused and frightened by theoretical outcomes. Thus, language must be individualized to the patient's educational level, and initiated within the framework of the patient's family vision and cultural background.

For example, one study examined miscommunication between genetic service providers and patients, particularly patients of Mexican origin. The authors were able to identify five common sources of miscommunication: (1) medical jargon, (2) the nondirective nature of counseling, (3) the inhibitions of counselors stemming from misplaced cultural sensitivity, (4) problems of translation, and (5) problems of trust.[18] These and other barriers must be overcome to achieve meaningful and effective counseling.

Key Messages

- The risk of chromosomal abnormality in the fetus increases with increasing maternal age; trisomy 21 accounts for approximately half of cases.

- Invasive diagnosis of chromosomal abnormalities can be performed using a variety of techniques, such as CVS and amniocentesis.

- Sonographic measurement of nuchal translucency between 11 and 14 weeks' estimated gestational age combined with maternal age and biochemical parameters allows individualized risk calculation for some aneuploidies, such as trisomy 21 and 18.

- In the presence of ultrasound abnormalities in the first trimester and/or a positive first-trimester screening result, CVS should be offered as the most rapid invasive diagnostic method between 10 and 12 weeks' estimated gestational age.

- At a constant false-positive rate, detection rates of Down syndrome are similar in first- and second-trimester screening.

- The role of the physician is to identify patients appropriate for genetic referral; one tool to assist in this role is the "SCREEN" mnemonic.

- Patients are protected under the GINA act to prevent genetic discrimination.

- Physicians must develop a method to relay scientific genetic advances in a manner sensitive to the social, economic, and cultural context of individual patients.

Glossary	
Term	**Definition**
Genetic terms	
Aneuploidy	Any variation in chromosomes that involves single chromosomes instead of complete sets
Genotype	The genetic blueprint
Phenotype	The translation of the genotype in the physical or biochemical manifestation in an individual
Proband	The subject (person or animal) being studied or reported
Trisomy	The presence of three copies of a chromosome instead of two
Autosomal chromosomes	
Allele	Each of the pair of genes of the homologous chromosomes
Homozygous	When both of the paired alleles have the mutation
Heterozygous	When the mutation occurs on only one of the allele pairs
Sex-linked chromosome	The X and Y chromosomes; XX in females, XY in males
Modes of inheritance	
Multifactorial	A constellation of genetic and environmental factors that interact to produce a specific condition
Mendelian Inheritance	Autosomal dominant and recessive inheritance, and X-linked inheritance
Autosomal dominant inheritance	When a disorder can result if one of a specific pair of genes has a mutation
Autosomal recessive inheritance	When a disorder can result only if both genes in a specific pair have a mutation
X-linked inheritance	Mutation exists on X chromosome
Non-mendelian Inheritance	
Polygenic	When more than one gene is involved in producing a condition
Types of genetic testing	
Cytogenetics	The branch of genetics concerned with the study and structure of the cell, especially the chromosome
Prenatal testing	Assessment of fetal DNA sequence or structure for specific disease-causing alleles or karyotypes
Newborn screening	A variety of genetic and metabolic tests performed in the newborn period for the purposes of early identification of children with disease-causing genotypes
Biochemical	
Analyte	Quantitative analysis of a substance in the body when increased or decreased amounts may be indicative of a genetic disorder
Down syndrome screening terms	
Nuchal translucency measurement	The width of translucent space at the back of the neck determined by ultrasound
Combined test	First-trimester test based on sonographic and maternal serum measurements (nuchal translucency, free or total ß-hCG, and PAPP-A), together with maternal age
Quadruple test	Second-trimester test based on measurement of maternal serum AFP, unconjugated estriol, ß-hCG, and inhibin-A, together with maternal age.

Beyond learning how to counsel effectively, physicians must learn when to counsel. Parents receiving unfavorable results or experiencing adverse pregnancy outcomes show similar grief reactions to those who are seen after the death of a loved one: denial, anger, guilt, bargaining, and resolution. Physicians must pay deference to this sequence by providing supportive counseling once the family is ready. Discussing recurrence risks immediately after the birth of an abnormal child not only is insensitive but also adds weight to a burden.

The authors believe that the appropriate time for counseling should be chosen by the mother. Most couples can be reassured that nothing could have prevented a given abnormality in their child.

DISCUSSION

The authors respect the scientific complexity and promise of genetic diagnosis. Nevertheless, most patients in the authors' urban, underserved community practice decline genetic testing once the benefits and risks are explained. One of these cases involved a low-risk patient with a cranial abnormality discovered at a 12-week ultrasound performed for dating purposes. The mother refused consult for genetic counseling and further genetic investigation. The baby was born at term via Cesarean section with Apgar scores of 8 and 9 at 1 and 5 minutes, respectively (**Fig. 6**). The cranial defect is suspected to be related to an amniotic band. Currently, the baby is 8 months old.

REFERENCES

1. Ververs T, Kassenbrood H, Visser G, et al. Prevalence and patterns of antidepressant drug use during pregnancy. Eur J Clin Pharmacol 2006;62(10):863–70.
2. Andrade SE, Raebel MA, Brown J, et al. Use of antidepressant medications during pregnancy: a multisite study. Am J Obstet Gynecol 2008;198(2):194–5.
3. Cooper WO, Willy ME, Pont SJ, et al. Increasing use of antidepressants in pregnancy. Am J Obstet Gynecol 2007;196(6):544–5.
4. ACOG Committee on Practice Bulletins. ACOG Practice Bulletin No. 77: screening for fetal chromosomal abnormalities. Obstet Gynecol 2007;109(1): 217–27.
5. ACOG Committee Opinion #296; first trimester screening for fetal aneuploidy. Obstet Gynecol 2004;101:215–7.
6. Whitehead NS, Rasmussen SA, Cox S, et al. Prevalence and predictors of receipt of prenatal information about genetic screening. Prenat Diagn 2006;26(10): 944–50.
7. Kuppermann M, Learman LA, Gates E, et al. Beyond race or ethnicity and socioeconomic status: predictors of prenatal testing for Down syndrome. Obstet Gynecol 2006;107(5):1087–97.
8. SCREEN: taking a family for familial disease. American Academy of Family Physicians Web site. Available at: http://www.aaafp.org. Accessed September 19, 2011.
9. ACOG Committee Opinion #486:Update on Carrier Screening for Cystic Fibrosis. Obstet Gynecol 2011;117(4):1028–31.
10. Saari-Kemppainen A, Karjalainen I, Ylostalo P, et al. Fetal anomalies in a controlled one-stage ultrasound screening trial. A report from the Helsinki Ultrasound Trial. J Perinat Med 1994;22:279.

11. Saari-Kemppainen A, Karjalainen I, Ylostalo P, et al. Ultrasound screening and perinatal mortality: controlled one-stage ultrasound screening trial. The Helsinki Ultrasound trial. Lancet 1990;336:387.

12. Crane JP, LeFevre ML, Winborn RC, et al. A randomized trial of prenatal ultrasonographic screening: impact on the detection, management, and outcome of anomalous fetuses. The RADIUS Study Group. Am J Obstet Gynecol 1994;171: 392.

13. Abuhamad AZ. ACOG Committee on Practice Bulletins-Obstetrics. ACOG Practice Bulletin, clinical management guidelines for obstetrician-gynecologist number 98, October 2008. Ultrasonography in pregnancy. Obstet Gynecol 2008;112:951.

14. Cunningham FG, MacDonald PC, Gant NF, et al. Williams obstetrics. 20th edition. Stamford (CT): Appleton & Lange; 1997. p. 972.

15. Murken J. Pranattale diagnostik. In: Murken J, Grimm T, Holinski-Feder E, editors. Humangenetik. 7th edition. Sturttgart (Germany): Thierne Verlag; 2006. p. 386–411.

16. National Society of Genetic Counselors Web site. Available at: www.nsgc.org. Accessed September 15, 2011.

17. Clayton EW. Ethical, legal, and social implications of genomic medicine. N Engl J Med 2003;349:562.

18. Browner CH, Preloran HM, Casado MC, et al. Genetic counseling gone awry: miscommunication between prenatal genetic service providers and Mexican-origin clients. Soc Sci Med 2003;56:1933–46.

First Trimester Complications

A. Ildiko Martonffy, MD[a,b,]*, Kirsten Rindfleisch, MD[a,b],
Anne Marie Lozeau, MD[a,c], Beth Potter, MD[a,b]

KEYWORDS

- Early pregnancy bleeding • Threatened abortion • Miscarriage
- Ectopic pregnancy • Gestational trophoblastic disease
- Hydatidiform mole • Hyperemesis gravidarum

BLEEDING IN EARLY PREGNANCY

Background

Early pregnancy bleeding, defined as bleeding before 20 weeks' gestation, is a common presenting complaint. The reported incidence ranges from 21% to 27% in clinically recognized pregnancies, defined as a positive chemical test for pregnancy and missed menses.[1,2] The principal causes of early pregnancy bleeding include threatened abortion in a viable pregnancy, miscarriage, ectopic pregnancy, gestational trophoblastic disease (GVD), and various nonobstetric conditions.

Evaluation

Emergent evaluation, including ultrasonography and surgical referral, is indicated for women with findings suggestive of peritonitis. In the absence of such findings, evaluation may proceed at a more measured pace. The combination of the patient's history, serum β-human chorionic gonadotropin (hCG) level, and transvaginal ultrasonography (TVUS) images yields a definitive diagnosis in most cases. Although bimanual and speculum examination have traditionally been a fundamental component of this evaluation, their diagnostic utility may be limited. A 2009 review of published studies examining the sensitivity and specificity of the bimanual and speculum examinations found no evidence to support their routine use in the diagnosis of threatened abortion, miscarriage, or ectopic pregnancy.[3] Given the physical and emotional distress

This work received no grant funding.
The authors have nothing to disclose.
[a] Department of Family Medicine, University of Wisconsin School of Medicine and Public Health, 1100 Delaplaine Court, Madison, WI 53715, USA
[b] Access-Wingra Family Medical Center, 701 Dane Street, Madison, WI 53713, USA
[c] Northeast Family Medical Center, 3209 Dreyden Drive, Madison, WI 53704, USA
* Corresponding author. Department of Family Medicine, University of Wisconsin School of Medicine and Public Health, 1100 Delaplaine Court, Madison, WI 53715.
E-mail address: ildi.martonffy@fammed.wisc.edu

experienced by most women in this setting, clinicians may choose to defer this component of the evaluation when appropriate.

Bimanual and speculum examination should be performed if there is suspicion for a nonobstetric cause of bleeding. However, these conditions, including infection, neoplasia, and lower genital tract trauma, are uncommon diagnoses in the setting of early pregnancy bleeding. For example, cervical cancer occurs at a rate of 7.5 cases per 100,000 pregnancies.[4] Bimanual and speculum examination should also be undertaken to determine appropriate disposition in patients with minor bleeding, absent or mild pain, and detectable fetal heart tones by Doppler ultrasonography. In the absence of findings suggestive of incomplete abortion (open internal os, visible products of conception) or ectopic pregnancy (adnexal mass or significant adnexal tenderness), it is acceptable to proceed with close clinical follow-up without immediate imaging or intervention.

In stable patients with more significant pain, moderate to heavy bleeding, or absent fetal heart tones, TVUS is almost always indicated. Alternative approaches, including serial examinations and β-hCG level determination, may be appropriate for some patients with a history of passage of tissue followed by abatement of symptoms or in remote areas without ready access to ultrasonography services.

TVUS provides a definitive diagnosis in many cases. When the initial ultrasound examination does not yield a diagnosis, the serum β-hCG level should be determined. The predictable correlation between serum β-hCG levels and TVUS features in normal pregnancies, as shown in **Table 1**, can be used to distinguish between threatened abortion, spontaneous abortion, and early ectopic pregnancy (discussed elsewhere).[5,6]

Threatened Abortion

Once intrauterine pregnancy has been confirmed, viability can be determined through various approaches, depending on the patient's clinical situation and personal preferences. Before ultrasound documentation of cardiac activity and in the absence of significant ongoing bleeding or pain, valid strategies include repeat β-hCG at 48 hours, repeat ultrasonography at 1 week, or watchful waiting with documentation of Doppler fetal heart tones by 11 menstrual weeks. No data on patient preferences or cost-effectiveness exist to indicate that one approach is superior to another. Convention teaches that β-hCG level increases 66% every 48 hours, but more recent data show that viable pregnancies at this stage can demonstrate a 48-hour increase in β-hCG level of as little as 53%, with a median increase of 124%.[6]

The prognosis of threatened abortion depends on many factors. Many sources cite a 50% miscarriage rate for women who experience bleeding in the first trimester.[5,7] However, the original data are largely drawn from emergency department populations, and many women experiencing mild symptoms may not seek emergency care. Furthermore, as pointed out by Hasan and colleagues,[2] many such emergency room visits herald the actual miscarriage event, whereas patients who do not

Table 1 Discriminatory criteria in TVUS	
Gestational sac	Visible when serum β-hCG reaches 1000–2000 mIU/mL
Yolk sac	Visible when gestational sac measures 10 mm
Embryo	Visible when gestational sac measures 18 mm
Cardiac activity	Visible when embryo measures 5 mm

immediately go on to miscarry may have a different risk profile. The investigators' community-based study of more than 4500 women showed no association between short-lived episodes of spotting or mild bleeding and subsequent miscarriage. By contrast, heavy bleeding (defined as bleeding similar to the heavy days of a period) was associated with a 3-fold increase in miscarriage. Extremes of age are predictive of miscarriage in the setting of threatened abortion, with women younger than 20 years or older than 34 years at twice the average risk.[8] Several findings on ultrasonography can provide modified risk estimates. One prospective study demonstrated a baseline miscarriage risk of 6% with first trimester bleeding and documented fetal cardiac activity.[8] The risk increased with the findings of fetal bradycardia, discrepancy between gestational sac size and crown-rump length, and discrepancy between the menstrual and sonographic gestational age. There was an 84% chance of spontaneous abortion in pregnancies with all 3 findings present. A finding of subchorionic hemorrhage is of uncertain significance. Some studies have found an increased risk of miscarriage depending on hematoma size and location, whereas others have found no increased risk in this setting.[9–15] Some women who go on to have a normal pregnancy will have spotting before their missed menses. This is often thought to be caused by implantation bleeding.

Threatened abortion is also associated with several complications later in pregnancy. A 2010 systematic review documented increased risk for antepartum hemorrhage due to placenta previa and other causes, preterm delivery, low birth weight, and perinatal infant mortality.[13] Retrospective cohort data suggest that increased risk for complications, including recurrent early pregnancy bleeding and preterm labor, accrues to subsequent pregnancies as well.[16]

Bed rest, pelvic rest, and progesterone injections have been used in the management of threatened abortion, but no high-quality evidence supports these therapies, and they no longer constitute the standard of care.[17] There is more variability in practice regarding the administration of anti-D immune globulin to Rh-negative women for the prevention of alloimmunization. The American College of Obstetrics and Gynecology acknowledges the lack of evidence behind the use of RhoGAM (anti-D immune globulin). Their recommendation that "anti-D immune globulin prophylaxis should be considered if the patient has experienced threatened abortion" is classified as level C (based primarily on consensus and expert opinion).[18]

Spontaneous Abortion

Historically, many terms have been applied to the diagnosis of spontaneous abortion or miscarriage, depending on the stage of embryonic development at which pregnancy failure occurred together with clinical findings, including bleeding, cervical dilation, and passage of tissue. Complete abortion may be diagnosed by a history of passage of tissue followed by gradual cessation of bleeding and pain. Care in this setting is mainly supportive, and ultrasonography is only necessary to rule out retained products of conception in the event of prolonged bleeding or pain or if symptoms of infection develop. Commonly, however, patients present with ongoing symptoms. Once nonviability has been established with ultrasonography, together with β-hCG correlation as needed, 3 management options may be considered: expectant management, medical management, and surgical management.

Expectant management may be an attractive option for patients with incomplete abortion, whereby success rates as high as 79% to 86% have been observed.[19,20] By contrast, patients with a closed cervical os and intact gestational sac on ultrasonography had a success rate of only 28.9% compared with a success rate of 86.7% with vaginal misoprostol.[20] Expectant management carries an increased risk for unplanned surgical intervention and blood loss when compared with surgical management.[21]

Variable results have been seen in studies comparing medical management with surgical management, with success rates for medical management ranging from 13% to 93%, depending on medication protocols, selection criteria, and outcome definitions.[22] Anembryonic pregnancies may be more prone to treatment failure with medical versus surgical management.[23,24] Most current treatment protocols are based on a well-designed multicenter study from 2005, which randomized 652 women to either vaginal misoprostol or manual vacuum aspiration.[23] Women receiving medical management were given an initial dose of misoprostol, 800 μg intravaginally, then a second dose after 3 days if expulsion did not occur. Misoprostol treatment was successful after the first dose in 71% and after the second dose in 84% of patients. Those who failed medical treatment were offered vacuum aspiration at day 8. By comparison, initial vacuum aspiration was successful in 97% of patients. There was no difference between the 2 groups for infections, hemodynamically significant bleeding, or emergency room visits. Patients receiving misoprostol reported more pain, bleeding, nausea, and vomiting. Satisfaction with treatment was similarly high in both treatment groups. Seventy-three percent of women randomized to misoprostol who had undergone vacuum aspiration with a previous miscarriage reported that they would use misoprostol again if needed.

Only one large study has directly compared expectant, medical, and surgical management.[22] Based on randomization of 1200 women, researchers in the United Kingdom found that women who underwent surgical management had fewer unplanned hospital admissions, unplanned curettages, and blood transfusions than those in the expectant and medical management arms. There was no difference in outpatient visits, infections, time to resumption of activities, duration of sick leave, or follow-up depression and anxiety scores. The investigators detail the difficulties they faced in recruiting an adequate number of women for randomization and posit that another head-to-head comparison of all 3 treatment options is unlikely.

Based on existing data, women who have not yet completed miscarriage can make treatment decisions in collaboration with their health care provider and in accordance with their personal preferences. β-hCG levels should be followed to less than 10 mIU/mL. This common practice is supported by a single prospective study of 152 patients, in which 5.9% of patients with apparently complete miscarriage were ultimately diagnosed with an ectopic pregnancy.[25] The decrease in β-hCG levels to nonpregnant levels also helps rule out the presence of gestational trophoblastic disease (discussed later in this article). Surgical specimens should be examined for the presence of chorionic villi, and some states mandate formal pathologic evaluation. The finding of normal chorionic villi is highly suggestive of intrauterine pregnancy (except in rare cases of heterotopic pregnancy). The American College of Obstetrics and Gynecology recommends administering anti-D immune globulin to all Rh-negative women after first trimester pregnancy loss.[19] Attention to the emotional needs of the patient and her family is another fundamental aspect of care. Multiple studies document the psychological repercussions of miscarriage for women and their partners.[26–28]

ECTOPIC PREGNANCY

Ectopic pregnancy is any pregnancy that occurs outside the intrauterine cavity and is a high-risk, potentially life-threatening condition. It is the leading cause of maternal death in the first trimester and accounts for 6% of all maternal deaths.[29,30] The rate of ectopic pregnancy in North America increased from less than 0.5% of all pregnancies in 1970 to almost 2% in 1992 and has remained at this rate.[30,31] Although the rate increased, the mortality associated with ectopic pregnancy has decreased to 0.05% because of early diagnosis and treatment before rupture.[30]

Diagnosis

Women presenting to the emergency department with first trimester bleeding and abdominal pain have a prevalence of ectopic pregnancy as high as 18% and require careful evaluation.[32] Physical examination findings that increase the likelihood of an ectopic pregnancy include vaginal bleeding, pelvic pain with manipulation of the cervix, and a palpable adnexal mass. Despite this, it is important to remember that physical examination findings alone cannot reliably exclude the diagnosis of ectopic pregnancy. The most cost-effective strategy for diagnosing ectopic pregnancy is TVUS followed by quantitative β-hCG testing if needed. If TVUS reveals a gestation either inside or outside the uterus, this test alone can confirm the diagnosis of intra-uterine pregnancy or ectopic pregnancy. If the result of ultrasonography is nondiag-nostic, then serum quantitative β-hCG levels should be obtained. If the β-hCG level is greater than the discriminatory zone and the TVUS is nondiagnostic, then ectopic pregnancy is suspected. The discriminatory zone for β-hCG is greater than or equal to 1500 to 2000 mIU/mL, the level of β-hCG at which a normal singleton intrauterine pregnancy can be visualized.[33] TVUS and serial quantitative β-hCG measurements combined are approximately 96% sensitive and 97% specific for diagnosing ectopic pregnancy.[34–36] Other diagnostic tests include progesterone levels and culdocente-sis. Progesterone levels may be helpful in diagnosing an abnormal pregnancy but are not specific for diagnosing ectopic pregnancy, and culdocentesis is only to be considered if ultrasonography is unavailable. When considering the diagnosis of ectopic pregnancy, it is important to keep in mind the possibility of heterotopic preg-nancy or multiple gestations, both of which are more diagnostically challenging.

Risk Factors

The most common risk factor for developing an ectopic pregnancy is prior tubal injury.[37] Causes of tubal injury may include a history of tubal surgery, ectopic preg-nancy, genital tract infections, or in utero exposure to diethylstilbestrol.[37] Other risk factors include a history of infertility or being a current smoker. Contraceptive use reduces the risk for any pregnancy occurring.[38] However, in the situation of steriliza-tion failure or pregnancy occurring with an intrauterine device in place, the likelihood that the pregnancy is ectopic increases.[38,39]

Treatment

In the setting of a ruptured ectopic pregnancy in which the patient is potentially hemo-dynamically unstable, emergent laparotomy is needed. For stable, unruptured, ectopic pregnancy, treatment options include medical management with metho-trexate and surgical management, preferably salpingostomy, with no difference in overall outcomes between these 2 therapies.[40] There is also a role for expectant management; however, it is difficult to distinguish patients who will have spontaneous resolution of an ectopic pregnancy from those who will require intervention. To consider expectant management, the patient should have a β-hCG level less than 1000 mIU/mL that is declining, an ectopic mass less than 3 cm, and no fetal heartbeat, and must agree to comply with close and complete follow-up. Regardless of the treat-ment, β-hCG levels should be monitored after treatment until a nonpregnancy level is reached.

Prognosis

The prognosis is good for patients who receive appropriate treatment. Recurrence of ectopic pregnancy and rates of tubal patency are similar after medical and surgical treatment.[30] The overall conception rate after treatment of ectopic pregnancy is approximately 77% regardless of the treatment.[41] The rate of recurrent ectopic pregnancy is between 5% and 20% and increases to 32% in women who have had 2 consecutive ectopic pregnancies.[41]

GESTATIONAL TROPHOBLASTIC DISEASE

In addition to being warning signs of other first trimester complications, bleeding and hyperemesis gravidarum can occur in gestational trophoblastic disease. Gestational trophoblastic disease occurs when abnormal growth arises from the trophoblast, the layer that surrounds the blastocyst and normally develops into the amnion and chorion.[35] Abnormal cell growth ensues and a normal fetus does not form.

Gestational trophoblastic disease is classified morphologically as hydatidiform mole, invasive mole, choriocarcinoma, or placental site trophoblastic tumor. The types that metastasize or invade locally are often referred to as gestational trophoblastic neoplasia.[42] Frequencies of the different types of gestational trophoblastic disease vary regionally, but hydatidiform moles are the most common type.[43]

Hydatidiform Mole

In the United States, hydatidiform moles are thought to occur in 1 in 1500 pregnancies; the incidence in Asian countries is higher, approaching 1 in 200 pregnancies.[44,45] They are most common in women younger than 17 years or older than 35 years and in women who have had previous occurrences of gestational trophoblastic disease. Although 80% of hydatidiform moles are benign, 20% can behave malignantly, necessitating chemotherapy after uterine evacuation. About 2% to 3% can be followed by choriocarcinoma.[44,45]

The most common symptom leading to the diagnosis of a hydatidiform mole is abnormal vaginal bleeding, which occurs in 84% of patients with complete moles.[45,46] Other warning signs include uterine enlargement greater than expected based on gestational age, hyperemesis gravidarum, absent fetal heart tones when one would expect to hear them, an abnormally high serum hCG level, and new hyperthyroidism.[45,47] Early pregnancy-induced hypertension or preeclampsia can be warning signs as well. With the prevalence of first trimester ultrasonography, a pattern classically described as a snowstorm with a complete mole may be seen, but ultrasonography alone is not sufficient for making the diagnosis.[43] The characteristic ultrasonic appearance of a complete mole is attributed to the villi and intrauterine blood clots that replace the normal placenta, but this may not be seen in a partial mole or early in the imaging of a complete mole.[45]

Hydatidiform moles are classified as partial or complete, with different characteristics and clinical features. A complete hydatidiform mole arises when 1 or 2 sperm cells fertilize an abnormal egg that contains no nucleus or DNA (an empty egg). There is no fetal tissue present because all genetic material comes from the sperm; the most common karyotype is 46,XX or 46,XY.[45,46] A partial hydatidiform mole arises when 2 sperms fertilize a normal egg; therefore, some fetal tissue is present, but no viable fetus is formed from this fertilization. Most commonly, the karyotype is 69,XXX or 69,XXY.[46] With a complete mole, there is diffuse proliferation of the trophoblastic tissue and diffuse edema of the villi with no fetal cells.[45] In a partial mole, there can be a variable amount of villous edema with fetal cells usually present. The trophoblastic proliferation is less prominent than in a complete mole. Uterine size can be small for gestational age in a partial mole and large for gestational age in a complete mole.

In addition to having different morphology, complete and partial moles can behave differently. Complete moles are more likely than partial moles to progress to gestational trophoblastic neoplasia. However, evacuation of the mole via suction curettage of the uterus is the initial procedure to treat both partial and complete moles. Most partial moles are completely treated by surgical removal via suction curettage. Medical methods of uterine evacuation are not recommended because they are associated with a higher rate of need for postprocedure chemotherapy.[44,46,48–53]

The initial evaluation for a molar pregnancy should include investigations for anemia, preeclampsia, electrolyte abnormalities, and hyperthyroidism; a baseline chest radiography should be obtained to investigate for metastatic disease to the lungs.[48] After evacuation, patients must be followed up with serial serum hCG measurements. As long as serum hCG levels are decreasing steadily after evacuation of the uterus, chemotherapy is not needed.

There is no way, based solely on histology, to predict if a hydatidiform mole will behave in a benign or malignant manner. Ultimately, this is determined by a patient's clinical course, with benign behavior characterized by the serum hCG level returning to normal within 12 weeks of evacuation of the mole; this is the course for 80% of patients with complete hydatidiform moles and 97% of patients with partial moles.[42] In cases in which hCG levels plateau or increase, further evaluation and treatment of malignant postmolar gestational trophoblastic disease are needed. Other reasons for needing chemotherapy after evacuation of a mole include histologic evidence of invasive mole or choriocarcinoma on evaluation of the suction curettage specimen or evidence of metastasis clinically or on chest radiography.[45] Partial moles are less likely to behave malignantly than are complete moles; only 2% to 3% of partial moles becoming malignant, whereas up to 20% of complete moles can become malignant. If they do become malignant, hydatidiform moles can metastasize to the lungs; this occurs in 4% to 5% of cases of complete moles.[42]

If a hydatidiform mole has become malignant, it is classified as being high risk (conferring a poor prognosis) or low risk. Combination chemotherapy is necessary for the high-risk group; a single agent (usually methotrexate) can be used for those in the low-risk group. The World Health Organization and the International Federation of Gynecology and Obstetrics have scoring systems to determine risk categories; factors that confer increased risk include age greater than 40 years, longer interval (>4 months) from index pregnancy, higher hCG levels (>1000), increased number and sites of metastases, largest tumor size greater than 3 cm, and previously failed chemotherapy.[46,48]

Women who have experienced a molar pregnancy are advised to wait at least 1 year before trying to conceive again. Conceiving at shorter intervals can make it difficult to determine if an increase in serum β-hCG level is from a normal subsequent pregnancy or from the hydatidiform mole behaving in a malignant manner. In addition, in patients with a history of previous pregnancy affected by gestational trophoblastic disease, serum hCG should be measured 6 weeks postpartum following any subsequent pregnancy to exclude gestational trophoblastic neoplasia.[42,45]

Invasive Mole (Chorioadenoma Destruens)

Most cases of persistent gestational trophoblastic disease are caused by invasive moles. An invasive mole occurs when a hydatidiform mole grows into the myometrium. Risk factors include maternal age greater than 40 years, longer than 4 months between the last menstrual period and treatment of the mole, a greatly enlarged uterus, and a previous history of gestational trophoblastic disease. A woman is at risk of significant bleeding if the invasive mole grows through the myometrium. Fifteen percent of invasive moles are metastatic. Treatment is with methotrexate or other combination chemotherapy regimens.[42,45]

Choriocarcinoma

Choriocarcinoma is a form of gestational trophoblastic neoplasia that is characterized by early hematogenous spread to the lung. Because of this spread, symptoms on presentation include shortness of breath, chest pain, and hemoptysis as well as vaginal bleeding. It may also be initially detected on routine obstetric ultrasonography. Half of the cases develop from a complete hydatidiform mole; choriocarcinoma can also develop from a pregnancy that ends in elective or spontaneous abortion as well as from a pregnancy that results in a normal term delivery (20%–30% of cases), with the prognosis usually worse if it develops after a normal delivered pregnancy.[42,45] Chemotherapy is the mainstay of treatment, with a cure rate of 90% to 95% even when lung metastases are present. Single-agent (methotrexate or actinomycin D) regimens are used for low-risk disease, and combination regimens are used for high-risk disease. Risk factors for high-risk disease are similar to the high-risk predictors in other forms of gestational trophoblastic disease. Hysterectomy may be necessary for patients having uncontrolled bleeding or those with severe infection. Choriocarcinoma that has metastasized to the brain or liver is usually fatal.[42,45]

Placental Site Trophoblastic Tumor

A placental site trophoblastic tumor is a rare tumor that occurs in the location of placental attachment to the uterus. It most commonly develops after a normal pregnancy (75% of cases) or after abortion but can develop after uterine evacuation of a complete or partial hydatidiform mole. This tumor does not spread to other sites but invades the uterine myometrium. Treatment is surgery (hysterectomy) rather than chemotherapy.[46]

NAUSEA AND VOMITING IN PREGNANCY

Between 50% and 75% of all pregnancies are complicated by nausea and vomiting. About 25% of women experience only nausea, and 50% have both nausea and vomiting.[54] For more than 90% of women, these symptoms resolve by 21 weeks. Experiencing nausea and vomiting in early pregnancy is associated with decreased risk of miscarriage.[54]

Approximately 1 in 200 women develop hyperemesis gravidarum.[55] This is defined by persistent vomiting, weight loss of more than 5%, ketones present in urine, and dehydration that is confirmed by increased specific gravity of the urine.[54] Hyperemesis can lead to severe complications such as Wernicke encephalopathy and liver and kidney damage.[56] It is rare to have neonatal complications (low birth weight and preterm birth) as long as women gain more than 6.8 kg (15 lb) during pregnancy.[54]

The cause of nausea and vomiting in pregnancy has not been clearly defined. It seems to be associated with higher levels of hCG, perhaps causing more estrogen to be released. Low levels of vitamin B may be another factor because vitamin B supplements help decrease nausea and vomiting.[54]

Evaluation of Women with Nausea and Vomiting

Most women do not need any further evaluation for the cause of nausea and vomiting. For persistent or severe nausea and vomiting causing weight loss and dehydration, some tests should be completed. Levels of electrolytes, liver enzymes, and thyrotropin should be evaluated to rule out other medical causes of nausea and vomiting, such as liver disease and hyperthyroidism. Also, women should undergo ultrasonography to evaluate for molar pregnancy or twins, which have been associated with hyperemesis.[54] There is some suggestion that *Helicobacter pylori* may cause hyperemesis, and it is reasonable to test for this in women who have intractable nausea and vomiting.[56]

Treatment

Less than 10% of women require medical treatment of nausea and vomiting during pregnancy.[54] Women are encouraged to avoid exposure to strong odors and foods that trigger the nausea. Women should have food at the bedside and avoid an empty stomach. It is also thought that a bland diet with lots of protein and small frequent meals are helpful. There are no data to support any of these interventions.[54]

Acupressure and acupuncture have been recommended to treat nausea and vomiting. There is some evidence to support the use of acupressure to reduce the symptoms for women with nausea and vomiting. There are no data to support the use of acupuncture to treat nausea and vomiting or hyperemesis.[55]

There is some evidence that ginger reduces nausea and vomiting for women. The dosages range from 250 mg 4 times a day to 350 mg 3 times a day.[56] It seems to be better than placebo for treating nausea and vomiting. Pyridoxine (vitamin B_6) also improves nausea and vomiting. The dosage ranges from 10 to 25 mg 3 times a day.[55]

Antihistamines have been shown to decrease nausea and vomiting for some women. The medication doxylamine has been associated with decreased hospitalizations for nausea and vomiting. In 1983, the medication Bendectin (doxylamine succinate 10 mg and pyridoxine hydrochloride 10 mg) was removed from the market in the United States because of concerns about teratogenicity, which were not supported by evidence.[54] In Canada, this medication is combined with vitamin B_6 and used frequently for treatment of nausea and vomiting in early pregnancy. In the United States, this medication is the active ingredient in Unisom doxylamine.[55]

Antiemetic medications have been used to treat severe cases of nausea and vomiting. Metoclopramide and prochlorperazine have not been shown to be much better than placebo in the treatment of nausea and vomiting. There are no data suggesting fetal malformation from the use of antiemetics, but there is concern about tardive dyskinesia with the long-term use of metoclopramide.[55] The newer antiemetic ondansetron (Zofran) is used more often for treatment of nausea and vomiting, but there are little data on improvement in symptoms. The medication inapsine (Droperidol) has also been used for the treatment of nausea and vomiting in pregnancy. However, this medication was given a black box warning by the US Food and Drug Administration in 2001 because of cardiac arrhythmias.

For refractory cases of hyperemesis, steroids have been used to reduce hospital readmissions. The use of methylprednisolone and hydrocortisone has been shown to reduce symptoms for some women. If steroids are given during the first trimester, there is an association with cleft lip and palate. The recommendation is to avoid usage during this period.[55]

SUMMARY

Vaginal bleeding in the first trimester of pregnancy is a common presenting complaint. Although it is often self-limited with no cause found, it can herald serious complications, such as miscarriage, ectopic pregnancy, or gestational trophoblastic disease. TVUS combined with quantitative serum β-hCG levels usually allow a diagnosis to be made. Once a diagnosis is made, treatment should follow in a timely manner. Nausea and vomiting in pregnancy may also be self-limited and may occur in a normal pregnancy, but hyperemesis should prompt the medical provider to consider the possibility of gestational trophoblastic disease. Emotional support should be provided to the patient during any pregnancy, especially a pregnancy that is made more difficult by these first trimester complications.

REFERENCES

1. Everett C. Incidence and outcome of bleeding before the 20th week of pregnancy: prospective study from general practice. BMJ 1997;315:32–4.
2. Hasan R, Baird DD, Herring AH, et al. Association between first-trimester vaginal bleeding and miscarriage. Obstet Gynecol 2009;114(4):860–7.
3. Isoardi K. Review article: the use of pelvic examination within the emergency department in the assessment of early pregnancy bleeding. Emerg Med Australas 2009;21(6):440–8.
4. Norstrom A, Jansson I, Anderson H. Carcinoma of the uterine cervix in pregnancy. A study of the incidence and treatment in the western region of Sweden 1973-1992. Acta Obstet Gynecol Scand 1997;76:583–9.
5. Paspulati RM, Bhatt S, Nour SG. Sonographic evaluation of first trimester bleeding. Radiol Clin N Am 2004;42(2):297–314.
6. Barnhart KT, Sammel MD, Rinaudo PF, et al. Symptomatic patients with an early viable intrauterine pregnancy: HCG curves redefined. Obstet Gynecol 2004; 104(1):50–5.
7. Deutchman M, Tubay AT, Turok D. First trimester bleeding. Am Fam Physician 2009;79(11):985–94.
8. Gracia CR, Sammel MD, Chittams J, et al. Risk factors for spontaneous abortion in early symptomatic first-trimester pregnancies. Obstet Gynecol 2005;106(5 Pt 1): 993–9.
9. Maso G, D'Ottavio G, De Seta F, et al. First-trimester intrauterine hematoma and outcome of pregnancy. Obstet Gynecol 2005;105(2):339–44.
10. Nagy S, Bush M, Stone J, et al. Clinical significance of subchorionic and retroplacental hematomas detected in the first trimester of pregnancy. Obstet Gynecol 2003;102(1):94–100.
11. Johns J, Hyett H, Jauniaux E. Obstetric outcome after threatened miscarriage with and without a hematoma on ultrasound. Obstet Gynecol 2003;102(3):483–7.
12. Bennett GL, Bromley B, Lieberman E, et al. Subchorionic hemorrhage in first-trimester pregnancies: prediction of pregnancy outcome with sonography. Radiology 1996;200(3):803–6.
13. Falco P, Milano V, Pilu G, et al. Sonography of pregnancies with first-trimester bleeding and a viable embryo: a study of prognostic indicators by logistic regression analysis. Ultrasound Obstet Gynecol 1996;7(3):165–9.
14. Pedersen JF, Mantoni M. Prevalence and significance of subchorionic hemorrhage in threatened abortion: a sonographic study. AJR Am J Roentgenol 1990;154(3):535–7.

15. Dickey RP, Olar TT, Curole DN, et al. Relationship of first-trimester subchorionic bleeding detected by color Doppler ultrasound to subchorionic fluid, clinical bleeding, and pregnancy outcome. Obstet Gynecol 1992;80(3 Pt 1):415–20.
16. Saraswat L, Bhattacharya S, Maheshwari A, et al. Maternal and perinatal outcome in women with threatened miscarriage in the first trimester: a systematic review. BJOG 2010;117(3):245–57.
17. Lykke JA, Dideriksen KL, Lidegaard O, et al. First-trimester vaginal bleeding and complications later in pregnancy. Obstet Gynecol 2010;115(5):935–44.
18. Sotiriadis A, Papatheodorou S, Makrydimas G. Threatened miscarriage: evaluation and management. BMJ 2004;329:152–5.
19. ACOG practice bulletin. Prevention of Rh D alloimmunization. Number 4, May 1999. Int J Gynaecol Obstet 1999;66(1):63–70.
20. Nielsen S, Hahlin M. Expectant management of first-trimester spontaneous abortion. Lancet 1995;345:84–6.
21. Bagratee JS, Khullar V, Regan L, et al. A randomized controlled trial comparing medical and expectant management of first trimester miscarriage. Hum Reprod 2004;19(2):266–71.
22. Nanda K, Peloggia A, Grimes D, et al. Expectant care versus surgical treatment for miscarriage. Cochrane Database Syst Rev 2006;2:CD003518.
23. Trinder J, Brocklehurst P, Porter R, et al. Management of miscarriage: expectant, medical, or surgical? Results of randomised controlled trial (miscarriage treatment (MIST) trial). BMJ 2006;332(7552):1235–40.
24. Zhang J, Giles JM, Barnhart K, et al. A comparison of medical management with misoprostol and surgical management for early pregnancy failure. N Engl J Med 2005;353(8):761–9.
25. Condous G, Okaro E, Khalid A, et al. Do we need to follow up complete miscarriages with serum human chorionic gonadotropin levels? BJOG 2005;112(6): 827–9.
26. Weeks A, Alia G, Blum J, et al. A randomized trial of misoprostol compared with manual vacuum aspiration for incomplete abortion. Obstet Gynecol 2005;106(3): 540–7.
27. Lok IH, Yip AS, Lee DT, et al. A 1-year longitudinal study of psychological morbidity after miscarriage. Fertil Steril 2010;93:1966–75.
28. Kong G, Chung T, Lai B, et al. Gender comparison of psychological reaction after miscarriage—a 1-year longitudinal study. BJOG 2010;117:1211–9.
29. Chang J, Elam-Evans LD, Berg CJ, et al. Pregnancy-related mortality surveillance—United States, 1991-1999. MMWR Surveill Summ 2003;52:1–8.
30. Barnhart KT. Ectopic pregnancy. N Engl J Med 2009;361:379–87.
31. Lozeau AM, Potter B. Diagnosis and management of ectopic pregnancy. Am Fam Physician 2005;72:1707–14.
32. Barnhart KT, Sammel MD, Gracia CR, et al. Risk factors for ectopic pregnancy in women with symptomatic first-trimester pregnancies. Fertil Steril 2006;86: 36–43.
33. Kadar N, Bohrer M, Kemmann E, et al. The discriminatory human chorionic gonadotropin zone for endovaginal sonography: a prospective, randomized study. Fertil Steril 1994;61:1016–20.
34. Mol BW, Van der Veen F, Bossuyt PM. Implementation of probabilistic decision rules improves the predictive values of algorithms in the diagnostic management of ectopic pregnancy. Hum Reprod 1999;14:2855–62.
35. Gracia CR, Barnhart KT. Diagnosing ectopic pregnancy: decision analysis comparing six strategies. Obstet Gynecol 2001;97:464–70.

36. Buckley RG, King KJ, Disney JD, et al. Derivation of a clinical prediction model for the emergency department diagnosis of ectopic pregnancy. Acad Emerg Med 1998;5:951–60.
37. Ankum WM, Mol BW, Van der Veen F, et al. Risk factors for ectopic pregnancy: a meta-analysis. Fertil Steril 1996;65:1093–9.
38. Sivin I. Dose- and age-dependent ectopic pregnancy risks with intrauterine contraception. Obstet Gynecol 1991;78:291–8.
39. Peterson HB, Xia Z, Hughes JM, et al. The risk of ectopic pregnancy after tubal sterilization. U.S. Collaborative Review of Sterilization Working Group. N Engl J Med 1997;336:762–7.
40. ACOG Practice Bulletin No. 94. Medical management of ectopic pregnancy. Obstet Gynecol 2008;111:1479–85.
41. Tay JI, Moore J, Walker JJ. Clinical review: ectopic pregnancy [published correction appears in BMJ 2000;321:424]. BMJ 2000;329:916–9.
42. Hernandez E. Gestational trophoblastic neoplasia. Updated March, 2010. Available at: http://emedicine.medscape.com/article/279116-overview. Accessed March 10, 2011.
43. Dresang LT. A molar pregnancy detected by following {beta}-human chorionic gonadotropin levels after a first trimester loss. J Am Board Fam Pract 2005;18: 570–3.
44. Gershenson DM, Ramirez PT. Gynecological tumors. Merck Manual Online; 2008. Available at: http://www.merckmanuals.com/professional/sec18/ch254/ch254f.html. Accessed March 10, 2011.
45. Soper JT, Mutch DG, Schink JC. Diagnosis and treatment of gestational trophoblastic disease: ACOG Practice Bulletin No. 53. Gynecol Oncol 2004;93(3):575–85.
46. Gerulath AH, Ehlen TG, Bessette P, et al. Gestational trophoblastic disease, SOGC clinical practice guidelines. Available at: http://www.sogc.org/guidelines/public/114E-CPG-May2002.pdf. Accessed March 10, 2011.
47. ARUP Consult. The physician's guide to laboratory test selection and interpretation. Gestational trophoblastic disease. Available at: http://www.arupconsult.com/Topics/GestationalTrophoblasticDz.html. Accessed March 10, 2011.
48. Leister AL, Aghajanian C. Evaluation and management of gestational trophoblastic disease. Community Oncol 2006;3:152–6.
49. Cancer.org. Gestational trophoblastic disease. 2010. Available at. http://www.cancer.org/Cancer/GestationalTrophoblasticDisease/DetailedGuide/gestational-trophoblastic-disease-what-is-g-t-d. Accessed March 10, 2011.
50. Seckl MJ, Sebire NJ, Berkowitz RS. Gestational trophoblastic disease. Lancet 2010;376:717–29.
51. Berkowitz RS, Goldstein DP. Clinical practice. Molar pregnancy. N Engl J Med 2009;360(16):1639–45.
52. Berkowitz RS, Goldstein DP. Current management of gestational trophoblastic diseases. Gynecol Oncol 2009;112(3):654–62.
53. Garner EI. Gestational trophoblastic disease. Management of hydatidiform mole. Reviewed September 2010. Available at: www.Uptodate.com. Accessed March 16, 2011.
54. Niebyl J. Nausea and vomiting in pregnancy. N Engl J Med 2010;363:1544–50.
55. Festin M. Nausea and vomiting in early pregnancy. Clin Evid. Web publication date: 3 Jun 2009 (based on May 2008 search). Available at: http://www.ncbi.nlm.nih.gov/pubmed/19454064. Accessed May 15, 2011.
56. Dynamed. Nausea and vomiting in pregnancy. Updated in February 22, 2011. Available at: http://dynamed.ebscohost.com/. Accessed March 9, 2011.

Update on Gestational Diabetes Mellitus

Ann E. Evensen, MD

KEYWORDS

- Gestational diabetes mellitus • Pregnancy • Prenatal care
- Obstetrics • Pregnancy complications • Glyburide • Insulin

DEFINITION

Gestational diabetes mellitus (GDM) is defined as carbohydrate intolerance that begins or is first recognized in pregnancy.[1] Historically, GDM has been labeled as classes A1 (non–insulin requiring) and A2 (insulin requiring).[2] Management of other classes such as diabetes diagnosed before conception (pregestational diabetes) or gestational diabetes insipidus is not covered in this review.

PATHOPHYSIOLOGY

All pregnant women develop some insulin resistance, which likely evolved to facilitate energy delivery to the fetus. Insulin resistance is proposed to occur in response to placental hormones. The role of placental hormones is consistent with the observed worsening of GDM throughout pregnancy (increasing placental size), the increased risk of GDM in pregnancies with multiple fetuses (larger total placental weight), and the rapid resolution of GDM with delivery of the placenta.[3] Insulin resistance may progress to GDM by revealing autoimmune-mediated or genetic abnormalities in pancreatic beta-cell function and/or worsening of chronic insulin resistance. Pregnant women with autoimmune beta-cell dysfunction may have more rapid escalation of blood glucose levels than women with chronic insulin resistance.[4]

PREVALENCE

The prevalence of GDM varies widely depending on the population studied, but the overall estimated prevalence in the United States is 2% to 10%.[5] The prevalence is increasing as rates of obesity increase.[4] The prevalence will also increase significantly if new screening recommendations are incorporated into clinical practice (see

This work received no grant funding.
The author has nothing to disclose.
Department of Family Medicine, University of Wisconsin School of Medicine and Public Health, 100 North Nine Mound Road, Verona, WI 53593, USA
E-mail address: ann.evensen@uwmf.wisc.edu

Prim Care Clin Office Pract 39 (2012) 83–94
doi:10.1016/j.pop.2011.11.011   **primarycare.theclinics.com**
0095-4543/12/$ – see front matter © 2012 Elsevier Inc. All rights reserved.

Screening section).[6] One-third of women with GDM have a recurrence in subsequent pregnancies. Risk factors for recurrence are weight gain between pregnancies, older maternal age, and greater parity.[7,8]

SCREENING

Women may have diabetes that existed but was undiagnosed before pregnancy. Patients at very high risk for preexisting diabetes (strong family history of type 2 diabetes, personal history of GDM, delivery of a large-for-gestational-age [LGA] infant, polycystic ovary syndrome, severe obesity, or glucosuria) should undergo a glucose tolerance test early in prenatal care.[8]

For patients not at high risk, there is debate about the need for universal screening.[9] Although there is consensus that treating GDM is beneficial, systematic reviews of the available evidence have not found sufficient evidence to support screening for GDM.[10–12]

Despite the lack of strong evidence for universal screening, it is routinely performed in US obstetric practice at 24 to 28 weeks' gestation. Screening before 24 weeks may miss cases of GDM, whereas screening later in pregnancy may delay treatment (although the benefits of early treatment have not been documented).

Selective screening is an alternative to universal screening. Selective screening uses certain criteria (**Box 1**) to avoid screening low-risk women. Selective screening is estimated to have very high sensitivity but only exempts a small percentage (3.5%) of the population from screening.[13] Because glucose intolerance occurs across a continuum, no cutoff identifies all persons with GDM, whether universal or selective screening is chosen.

A 2-step testing procedure is recommended for screening and diagnosis of GDM. This process is outlined in the most recent American College of Obstetricians and Gynecologists (ACOG) Practice Bulletin addressing GDM (published in 2001 and reaffirmed in 2011). This Practice Bulletin recommends screening with the O'Sullivan test—a 1-hour, nonfasting, 50-g glucose challenge.[1] A blood glucose level cutoff of either 130 or 140 mg/dL has been used to diagnose GDM. Using a cutoff of 130 mg/dL increases sensitivity and decreases specificity of the screening tool; the opposite is true for a cutoff of 140 mg/dL. The use of either cutoff is acceptable because the risks and benefits of each cutoff are unknown.[1] If the 1-hour screening test is abnormal, a 3-hour, fasting, 100-g glucose tolerance test is performed to diagnose

---

Box 1
Criteria for selective screening of women at low risk for GDM

You may choose not to screen low-risk women who meet ALL the following criteria:

1. Younger than 25 years

2. Not a member of an ethnic group at an increased risk for the development of type 2 diabetes mellitus (Hispanic, African, Native American, South or East Asian, or Pacific Islands ancestry)

3. Normal weight before pregnancy

4. No history of abnormal glucose tolerance

5. No history of adverse obstetric outcomes usually associated with GDM

6. No known diabetes in first-degree relatives

Data from American Diabetes Association. Standards of medical care in diabetes—2010. Diabetes Care 2010;33(Suppl 1):S11–61.

GDM. Either the Carpenter/Coustan or the National Diabetes Data Group criteria can be used for interpreting the 3-hour test results. As with the 1-hour challenge, there are no data from clinical trials demonstrating superiority of either criterion.[13]

In 2010, the International Association of Diabetes and Pregnancy Study Group (IADPSG) recommended abandoning the 2-step screening process and adopting a 2-hour, fasting, 75-g glucose tolerance test for all women.[6] This method would allow for screening and diagnosis with a single glucose tolerance test. The cutoffs recommended by the IADPSG are much more stringent than the 2-hour, fasting, 75-g glucose tolerance test previously endorsed by the World Health Organization. The IADPSG reported that the new cutoffs were chosen based on the landmark Hyperglycemia and Adverse Pregnancy Outcomes (HAPO) study but acknowledged that no trial has been performed to document benefit to mothers or infants if this method of screening were to be adopted.[14] At this time, the ACOG recommends the 2-step testing because of the costs of treatment and monitoring for an estimated 18% of all pregnancies (more than double the incidence of GDM based on the 2-step testing) without documented benefits and improvements in maternal or neonatal outcomes.[15] **Table 1** compares testing methods and cutoffs for screening and diagnosis of GDM.

Regardless of the choice of test, venous samples are recommended over capillary measurements (point-of-care "fingerstick"). Capillary samples overestimate blood glucose levels compared with venous samples.[16] The use of food (such as jelly beans) instead of a standard glucose solution is not recommended because of the decreased test sensitivity.[17]

MATERNAL, FETAL, AND NEONATAL RISKS OF GDM

The risks of GDM are numerous for both the mother and the infant (**Box 2**). It is unclear as to what proportion of the risk is from the conditions that coexist with GDM such as obesity or older maternal age and what proportion is from the GDM itself.[1] The HAPO

Table 1					
Comparison of glucose tolerance tests used for screening and diagnosis of GDM					
Test or Criterion Name	Glucose Challenge (g)	Fasting	Time Measurement	Cutoffs (mg/dL)	Number of Abnormal Results Required for a Positive Test Result
O'Sullivan	50	No	At 1 h	>140 or >130	1
IADPSG	75	Yes	Fasting At 1 h At 2 h	≥92 ≥180 ≥153	1
World Health Organization	75	Yes	Fasting At 2 h	>126 >140	1
National Diabetes Data Group	100	Yes	Fasting At 1 h At 2 h At 3 h	≥105 ≥190 ≥165 ≥145	2
Carpenter/Coustan criteria	100	Yes	Fasting At 1 h At 2 h At 3 h	≥95 ≥180 ≥155 ≥140	2

Data from Refs.[1,4,33]

Box 2
Maternal, fetal, and neonatal complications of GDM

Maternal

    Gestational hypertension and preeclampsia

    Polyhydramnios

    Risks associated with increased rates of induction (operative delivery, chorioamnionitis, tachysystole, uterine rupture, cord prolapse, and hemorrhage)

    Need for cesarean delivery

    Maternal trauma from operative delivery

    Preterm labor

Fetal

    Macrosomia: birthweight exceeding 4000 to 4500 g

    Shoulder dystocia

    Preterm delivery

    Fetal cardiomyopathy

    Stillbirth

    Congenital malformations (if diabetes was not diagnosed before pregnancy)

    Risks of operative delivery (shoulder dystocia, brachial plexus injury, and birth trauma)

Neonatal

    Respiratory distress syndrome and lung immaturity

    Cardiomyopathy

    Small-for-gestational-age (SGA)

    Increased lifetime risk of developing diabetes mellitus and obesity

    Changes in neurodevelopment including attention and motor skills

    Hyperbilirubinemia

    Hypoglycemia

    Hypocalcemia and hypomagnesemia

    Erythremia (increased red blood cells)

    Poor feeding

Data from Refs.[1,4,18–22]

---

study found a linear relationship between complications (fetal macrosomia and the need for primary cesarean delivery) and glucose intolerance. This linear relationship was seen even at levels of glucose intolerance that did not meet the criteria for GDM.[14]

Elevated maternal blood glucose levels clearly result in some increased risk. Glucose crosses the placenta but insulin does not, and the fetus produces its own insulin in response to the glucose entering the placental circulation. Fetal insulin allows for the storage of excess glucose as fetal fat deposits. In addition, fetal insulin acts as a growth factor, causing macrosomia. Macrosomia, in turn, increases the risk of an operative delivery and incidence of shoulder dystocia. These delivery complications increase the risk of maternal and fetal trauma, including injury to maternal internal organs, maternal hemorrhage and infection, perineal laceration, brachial plexus injury, and cephalohematoma.

Other risks are less obviously related to hyperglycemia but are found at increased rates in pregnancies complicated by GDM (eg, preeclampsia, fetal cardiomyopathy, delayed fetal lung maturation, and abnormal pediatric psychomotor development).[18–20,22]

Two potential iatrogenic risks of managing pregnancies complicated by GDM are respiratory distress syndrome and SGA neonates. Aggressive lowering of maternal blood glucose levels during pregnancy increases the risk of SGA infants.[4] Inducing labor before 38 to 39 weeks increases the already-elevated risk of neonatal lung immaturity in infants of mothers with GDM.

ANTEPARTUM MANAGEMENT OF GDM

Although there is debate about the ideal method of screening for GDM, there is agreement that once diagnosed, patients with GDM should be treated with diet and, if needed, medication. The authors of a systematic review of the benefits of treating GDM with diet and insulin (added to diet if needed) found that treatment reduced risk of shoulder dystocia, preeclampsia, and macrosomia. More intensive treatment was more effective than less-intensive treatment in reducing the risk of shoulder dystocia. Treatment of GDM had no effect on the rates of SGA infants and perinatal or neonatal mortality.[11,20,23]

The 3 primary goals in antenatal management of GDM are to prevent macrosomia, avoid ketosis, and detect pregnancy complications (eg, hypertension, intrauterine growth restriction, and fetal distress). Despite agreement on these goals, there is no evidence to support specific management recommendations. Diet, exercise, oral hypoglycemic medications, and insulin may be used to treat GDM.

The goals of diet therapy in GDM are to avoid ketosis, achieve normal blood glucose levels, obtain proper nutrition, and gain weight appropriately. The American Diabetes Association recommends nutrition counseling, preferably with a registered dietician.[24] Counseling should be individualized, combined with recommendations for exercise, and culturally appropriate. The amount and distribution of carbohydrate should be based on clinical outcome measures (eg, hunger, blood glucose levels, weight gain, and [rarely used] ketone levels), but a minimum of 175 g of carbohydrate per day should be provided.[24] Carbohydrate should be distributed throughout the day in 5 to 7 meals and snacks. Carbohydrate is generally less well tolerated at breakfast than at other meals. Use of a low–glycemic index diet decreases the need for insulin to maintain euglycemia.[25,26] Fiber supplementation is not known to benefit patients with GDM.[24]

Experts recommend that women with GDM should exercise regularly to control blood glucose levels, but an improvement in clinical outcomes has not been demonstrated from compliance with this recommendation.[1,4,27]

Weight loss during pregnancy is not recommended, but the ideal weight gain for patients with GDM is unknown.[4,24] The Institute of Medicine (IOM) has published recommendations for weight gain in pregnancy, but the guidelines are the same for patients with and without GDM.[28] A cohort study showed that women with GDM who gained more weight than was recommended by the IOM had an increased risk of preterm delivery, macrosomic neonates, and cesarean delivery. Women with GDM who gained less weight than was recommended had an increased rate of SGA infants.[29]

TREATMENT WITH INSULIN

Traditionally, insulin is used if dietary management does not maintain fasting blood glucose level measurements less than 96 mg/dL, 1-hour measurements less than 130 to 140 mg/dL, and 2-hour measurements less than 120 mg/dL.[4] Another gauge that is used to determine the need for insulin is the fetal abdominal circumference measured at 29 to 33 weeks. If this measurement exceeds the 75th percentile, adding insulin to a management regimen will decrease the incidence of LGA infants.[30]

Insulin does not cross the placenta. Humalog, neutral protamine Hagedorn (NPH), and insulin lispro are used because of their rapid action and documented safety.[31] Long-acting glargine and detemir may be more convenient to use but may not adequately manage postprandial hyperglycemia. A recent systematic review and meta-analysis of retrospective cohort studies evaluating the use of glargine in the treatment of GDM found no adverse fetal outcomes.[4,31,32] However, no prospective studies of glargine or detemir have been carried out.

Two large randomized controlled trials of GDM treatment using diet and insulin (if needed) showed benefits including decreased incidence of fetal overgrowth, shoulder dystocia, cesarean delivery, hypertensive disorders, and serious perinatal complications (defined as death, shoulder dystocia, bone fracture, and nerve palsy).[20,23]

Insulin may be initiated at 0.7 U/kg actual body weight/d given in divided dosages: two-thirds of the daily dosage before breakfast (given as two-thirds NPH and one-third regular insulin) and the remainder of the dosage before dinner (given as half regular insulin and half NPH). It is also acceptable to use rapid-acting insulin with each meal instead of the twice-daily regular insulin. All regimens require close monitoring and adjustment based on blood glucose levels, meal choices, and activity levels.[33]

TREATMENT WITH ORAL HYPOGLYCEMIC AGENTS

The use of oral hypoglycemic agents (OHAs) instead of insulin is controversial.[34–36] OHA therapy was initially rejected when early-generation sulfonylureas were found to cross the placenta and cause fetal hyperinsulinemia.[1] There was also concern that OHAs would not be sufficient to manage postprandial hyperglycemia. However, glyburide was subsequently found to be safe and effective in randomized, prospective, cohort studies.[37] Metformin has also been evaluated in randomized prospective studies comparing it with insulin and glyburide. These studies have found no difference in perinatal complications.[38–41] A 2010 systematic review and meta-analysis of OHAs compared with insulin showed no significant difference in maternal fasting or postprandial glycemic control. The use of OHAs was not associated with the risk of neonatal hypoglycemia, increased birth weight, incidence of cesarean section, or incidence of LGA infants.[40]

An appropriate starting dosage of glyburide is 1.25 to 2.5 mg/d, which can be gradually increased to a maximum of 10 mg twice a day. Metformin can be started at 500 mg/d and increased to a maximum of 2000 mg/d. Long-acting formulations of both glyburide and metformin are available but were not used in the trials evaluating safety and effectiveness. OHAs should be initiated only if there is a willingness to abandon them. Failure of OHAs occurs more often in pregnancies complicated by early diagnosis of GDM, older age, higher parity, and higher fasting blood glucose levels[34] and is more common in pregnancies managed with metformin (25%–46%) than in those managed with glyburide (16%–24%).[38,39,41,42]

It is unclear whether the use of OHAs during the first trimester of pregnancy is safe. In Dhulkotia's[40] systematic review, none of the trials evaluated women who required treatment before 11 weeks. A Cochrane study group attempted to review the safety of OHA use in the treatment of women with diabetes and glucose intolerance diagnosed before pregnancy. However, no well-designed trial could be identified for analysis.[36] The use of OHAs other than glyburide and metformin (such as thiazolidinediones, alpha-glucosidase inhibitors, meglitinides, and peptide analogs) is untested and not recommended at this time. **Table 2** shows the safety of GDM medications in pregnant and lactating women.

WHEN TO TEST?

The growth and well-being of a fetus is more sensitive to hyperglycemia than hypoglycemia. To detect and avoid postprandial hyperglycemia, it is recommended that patients test blood glucose levels after meals. A study of patients with insulin-requiring GDM documented improved outcomes (improved glycemic control and decreased risk of neonatal hypoglycemia, macrosomia, and cesarean delivery) with postprandial testing rather than with testing when fasting.[43]

HOW OFTEN TO TEST?

Since treatment of GDM is beneficial and more intensive treatment results in better perinatal outcomes, it is assumed that frequent self-monitoring of blood glucose levels is necessary.[11,20,23] Studies of high-frequency testing (self-testing 7 times a day for insulin-requiring patients and once a day for diet-controlled patients) found better maternal and fetal outcomes when compared to low-frequency testing.[43–45] The optimal frequency of testing for patients on OHAs is unknown, but a reasonable frequency may be 4 to 6 times daily.[3,34]

Laboratory studies, ultrasonographies, and assessments of fetal well-being are used to monitor pregnancies complicated by GDM. Patients should undergo baseline urine protein (because of the increased risk of preeclampsia) and baseline hemoglobin A1c (HbA1c) assessments.[4] An initial HbA1c level of more than 7 or an initial fasting blood glucose level of more than 120 should be assumed to be undiagnosed,

Table 2		
Safety of GDM medications in pregnancy and breastfeeding		
Drug	**Pregnancy Class**	**Breastfeeding Class**
Insulin	B (regular, lispro, NPH) C (glargine, detemir)	All forms safe in breastfeeding (infants cannot absorb insulin intact through their gastrointestinal tracts)
Glyburide	B/C (manufacturer dependent)	Does not enter breast milk, but breastfeeding is not recommended by the manufacturer
Glipizide	C	Does not enter breast milk, but breastfeeding is not recommended by the manufacturer
Metformin	B	Small amount (<1% weight-adjusted maternal dose) enters breast milk, but breastfeeding is not recommended by the manufacturer

Experts consider insulin, glyburide, glipizide, and metformin safe to use in women who are breastfeeding despite the manufacturers' cautions.

Data from Metzger BE, Buchanan TA, Coustan DR, et al. Summary and recommendations of the Fifth International Workshop—Conference on Gestational Diabetes Mellitus. Diabetes Care 2007;30(Suppl 2):S251–60; and Lexi-Comp [Internet]. Ohio: Lexi-Comp, Inc.; 2011. Available at: http://www.lexi.com/. Accessed November 3, 2011.

preexisting diabetes mellitus rather than GDM. Preexisting diabetes increases the risk of many congenital malformations, especially in the cardiovascular and central nervous systems. An ultrasonography that includes careful assessment of fetal cardiac structures and screening for other anomalies should be offered to these patients.

Measurement of ketones in the blood or urine may aid in the management of a pregnancy complicated by severe hyperglycemia or weight loss, but there is no evidence that this monitoring improves outcomes in less-complicated pregnancies.[4]

Ultrasonography is commonly performed early in the second trimester and repeated to evaluate excessive or inadequate growth.[4] Ultrasonography may be performed more frequently for patients treated with insulin or OHAs. A study showed that having 2 second- or third-trimester ultrasounds demonstrating fetal abdominal circumference below the 90th percentile reliably excluded the risk of having an LGA newborn.[46]

In contrast, ruling in the diagnosis of macrosomia is difficult. A systematic review reported ultrasonography underestimating or overestimating the fetal weight by a no better than 14%.[47] In pregnancies not complicated by diabetes, suspected fetal macrosomia is not an indication for cesarean delivery.[21] However, suspected fetal macrosomia is taken into consideration in the management of pregnancies complicated by GDM. When comparing deliveries of fetuses of similar weights, a woman with diabetes has an increased risk of shoulder dystocia, even if the fetus is not macrosomic.[48] If fetal weight is estimated to be more than 4500 g, a trial of labor is not recommended; instead, a cesarean delivery should be offered. If the fetal weight is estimated to be 4000 to 4500 g, a clinician should consider the patient's delivery history, clinical pelvimetry, and progress of labor in determining the best delivery method. A cesarean delivery should be offered to a patient with GDM who has a prolonged second stage or arrest of descent in the second stage of labor.[1]

The frequency of assessments of maternal and fetal well-being such as office visits (including discussion of blood glucose level management), nonstress testing (NST), fetal kick counts, contraction stress testing (CST), amniotic fluid index (AFI) measurements, and biophysical profiles (BPPs) may be decided according to local obstetric practice. There is no evidence of better outcomes with any particular monitoring pattern. Patients who require medication to control GDM are seen every 1 to 2 weeks in the office. Assessments of fetal well-being (NSTs, AFIs, and BPPs, or CSTs when interpretation of NST or BPP is unclear) begin at 32 weeks' gestation and are scheduled 2 times per week. Monitoring of very high–risk patients can be started at 26 to 28 weeks' gestation.[1,4,34,49] Patients with GDM who control blood glucose levels with diet should have antenatal testing beginning at 40 weeks.[3]

DECISION TO DELIVER

The goal of intrapartum GDM management is to avoid operative delivery, shoulder dystocia, birth trauma, and neonatal hypoglycemia. For patients who have maintained excellent control of blood glucose levels with diet and exercise, delivery is recommended at 40 weeks (or antenatal testing should begin at that time). For patients with medication-requiring GDM, induction at 38 to 39 weeks' gestation is recommended based on the results of a single trial of patients with insulin-requiring diabetes who were randomized to induction at 38 to 39 weeks versus expectant management. There was no difference in cesarean delivery between the 2 groups, and fewer shoulder dystocias occurred in the induction group.[50] A clinician may choose to assess fetal lung maturity before induction at 39 weeks.[1]

INTRAPARTUM MANAGEMENT OF GDM

For patients with diet-controlled GDM, a random blood glucose level may be measured on admission to the labor ward.[33] If the blood glucose levels are normal, routine glucose measurements are not required. If a patient with GDM was treated with OHAs or insulin before admission, intrapartum blood glucose level monitoring and dextrose and/or insulin intravenous infusions may be required. Long-acting and subcutaneous insulins are not used in labor because of the slower onset of action and risk of hypoglycemia. Maintaining maternal euglycemia may prevent fetal hypoxia and neonatal hypoglycemia. The ideal intrapartum glucose target is unknown.[4] Intrapartum insulin, dextrose, and monitoring regimens are reviewed elsewhere.[3,51]

POSTPARTUM MANAGEMENT OF GDM AND INTERCONCEPTION CARE

In most women with GDM, hyperglycemia rapidly resolves shortly after delivery. It is reasonable to measure a single random (normal level <200 mg/dL) or fasting (normal level <126 mg/dL) blood glucose level before discharge from the hospital.

With few exceptions, women with GDM should be encouraged to exclusively breast-feed their infants. In addition to the many advantages of breastfeeding to mothers and infants, breastfeeding decreases the risk of obesity in children of mothers with GDM and lowers the rates of postpartum diabetes and fasting blood glucose levels in mothers with prior GDM.[4,52,53] Experts consider insulin, glyburide, glipizide, and metformin safe to use in women who are breastfeeding despite the manufacturers' cautions (see **Table 2**).[4]

Contraception choices for women with GDM are not limited unless the patient is determined to be at an increased risk for cardiovascular diseases (in this situation, estrogen-containing contraceptives should be avoided). Hormonal contraception does not increase blood glucose levels.[54] However, patients should be counseled about the risk of weight gain with injectable medroxyprogesterone (DepoProvera).[4] Patients should also be counseled about the risk of miscarriage and congenital malformations because of maternal hyperglycemia and encouraged to be evaluated for hyperglycemia before their next conception.

Postpartum glucose tolerance testing is exceptionally important for women who had GDM. Women with GDM have a 7-fold increased risk of developing type 2 diabetes mellitus compared with those who had a normoglycemic pregnancy.[55] At 6 to 12 weeks postpartum, only one-third of women with persistent glucose intolerance have an abnormal fasting blood glucose level.[4] Therefore, to detect all women with glucose intolerance, a 75-g, fasting, 2-hour, oral glucose tolerance test is recommended.[6] Blood glucose norms for nonpregnant patients should be used to interpret the results. If the 6 to 12 weeks' postpartum test findings are normal, repeating an assessment (oral glucose tolerance test, fasting blood glucose level, or HbA1c) every 3 years is recommended.[6] A clinician should evaluate other cardiovascular risk factors (lipid disorders, blood pressure, tobacco use, etc) based on the standard population screening guidelines.[6]

TREATMENT OF THE NEWBORN

Children born to mothers with GDM are at an increased risk for immediate and long-term complications. Management of GDM-exposed neonates in the immediate newborn period is reviewed elsewhere. After discharge from the hospital, the newborn's physician should be aware of the mother's diagnosis of GDM, which allows for family counseling about weight gain, screening for diabetes and lipid disorders, and monitoring for abnormalities in neurodevelopment including attention and motor skills.[18,19]

REFERENCES

1. American College of Obstetricians and Gynecologists Committee on Practice Bulletins—Obstetrics. ACOG Practice Bulletin. Clinical management guidelines for obstetrician-gynecologists. Number 30, September 2001 (replaces Technical Bulletin Number 200, December 1994). Gestational diabetes. Obstet Gynecol 2001;98:525–38.
2. White P. Pregnancy complicating diabetes. Am J Med 1949;7:609–16.
3. Cheng YW, Caughey AB. Gestational diabetes: diagnosis and management. J Perinatol 2008;28:657–64.
4. Metzger BE, Buchanan TA, Coustan DR, et al. Summary and recommendations of the Fifth International Workshop—Conference on Gestational Diabetes Mellitus. Diabetes Care 2007;30(Suppl 2):S251–60.
5. National Diabetes Information Clearinghouse [Internet]. Maryland: National Institutes of Health 2011. Available at: http://diabetes.niddk.nih.gov/dm/pubs/statistics/#Gestational. Accessed November 3, 2011.
6. American Diabetes Association. Standards of medical care in diabetes—2011. Diabetes Care 2011;34(Suppl 1):S11–61.
7. Moses RG. The recurrence rate of gestational diabetes in subsequent pregnancies. Diabetes Care 1996;19:1348–50.
8. American Diabetes Association. Standards of medical care in diabetes—2010. Diabetes Care 2010;33(Suppl 1):S11–61.
9. Hieronimus S, Le Meaux JP. Relevance of gestational diabetes mellitus screening and comparison of selective with universal strategies. J Gynecol Obstet Biol Reprod (Paris) 2010;39:S200–13 [in French].
10. Tieu J, Middleton P, McPhee AJ, et al. Screening and subsequent management for gestational diabetes for improving maternal and infant health. Cochrane Database Syst Rev 2010;7:CD007222.
11. Horvath K, Koch K, Jeitler K, et al. Effects of treatment in women with gestational diabetes mellitus: systematic review and meta-analysis. BMJ 2010;340:c1395.
12. Hillier TA, Vesco KK, Pedula KL, et al. Screening for gestational diabetes mellitus: a systematic review for the U.S. Preventive Services Task Force. Ann Intern Med 2008;148:766–75.
13. Teh WT, Teede HJ, Paul E, et al. Risk factors for gestational diabetes mellitus: implications for the application of screening guidelines. Aust N Z J Obstet Gynaecol 2011;51:26–30.
14. HAPO Study Cooperative Research Group, Metzger BE, Lowe LP, et al. Hyperglycemia and adverse pregnancy outcomes. N Engl J Med 2008;358: 1991–2002.
15. Committee Opinion No. 504: screening and diagnosis of gestational diabetes mellitus. Obstet Gynecol 2011;118:751–3.
16. Carr SR, Slocum J, Tefft L, et al. Precision of office-based blood glucose meters in screening for gestational diabetes. Am J Obstet Gynecol 1995;173:1267–72.
17. Lamar ME, Kuehl TJ, Cooney AT, et al. Jelly beans as an alternative to a fifty-gram glucose beverage for gestational diabetes screening. Am J Obstet Gynecol 1999;181:1154–7.
18. Weintrob N, Karp M, Hod M. Short- and long-range complications in offspring of diabetic mothers. J Diabetes Complications 1996;10:294–301.

19. Rizzo TA, Dooley SL, Metzger BE, et al. Prenatal and perinatal influences on long-term psychomotor development in offspring of diabetic mothers. Am J Obstet Gynecol 1995;173:1753–8.
20. Crowther CA, Hiller JE, Moss JR, et al. Effect of treatment of gestational diabetes mellitus on pregnancy outcomes. N Engl J Med 2005;352:2477–86.
21. ACOG Committee on Practice Bulletins—Obstetrics. ACOG Practice Bulletin No. 107: induction of labor. Obstet Gynecol 2009;114:386–97.
22. Mitanchez D. Foetal and neonatal complications in gestational diabetes: perinatal mortality, congenital malformations, macrosomia, shoulder dystocia, birth injuries, neonatal complications. Diabetes Metab 2010;36:617–27.
23. Landon MB, Spong CY, Thom E, et al. A multicenter, randomized trial of treatment for mild gestational diabetes. N Engl J Med 2009;361:1339–48.
24. American Diabetes Association, Bantle JP, Wylie-Rosett J, et al. Nutrition recommendations and interventions for diabetes: a position statement of the American Diabetes Association. Diabetes Care 2008;31(Suppl 1):S61–78.
25. Tieu J, Crowther CA, Middleton P. Dietary advice in pregnancy for preventing gestational diabetes mellitus. Cochrane Database Syst Rev 2008;2:CD006674.
26. Moses RG, Barker M, Winter M, et al. Can a low-glycemic index diet reduce the need for insulin in gestational diabetes mellitus? A randomized trial. Diabetes Care 2009;32:996–1000.
27. Ceysens G, Rouiller D, Boulvain M. Exercise for diabetic pregnant women. Cochrane Database Syst Rev 2006;3:CD004225.
28. Rasmussen KM, Yaktine AN. Weight Gain During Pregnancy: Reexamining the Guidelines. Committee to Reexamine IOM Pregnancy Weight Guidelines; Institute of Medicine; National Resource Council. The National Academies Press 2009. Available at: http://books.nap.edu/openbook.php?record_id=12584. Accessed November 3, 2011.
29. Cheng YW, Chung JH, Kurbisch-Block I, et al. Gestational weight gain and gestational diabetes mellitus: perinatal outcomes. Obstet Gynecol 2008;112:1015–22.
30. Buchanan TA, Kjos SL, Montoro MN, et al. Use of fetal ultrasound to select metabolic therapy for pregnancies complicated by mild gestational diabetes. Diabetes Care 1994;17:275–83.
31. Torlone E, Di Cianni G, Mannino D, et al. Insulin analogs and pregnancy: an update. Acta Diabetol 2009;46:163–72.
32. Pollex E, Moretti ME, Koren G, et al. Safety of insulin glargine use in pregnancy: a systematic review and meta-analysis. Ann Pharmacother 2011;45:9–16.
33. Patel P, Macerollo A. Diabetes mellitus: diagnosis and screening. Am Fam Physician 2010;81:863–70.
34. Pridjian G, Benjamin TD. Update on gestational diabetes. Obstet Gynecol Clin North Am 2010;37:255–67.
35. Alwan N, Tuffnell DJ, West J. Treatments for gestational diabetes. Cochrane Database Syst Rev 2009;3:CD003395.
36. Tieu J, Coat S, Hague W, et al. Oral anti-diabetic agents for women with pre-existing diabetes mellitus/impaired glucose tolerance or previous gestational diabetes mellitus. Cochrane Database Syst Rev 2010;10:CD007724.
37. Rosenn BM. The glyburide report card. J Matern Fetal Neonatal Med 2010;23:219–23.
38. Moore LE, Clokey D, Rappaport VJ, et al. Metformin compared with glyburide in gestational diabetes: a randomized controlled trial. Obstet Gynecol 2010;115:55–9.
39. Silva JC, Pacheco C, Bizato J, et al. Metformin compared with glyburide for the management of gestational diabetes. Int J Gynaecol Obstet 2010;111:37–40.

40. Dhulkotia JS, Ola B, Fraser R, et al. Oral hypoglycemic agents vs insulin in management of gestational diabetes: a systematic review and metaanalysis. Am J Obstet Gynecol 2010;203:457.e1–457, e9.
41. Ijas H, Vaarasmaki M, Morin-Papunen L, et al. Metformin should be considered in the treatment of gestational diabetes: a prospective randomised study. BJOG 2011;118(7):880–5.
42. Rowan JA, Hague WM, Gao W, et al, MiG Trial Investigators. Metformin versus insulin for the treatment of gestational diabetes. N Engl J Med 2008;358:2003–15.
43. de Veciana M, Major CA, Morgan MA, et al. Postprandial versus preprandial blood glucose monitoring in women with gestational diabetes mellitus requiring insulin therapy. N Engl J Med 1995;333:1237–41.
44. Jovanovic LG. Using meal-based self-monitoring of blood glucose as a tool to improve outcomes in pregnancy complicated by diabetes. Endocr Pract 2008; 14:239–47.
45. Hawkins JS, Casey BM, Lo JY, et al. Weekly compared with daily blood glucose monitoring in women with diet-treated gestational diabetes. Obstet Gynecol 2009;113:1307–12.
46. Schaefer-Graf UM, Wendt L, Sacks DA, et al. How many sonograms are needed to reliably predict the absence of fetal overgrowth in gestational diabetes mellitus pregnancies? Diabetes Care 2011;34:39–43.
47. Dudley NJ. A systematic review of the ultrasound estimation of fetal weight. Ultrasound Obstet Gynecol 2005;25:80–9.
48. Acker DB, Sachs BP, Friedman EA. Risk factors for shoulder dystocia. Obstet Gynecol 1985;66:762–8.
49. ACOG Practice Bulletin. Antepartum fetal surveillance. Number 9, October 1999 (replaces Technical Bulletin Number 188, January 1994). Clinical management guidelines for obstetrician-gynecologists. Int J Gynaecol Obstet 2000;68:175–85.
50. Kjos SL, Henry OA, Montoro M, et al. Insulin-requiring diabetes in pregnancy: a randomized trial of active induction of labor and expectant management. Am J Obstet Gynecol 1993;169:611–5.
51. Caplan RH, Pagliara AS, Beguin EA, et al. Constant intravenous insulin infusion during labor and delivery in diabetes mellitus. Diabetes Care 1982;5:6–10.
52. Schaefer-Graf UM, Hartmann R, Pawliczak J, et al. Association of breast-feeding and early childhood overweight in children from mothers with gestational diabetes mellitus. Diabetes Care 2006;29:1105–7.
53. Horta BL, Bahl R, Martines JC, et al. Evidence on the long-term effects of breast-feeding: systematic reviews and meta-analyses. Geneva (Switzerland): World Health Organization, Department of Child and Adolescent Health and Development; 2007.
54. Kerlan V. Postpartum and contraception in women after gestational diabetes. Diabetes Metab 2010;36:566–74.
55. Bellamy L, Casas JP, Hingorani AD, et al. Type 2 diabetes mellitus after gestational diabetes: a systematic review and meta-analysis. Lancet 2009;373:1773–9.

Third-Trimester Pregnancy Complications

Emily Newfield, MD, MS

KEYWORDS

- Abruptio placentae • Antenatal • Hypertension
- Placenta previa • Preeclampsia • Pregnancy
- Preterm birth • Preterm labor

Complications arising in the third trimester often challenge the clinician to balance the concern for maternal well-being with the consequences of infant prematurity. The most serious and challenging antepartum issues relate to preterm labor and birth, hypertensive disorders, and bleeding events. The article guides the practitioner through decision-making and management of these problems.

PRETERM BIRTH
Background

Preterm birth (delivery <37 weeks' gestation) is considered the leading cause of infant morbidity and mortality worldwide. The consequences of prematurity can be lifelong and include complicated medical conditions, developmental concerns, and poor performance in school. In addition, the cost of neonatal intensive care and management of chronic health conditions can be enormous. A 2006 Institute of Medicine report estimated the annual costs of evaluation and care associated with preterm birth to be approximately $26.2 billion in 2005, or $51,600 per infant born preterm.[1]

In 2009 there were more than 500,000 preterm deliveries in the United States with a rate of 12.18%, down from 12.3% in 2006.[2] Approximately 23% of all preterm births were recurrent. There are clear racial disparities in the incidence of preterm birth in the United States. African American women experience the highest rates of preterm birth (17.5% in 2009) and Asian/Pacific Islander women the lowest (10.7%). The differences in preterm birth observed between racial groups have not been explained by socioeconomic factors or other risk factors, including tobacco or drug use. The greatest risk factor for preterm birth is a history of preterm birth in a prior pregnancy; approximately 15% of all preterm births occur in women with this history.[3] Other risk

The author has nothing to disclose.
Department of Obstetrics and Gynecology, Contra Costa Regional Medical Center, 2500 Alhambra Avenue, Martinez, CA 94543, USA
E-mail address: dr.emily.newfield@gmail.com

Prim Care Clin Office Pract 39 (2012) 95–113
doi:10.1016/j.pop.2011.11.005
primarycare.theclinics.com

factors include multiple gestation and low prepregnancy weight (body mass index [BMI] <20, calculated as the weight in kilograms divided by height in meters squared).

Many clinical management strategies have been developed and tested to assist women at risk for preterm birth. The role of prenatal care providers is to identify patients at greatest risk for preterm birth, offer safe interventions to patients to prevent recurrent preterm birth, and identify early symptoms of preterm parturition to manage the pregnancy effectively and efficiently.

Women with a History of Preterm Birth

Any woman with a history of any delivery between 16 0/7 and 36 6/7 weeks is at high risk of recurrent preterm birth. Women with a history of more than 1 preterm birth and a history of preterm birth at less than 32 weeks' gestation are at greatest risk of recurrence. Women with a history of stillbirth are also at increased risk of future preterm birth.

Understanding the sequence of events that led to a prior preterm birth is important for helping to establish the risk of recurrence. The physical changes and symptoms of preterm birth are different from those that occur at term. In most preterm births, the cervix shortens (ripens), followed by decidual-membrane activation (commonly detected by the fetal fibronectin test), followed by uterine contractions. Most women experience these changes as increasing vaginal and/or pelvic pressure, mild pelvic cramping or low back pain, and increasing vaginal discharge. These early changes and symptoms can precede preterm labor by 3 to 6 weeks.[4]

Determining the series of events that preceded a spontaneous preterm birth is critical for effective counseling regarding the risk of reoccurring preterm birth. For example, if the woman describes a history of vaginal spotting (from vanishing twin or diagnostic amniocentesis) followed by ruptured membranes and preterm delivery, this may represent a lower risk of recurrent preterm birth. Acute events, such as placental abruption or chorioamnionitis, may provoke preterm labor and birth and, depending on the cause of the event, may be less likely to repeat themselves.

Prior preterm delivery of twin pregnancy is associated with increased risk of recurrent preterm birth, but the degree of risk depends on the gestational age at time of preterm delivery. If the twins are delivered after 34 weeks the risk of recurrent preterm birth is small, but can be up to 40% if the twins are delivered earlier than 30 weeks' gestation.

Prevention Strategies

Counseling

An in-depth review and discussion of the patient's obstetric and gynecologic history and associated risk of preterm birth is recommended in the first trimester. Obtaining the obstetric records, including operative and pathology reports, regarding any preterm birth is paramount to appropriate counseling and management of the current pregnancy. Surgical procedures on the cervix, that is, loop electrosurgical excision procedure and cold knife cone, are risk factors for preterm birth. Because assisted reproductive technology (including ovulation induction using clomiphene citrate and in vitro fertilization) is associated with an increased risk of preterm birth, it is important to know the circumstances regarding conception of the current pregnancy.

Primary prevention

At present there are no recommended interventions for primary prevention of preterm birth, but support for smoking-cessation efforts can be influential. Women at high risk of preterm birth (African American, low prepregnancy weight) should be counseled regarding the signs and symptoms of preterm labor. Patients who have a shortened cervix identified by midtrimester ultrasonography (US) may benefit from cerclage placement and/or vaginal progesterone (200 mg per vagina at bedtime).[5]

Prevention of recurrent preterm birth

Progesterone 17α-Hydroxyprogesterone caproate (250 mg weekly) intramuscular (IM) injections from 16 to 36 weeks' gestation have been demonstrated in several large randomized controlled trials to reduce the rate of recurrent preterm birth by approximately 33%.[6] Some practitioners do not suggest progesterone treatment if not already initiated before 24 to 26 weeks' gestation, because patients in the original research trials were enrolled up to 26 6/7 weeks. Patients with a history of delivery between 16 and 20 weeks may benefit from weekly progesterone treatment and should be offered this care. Oral and vaginal preparations are considered less effective than the IM preparation in patients with a history of preterm birth at greater than 20 weeks' gestation and should not be used. Progesterone treatment does not prevent preterm birth in twin gestations.[7,8]

Smoking Smoking-cessation programs have shown an effect in reducing recurrent preterm delivery.

Cerclage Prophylactic vaginal cerclage in patients with a history of 3 or more second-trimester losses reduces the risk of preterm birth. In patients with a history of preterm birth, serial transvaginal US examinations beginning at 16 weeks have been helpful in identifying patients with shortened cervix (measuring less than 25 mm); these women may also benefit from vaginal cerclage placement.[4] If a patient has failed vaginal cerclage in the past, transabdominal (open or laparoscopic) cerclage can be placed in early pregnancy (**Figs. 1** and **2**).

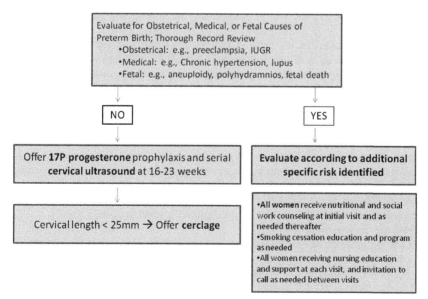

Fig. 1. Prenatal care algorithm for women with a prior preterm birth at 16 to 34 weeks. IUGR, intrauterine growth retardation. (*Adapted from* Iams JD, Berghella V. Care for women with prior preterm birth. Am J Obstet Gynecol 2010;203(2):89–100; with permission.)

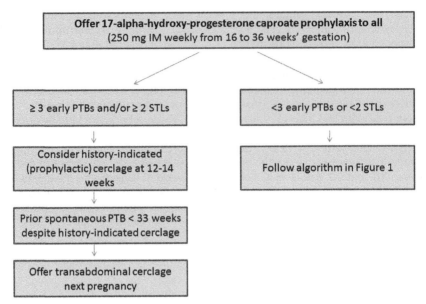

Fig. 2. Care algorithm for asymptomatic women with multiple prior preterm births (PTBs) or second-trimester losses (STLs). (*Adapted from* Iams JD, Berghella V. Care for women with prior preterm birth. Am J Obstet Gynecol 2010;203(2):89–100; with permission.)

Evaluation of Preterm Labor

Patients who present for evaluation of pelvic pressure, vaginal discharge, vaginal bleeding, or low-back pain between 16 0/7 and 36 6/7 weeks should be assessed for possible preterm labor. Many hospital systems require patients with pregnancies less than 20 weeks' gestation to be evaluated in the emergency department, whereas rapid assessment of possible preterm labor and development of an intervention strategy may be delayed. A detailed history of symptoms can help differentiate between spontaneous and evoked preterm labor. A complete obstetric history is important to determine the risk for possible recurrent preterm birth.

1. Accurate calculation of gestational age. Many of the tests and interventions associated with the management of preterm labor and birth are gestational-age dependent. Thus, immediate determination of fetal gestational age assists one in identifying which patients require what particular tests and/or interventions. If no prior US has been performed in the pregnancy, consider informal or formal US to assist in calculation of gestational age, estimated fetal weight, and fetal position.
2. Maternal vital assessment. Evaluation of the maternal condition is essential. For example, fever could represent chorioamnionitis, pyelonephritis, appendicitis, or influenza. Hypertension could represent pain or preeclampsia.
3. Fetal vital assessment
   a. Documentation of normal fetal heart tones is sufficient for fetuses less than 23 6/7 weeks.
   b. Continuous external fetal heart rate monitoring should be performed for all viable fetuses (24 0/7 weeks and more).
   c. Continuous tocometry is recommended.
   d. Informal (bedside) US should be performed to document fetal position, estimated fetal weight, placental location, cervical length, and quantity and quality

of amniotic fluid. Shortened cervical length (<2 cm) is strongly associated with risk of preterm delivery.[8]

4. Physical examination. Complete physical assessment of the mother, including cardiovascular, pulmonary, abdominal, and neurologic examinations, is important. Pelvic examination is mandatory. Informal bedside US or review of prior US reports/images should be undertaken to determine placental location before sterile vaginal examination is performed. If placenta previa or vasa previa is present, avoid digital examination. Careful examination for the presence of blood is important because the presence of blood may represent abruptio placentae, a known promoter of preterm labor.

   a. Sterile speculum examination should be performed first, before any sterile vaginal examination, because the fetal fibronectin test is invalid if the cervix has been manipulated in the prior 24 hours.

   b. Visual inspection of the vaginal vault and cervix can determine the presence of significant discharge or cervical shortening. Prolapsed membranes should not be manipulated digitally until confirmation of gestational age and determination of fetal presentation. Cervical bleeding can originate from the ectocervix (hemangioma, polyp, laceration, lesion) or from the cervical os itself.

   c. Tests
   - Fetal fibronectin: a glycoprotein present at the maternal-fetal interface, absent between 24 and 34 weeks' gestation. The presence of fetal fibronectin in symptomatic patients is the most effective predictor of preterm labor. The negative predictive value of the test approximates to 99%; symptomatic patients with a negative result of fetal fibronectin test are very unlikely to deliver in the following 7 days. The positive predictive value ranges from 75% to 85%. The test is invalid if performed before 24 0/7 or after 34 0/7 weeks, and cannot be performed if the patient has had intercourse or sterile vaginal examination in the past 24 hours or if significant vaginal bleeding is present.
   - Evaluation of any pooled fluid should be performed to exclude spontaneous rupture of membranes.
   - *Neisseria gonorrhoeae* and *Chlamydia trachomatis* infections are the most common bacterial infections resulting in cervicitis and associated with preterm labor.
   - Microscopic evaluation of any vaginal discharge can determine the presence of bacterial vaginosis, trichomoniasis, or *Candida* infection. Bacterial vaginosis is associated with increased risk of preterm delivery, and although screening and treating asymptomatic patients has not been effective at preventing preterm delivery, treating symptomatic patients is recommended. Trichomoniasis should be treated, and the patient's partner should be offered treatment as well. Microscopy can also determine if amniotic fluid is present in the vaginal vault, signifying preterm premature rupture of membranes (PPROM). Placental abruption and PPROM often coexist, with resultant uterine contractions because blood functions as a uterine irritant.
   - Urine analysis and culture is recommended. If patient cannot reliably perform a sterile urine sample, a catheter-obtained sample is appropriate.
   - Cocaine and amphetamines are associated with preterm labor, often secondary to placental abruption. Urine toxicology screening, with confirmatory testing on any positive result, should be obtained for all patients who present for evaluation of preterm labor.

- Group B *Streptococcus* (GBS) testing should be performed on all women at the time of sterile speculum examination. Patients allergic to penicillin have to inform the laboratory, so that appropriate sensitivity testing can be performed on any isolates.
- The sterile vaginal examination is critical to the diagnosis of preterm labor, provided the fetal membranes are intact and fetal fibronectin testing has been performed. Patients who present with cervical dilation of 3 cm or more with 80% cervical effacement are in active preterm labor and should be admitted for management. Patients with dilation of 2 to 3 cm and less than 80% cervical effacement are likely in preterm labor and should have the sterile vaginal examination repeated in 30 to 60 minutes. Patients with cervical dilation of less than 2 cm and less than 80% cervical effacement should be monitored for the following 1 to 2 hours to determine the rate of cervical change. If fetal fibronectin test result is negative in these patients, the likelihood of preterm delivery in the subsequent 7 days is less than 2%, and patients can be monitored in the outpatient setting.

Management of Preterm Labor

Steroids
If a patient shows evidence of preterm labor between 23 5/7 and 34 0/7 weeks' gestation, she requires immediate administration of steroids to promote fetal lung maturity. Treatment options include:

a. Betamethasone (12 mg IM × 2 doses at 24-hour intervals)
b. Dexamethasone (6 mg IM × 4 doses at 12-hour intervals).

Tocolytics
Medications to slow or stop contractions are the mainstay of treatment of preterm labor, although no data exist to suggest that these treatments prolong pregnancy for greater than 48 hours. These medications, including nonsteroidal anti-inflammatory drugs (NSAIDs), β-mimetics, magnesium sulfate, and calcium-channel blockers, can be used to prolong the pregnancy in order to complete the steroid administration and if necessary, to allow for transport to an appropriate clinical setting. All medications are equally efficacious, although calcium-channel blockers appear to have the lowest maternal safety profile. NSAIDs are associated with fetal oliguria and premature closure of the ductus arteriosus. Magnesium sulfate is associated with maternal respiratory distress and should not be used in patients with renal insufficiency. β-Mimetics can provoke maternal cardiovascular events and metabolic derangements. All tocolytics should be used cautiously and not in combination.[9] Tocolytic therapy should be discontinued when labor is halted or after 48 hours, and multiple agents should not be used simultaneously. Tocolytics should not be used in patients with preterm labor preceded by ruptured membranes.

Magnesium sulfate for neuroprotection
Current evidence suggests that 24 hours of magnesium sulfate exposure in fetuses less than 32 weeks gestational age reduces the risk of cerebral palsy. This treatment should be offered to patients in preterm labor presenting between 24 0/7 and 32 0/7 weeks' gestation who appear to be at high risk for imminent delivery. Use of magnesium sulfate for neuroprotection and a separate agent for tocolysis is not recommended. Based on the data from available randomized controlled trials, the recommended dose for magnesium sulfate for neuroprotection is 4 g intravenous (IV) loading dose followed by a maintenance dose of 1 g IV per hour for a total of

24 hours. The medication is discontinued if no delivery has occurred within 24 hours or following delivery. There is no recommendation for readministration of magnesium sulfate for neuroprotective purposes.[10,11]

Penicillin

Although antibiotic therapy has not been demonstrated to stall progression of preterm labor, penicillin for GBS prophylaxis should be administered if delivery appears imminent. If the patient has experienced an allergic reaction to penicillin or cephalosporins that includes anaphylaxis, angioedema, respiratory distress, or urticaria, the 2010 *Guidelines for Prevention of Perinatal Group B Streptococcal Disease* by the Centers for Disease Control and Prevention recommends the use of clindamycin or vancomycin for GBS prophylaxis (refer to the guidelines at http://www.cdc.gov/groupbstrep/guidelines/guidelines.html).

Transfer of care

Depending on the level of care offered by a pediatric staff and the services available in the hospital, the patient may be served by transfer to a facility that can accommodate her preterm baby. Consultation with a perinatologist can be useful while managing a patient in preterm labor.

Mode of delivery

Vaginal delivery is appropriate for preterm infants, provided there is no evidence of fetal distress with contractions. Cesarean delivery may be considered for preterm infants who demonstrate evidence of fetal growth restriction or if serious maternal conditions coexist, such as severe preeclampsia or eclampsia.[12]

Postpartum management

Mothers of preterm infants should be encouraged to breastfeed provided there are no contraindications. Patients who experience preterm birth require counseling in the immediate postpartum period regarding their risk for recurrent preterm birth. The recommended pregnancy interval for patients with a history of preterm birth is greater than 18 months, to limit recurrent adverse outcomes.[13]

HYPERTENSIVE DISORDERS

Hypertensive disorders complicate approximately 6% of all pregnancies[14] and account for 15% of all maternal deaths, being the second leading cause of maternal mortality in the United States. Women with hypertensive disorders in pregnancy are at risk for significant complications, including placental abruption, cerebral hemorrhage, hepatic dysfunction, renal insufficiency, and disseminated intravascular coagulation (DIC). The fetal consequences of hypertension include growth restriction, premature birth, and fetal demise.

There are 4 categories of hypertensive disorders in pregnancy: chronic hypertension, preeclampsia/eclampsia, gestational hypertension, and preeclampsia superimposed on chronic hypertension.

Chronic Hypertension

Hypertension is defined as a systolic blood pressure (SBP) of 140 mm Hg or more, a diastolic blood pressure (DBP) of 90 mm Hg or more, or both. It is important to differentiate hypertension that precedes pregnancy (chronic hypertension) from hypertension that develops during pregnancy (gestational hypertension or preeclampsia). According to the National High Blood Pressure Education Program Working Group on High Blood Pressure in Pregnancy, hypertension that is identified before 20 weeks' gestation is chronic hypertension.[14] Chronic hypertension is classified as mild (blood pressure >140/90 mm Hg) or severe (blood pressure >180/110 mm Hg). It may be challenging to identify women with chronic hypertension if they initiate prenatal care after 20 weeks' gestation, because the physiologic decrease in blood pressure that occurs in the second trimester may delay accurate diagnosis.

Women with chronic hypertension are at increased risk of severe pregnancy complications, including intrauterine growth retardation (IUGR), preterm delivery, placental abruption, and fetal demise. This risk seems higher when patients have evidence of significant proteinuria (≥300 mg protein on 24-hour urine collection in early pregnancy). These women may also have end-organ damage (left ventricular hypertrophy, cardiomegaly, ischemic heart disease, chronic renal insufficiency) from the effects of long-standing hypertension. Cardiac disease can result in cardiac decompensation during the third trimester and parturition.

The current available data suggest that antihypertensive medications do not improve perinatal outcomes in patients with chronic hypertension. It is unclear whether patients treated with antihypertensive medication at the start of pregnancy should continue their medication, because continued use does not seem to prevent poor outcomes and may contribute to decreased placental perfusion. The current recommendation is to withhold antihypertensive medication in patients with mild hypertension unless blood pressures exceed 150/100 mm Hg, and to continue or initiate medication in patients with severe chronic hypertension (blood pressure ≥180/110 mm Hg).[15] Target blood pressure in patients without evidence of end-organ damage (chronic renal insufficiency, cardiac disease) should be 140 to 150/80 to 90 mm Hg and less than 140/90 mm Hg if end-organ damage exists.

Although methyldopa has been used historically and is proven as effective in pregnancy with no issues of fetal safety, it is often poorly tolerated by women and can be unpredictable. Labetalol is a combined α-blocker and β-blocker, which is effective and well tolerated and is suggested as a first-line agent to control hypertension in pregnancy. Nifedipine can also be used safely in pregnancy. Diuretics have been studied and appear safe unless there is documented uteroplacental insufficiency, whereby diminished blood volume may compromise fetal well-being. Angiotensin-converting enzyme inhibitors and angiotensin receptor blockers are contraindicated in the second and third trimesters because of severe fetal consequences including underdeveloped calvarium, anuria, renal dysgenesis, IUGR, and fetal death.[16,17]

Antepartum management

Initial evaluation of a pregnant patient with chronic hypertension should include a baseline 24-hour urine collection and blood tests of renal function. Renal dysfunction in early pregnancy is associated with poor pregnancy outcomes; patients with a serum creatinine level of more than 2.5 at the start of pregnancy have a 40% risk of developing end-stage renal disease requiring dialysis during pregnancy or in the postpartum period.[17] Determining whether patients have baseline renal dysfunction can also help interpret third-trimester changes that may represent superimposed preeclampsia. Women with chronic hypertension have a 10% to 25% risk of developing preeclampsia superimposed on baseline hypertension.

Because of the increased risk of intrauterine growth restriction, patients with chronic hypertension should receive a baseline US at 18 to 22 weeks' gestation with US being repeated at 28 to 32 weeks, and then monthly until delivery. Twice-weekly fetal testing should begin at 32 weeks and continue until delivery. There is little consensus as to whether patients with mild chronic hypertension require induction at gestational age less than 40 weeks. Given that patients with chronic hypertension are at increased risk for stillbirth and significant likelihood of developing superimposed preeclampsia, the American Congress of Obstetricians and Gynecologists Practice Bulletin on Chronic Hypertension in Pregnancy recommends induction of labor after 37 weeks for patients with mild chronic hypertension.[15] Patients with severe hypertension often deliver prematurely or require early intervention because of superimposed preeclampsia. Patients with severe preeclampsia superimposed on chronic hypertension who are at greater than 28 weeks' gestation should undergo delivery. If patients remain pregnant after 37 weeks' gestation, those with severe chronic hypertension should undergo delivery. Cesarean delivery should be reserved for maternal or fetal indications; the diagnosis of hypertension does not require cesarean delivery.

Preeclampsia/Eclampsia

This pregnancy-specific problem is defined as an increase in blood pressure of 140/90 mm Hg or more after 20 weeks' gestation with associated proteinuria of 300 mg or more protein in 24 hours. The disease typically manifests in the late third trimester, and risk factors include chronic hypertension, diabetes, extremes of maternal age, and history of preeclampsia in prior pregnancy. Preeclampsia is associated with severe maternal and fetal complications, including seizure, cerebral hemorrhage, acute kidney injury, pulmonary edema, liver hemorrhage (maternal) and fetal growth restriction, placental abruption, and complications of prematurity (fetal). Delivery is the only definitive treatment for preeclampsia. There is always maternal benefit to delivery because the risk for severe complications diminishes significantly and rapidly with delivery. The struggle for the obstetrician is to determine when the fetal consequences of delivery, that is, prematurity, are greater than the risk of prolonging a pregnancy complicated by preeclampsia.

Diagnosis

Hypertension Blood pressure elevations of 140/90 mm Hg or more should be measured on two separate occasions more than 4 hours apart but within 1 week. Patients at present using antihypertensives (for treatment of chronic hypertension) can be diagnosed with preeclampsia, if a single DBP of 110 mm Hg or more is observed.

Proteinuria The gold-standard test for the presence of significant proteinuria is the 24-hour urine collection for protein. Some practitioners advocate using the spot urine protein-to-creatinine ratio test to help determine if random elevations in blood pressure suggest the diagnosis of preeclampsia; a protein-to-creatinine ratio of greater than 0.19 is correlated with greater than or equal to 300 mg of protein in a 24-hour collection.[18,19] Clinical studies addressing perinatal outcomes related to preeclampsia have assigned the diagnosis of preeclampsia to women with blood pressure measurements of more than 140/90 mm Hg on two occasions and 2+ protein or more (≥100 mg/dL) on urinalysis on two separate occasions at least 4 hours apart without evidence of urinary tract infection. At this time there is no recommendation for replacement of the 24-hour urine collection as the definitive diagnostic test for the presence of significant proteinuria, but the spot urine protein-to-creatinine ratio may help screen patients who have a hypertensive disorder without proteinuria. Once the diagnosis of preeclampsia is made, there is no benefit to repeating the 24-hour urine collection because worsening proteinuria without other signs or symptoms of severe disease is not associated with adverse perinatal outcomes.

Preeclampsia is classified as mild or severe based on the blood pressure measurements, the degree of proteinuria, and evidence of laboratory abnormalities. The criteria are shown in **Box 1**.

> **Box 1**
> **Criteria for mild and severe preeclampsia**
>
> *Mild preeclampsia*
> - SBP $\geq$140 mm Hg
> - DBP $\geq$90 mm Hg
> - Proteinuria $\geq$300 mg/24-hour urine collection
>
> *Severe preeclampsia*
> - SBP $\geq$160 mm Hg
> - DBP $\geq$110 mm Hg
> - Proteinuria $\geq$5000 mg/24-hour urine collection
> - Oliguria <400 mL urine output in 24 hours
> - Cr $\geq$1.2
> - Aminotransferases (ALT and AST) 2 times the upper limit of normal
> - Thrombocytopenia <100,000
> - Hemolysis
> - Epigastric pain, nausea, and vomiting
> - Pulmonary edema
> - Visual disturbance
>
> *Abbreviations:* ALT, alanine aminotransferase; AST, aspartate aminotransferase; Cr, creatinine.

In the past, the presence of edema (lower extremity, hands, face) was considered part of the diagnostic criteria for preeclampsia, but it has become discarded, as these symptoms are common in the third trimester and a significant number of women with preeclampsia do not develop edema.

The HELLP syndrome (Hemolysis, Elevated Liver enzymes, Low Platelets) is considered a variant of severe preeclampsia but may present independently of hypertension and proteinuria. Patients may also exhibit only part of the syndrome, that is, low platelet count and transaminitis without evidence of hemolysis. DIC does not appear to coexist except in patients with abruptio placentae or subcapsular hematoma of the liver. Pregnancies complicated by HELLP are at risk for severe maternal and fetal complications; perinatal mortality has ranged from 7% to 60%[20] and maternal mortality is high. Attempts to prolong the pregnancy by increasing plasma volume and correcting laboratory abnormalities using high-dose steroids have had limited success; most patients deteriorate within 1 week of initiation of conservative management. The general recommendation is immediate delivery, although delay for administration of betamethasone to promote fetal lung maturity is acceptable.

Patients who develop atypical preeclampsia with onset of proteinuria and edema (capillary leak syndrome) or multisystem organ dysfunction, without coexistent hypertension (**Fig. 3**) should be managed in a similar way to patients with typical severe preeclampsia.

Several conditions mimic severe preeclampsia/HELLP, including acute fatty liver of pregnancy, viral hepatitis, idiopathic thrombocytopenic purpura, thrombotic thrombocytopenic purpura (TTP), gallbladder disease, diabetes mellitus, pyelonephritis, and systemic lupus erythematosus. When patients present with multiorgan dysfunction, consultation with a perinatologist is very helpful, and these patients often require

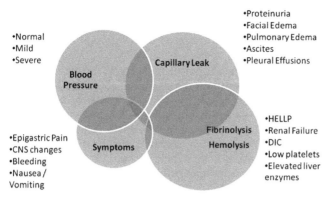

•Proteinuria
•Facial Edema
•Pulmonary Edema
•Ascites
•Pleural Effusions

•Normal
•Mild
•Severe

Capillary Leak

Blood Pressure

•HELLP
•Renal Failure
•DIC
•Low platelets
•Elevated liver enzymes

Fibrinolysis
Hemolysis

•Epigastric Pain
•CNS changes
•Bleeding
•Nausea /
Vomiting

Symptoms

Fig. 3. Overlapping role of hypertension, capillary leak, maternal symptoms, and fibrinolysis/hemolysis in the spectrum of atypical preeclampsia. CNS, central nervous system. (*Adapted from* Sibai BM, Stella CL. Diagnosis and management of atypical preeclampsia-eclampsia. Am J Obstet Gynecol 2009;200(5):481.e1–7; with permission.)

admission to the intensive care unit and may necessitate large-volume transfusion or plasmapheresis; these problems are often best managed in a tertiary care referral hospital.

Eclampsia is the presence of seizure activity in a patient with preeclampsia and no other known cause of seizure. Anyone who develops new-onset seizures during pregnancy should be presumed to have eclampsia, but the differential diagnosis of seizures in pregnancy includes cerebrovascular accidents, brain tumor, seizure disorder, drug ingestion, metabolic diseases, TTP, and reversible posterior leukoencephalopathy syndrome.

Evaluation

There is some evidence that the hypertension and symptoms associated with preeclampsia are late findings of a disorder that has been manifesting for days to weeks before diagnosis. Patients evaluated in the clinic with new-onset hypertension should undergo physical examination for signs or symptoms of preeclampsia. Laboratory evaluation for the evidence of severe disease should be ordered: complete blood count (CBC), blood urea nitrogen, creatinine, alanine aminotransferase, aspartate aminotransferase, uric acid, and L-lactate dehydrogenase. Patients should then complete a 24-hour urine collection for the diagnosis of proteinuria, differentiating gestational hypertensions from preeclampsia and from atypical preeclampsia. Patients should be referred for immediate fetal testing to evaluate evidence of preterm labor, fetal distress, or oligohydramnios. Assessment of fetal growth should be obtained, as well as umbilical artery Doppler velocimetry to evaluate placental function.

Women with a diagnosis of mild preeclampsia at 37 weeks' gestation or more can be considered for delivery. If patients are at less than 37 weeks' gestation, most guidelines recommend delivery for evidence of severe disease, fetal growth restriction, oligohydramnios, or nonreassuring fetal testing.[14]

Patients with severe preeclampsia well before term (28–32 weeks' gestation) can be managed expectantly but require hospitalization and a daily assessment of blood pressure, laboratory values, amniotic fluid volume, and umbilical artery Doppler velocimetry. If less than 34 weeks' gestation at the time of diagnosis, these patients should receive betamethasone to enhance fetal lung maturity given the high likelihood of preterm delivery caused by the worsening disease. Patients with severe preeclampsia at greater than 34 weeks' gestation should undergo delivery immediately.

Intrapartum management
Mode of delivery The diagnosis of preeclampsia does not require cesarean delivery, although patients with severe preeclampsia and compromised hepatic, renal, or hematologic function are best served by rapid delivery. Given the high risk of adverse maternal and fetal outcomes, many practitioners are uncomfortable with prolonged induction of labor in patients with severe disease and limit the time for cervical ripening to 24 hours. Correction of severe coagulopathy should be considered before cesarean delivery, and magnesium sulfate infusion can be halted before surgery and restarted in the immediate postpartum period. If concern exists for liver hemorrhage, alerting the available gynecologic oncologist or general surgeon/trauma surgeon in one's facility is wise.

Magnesium sulfate Magnesium sulfate is used for seizure prophylaxis in patients with preeclampsia; its mechanism of action seems to be stabilization of the cerebrovascular endothelium and reduction of the cerebral perfusion pressure in patients with high baseline perfusion pressure.[21] Magnesium sulfate therapy is associated with the risk of pulmonary edema and respiratory depression; it is particularly dangerous in patients with compromised renal function, as in severe preeclampsia. Although its efficacy is proven in patients with severe preeclampsia, its use as an anticonvulsant in patients with mild preeclampsia is controversial because of the high risk-to-benefit ratio.[22] The dose of magnesium sulfate is 4 g IV loading dose followed by 1 to 2 g/h IV based on renal function. Strict evaluation of fluid status should be maintained; although a Foley catheter is not required, patients receiving magnesium therapy should not ambulate. Some practitioners advocate for fluid restriction to 1 L per day to prevent pulmonary edema from developing, particularly in patients receiving magnesium therapy. Care should be taken to avoid generating acute kidney injury from volume depletion, because most patients with preeclampsia suffer from a capillary leak syndrome and are typically total body volume overloaded with a larger volume of fluid in the extravascular space.

Blood pressure control Patients with severe preeclampsia are at risk for hemorrhagic stroke. This risk seems to be related primarily not only to SBP but also to DBP and mean arterial pressure (MAP). Patients with SBP of persistently more than 160 mm Hg should receive medication to gradually lower SBP and MAP. Patients with symptoms of cerebrovascular irritability (headache, vision changes, somnolence, confusion) should be treated at lower thresholds with an SBP of 150 mm Hg or more and a DBP of 95 to 100 mm Hg or more. The recommended antihypertensives for parenteral treatment are labetalol and hydralazine. Acute changes in blood pressure can result in fetal distress caused by decreased placental perfusion pressure, and fetal cardiac monitoring should be continuous when adjusting antihypertensives.

Postpartum management
If patients have received magnesium sulfate therapy for seizure prophylaxis intrapartum, this treatment should continue for 24 hours postpartum because 25% of eclamptic seizures occur during the first 24 to 48 hours postpartum. Women may require continued blood pressure control in the postpartum period. If the patient is breastfeeding, care should be taken to avoid medications contraindicated in the newborn. β-Blockers and combined α-β–blockers (metoprolol, atenolol, and labetalol) have the least transfer to maternal milk, and calcium-channel blockers (nifedipine,

diltiazem) are also acceptable for breastfeeding women. If patients remain persistently volume overloaded, they may benefit from diuretic administration (furosemide) to acutely lower blood pressure, but care should be avoided to prevent volume depletion, which can interfere with milk production.

Postpartum preeclampsia may be diagnosed in women who were previously normotensive and asymptomatic. Often these patients require readmission to the hospital for blood pressure control, and if there is evidence of severe hypertension, magnesium sulfate therapy for 24 hours for seizure prophylaxis is provided. Care should be taken to ensure accurate diagnosis in postpartum patients. For example, severe preeclampsia can manifest as pulmonary edema caused by capillary leak syndrome, but pulmonary edema may represent postpartum cardiomyopathy in which magnesium sulfate therapy is contraindicated. Neurologic signs may be symptomatic of severe preeclampsia but may also represent complications, such as reversible posterior leukoencephalopathy syndrome. Patients who present to the emergency department in the postpartum period with symptoms consistent with severe preeclampsia should receive consultation and guidance from the available obstetrics team.

Eclampsia

Eclampsia is presence of seizures in a patient without other neurologic issues, with signs and symptoms consistent with preeclampsia. Women with eclampsia may demonstrate markedly high blood pressure and severe laboratory abnormalities, or minimal blood pressure changes and no symptoms of neuroirritability before seizure activity. This range of presentation makes it complicated to predict those at the greatest risk for seizure. Eclamptic seizures may occur at any point during the pregnancy; 50% of seizures occur antepartum, 25% intrapartum, and 25% postpartum.

Eclamptic seizures are controlled with magnesium sulfate; the treatment is a loading dose of 6 g IV over 15 to 20 minutes followed by a maintenance rate of 2 g IV per hour. Serum magnesium level should be checked 4 hours after the loading dose. If patients continue to seizure after administration of the loading dose, another dose of 2 g IV may be given. Benzodiazepines should not be administered, as they may contribute to decreased respiratory effort and risk of aspiration. Care should be instilled to avoid maternal injury (padded guard rails on bed, padded tongue blade to bedside). Laboratory evaluation should be performed to evaluate for metabolic acidosis and abnormalities related to severe preeclampsia or HELLP.

Fetal outcome is generally good after an eclamptic event, although placental abruption may occur after eclamptic seizure, and the fetus may be affected by transient hypoxia associated with convulsions. Patients with eclampsia who are less than 32 weeks' gestation with an unfavorable cervix should undergo cesarean delivery; these infants are at risk for complications related to prematurity as well as possible growth restriction. Patients at greater than 32 weeks' gestation are induced after stabilization, provided there are no fetal indications for emergent cesarean delivery. Continuous fetal monitoring during labor induction is essential. Maternal mortality from eclampsia is associated with antepartum seizure activity, fetal prematurity, and advanced maternal age. It is appropriate to consider transfer to a tertiary care center for management of the complicated fetal and maternal issues associated with eclampsia.

Future complications

Although most women with preeclampsia do not experience recurrent preeclampsia in future pregnancies, 15% develop preeclampsia in their second pregnancy. Women with preeclampsia in 2 prior pregnancies have a recurrence risk of 30%.[23,24] Women with a history of severe preeclampsia resulting in a preterm delivery are at greatest risk for recurrence, particularly if the prior pregnancy was complicated by abruptio placentae, and should receive frequent surveillance and fetal monitoring. Although several interventions, including low-dose aspirin, vitamin C, calcium, and magnesium, have been tested for the prevention of preeclampsia in patients at high risk of disease, there is no evidence that any of these treatments are effective in disease prevention.[14]

Women with a history of preeclampsia are at risk for development of chronic hypertension, ischemic heart disease, and end-stage renal disease.[24–26] Given that a woman's obstetric history is an important component to her risk assessment for future cardiovascular and renal disease, it is important to ensure adequate documentation of pregnancy-related complications for effective counseling and evaluation by her primary care physician.

Gestational Hypertension

Diagnostic criteria
This diagnosis is assigned to women who develop hypertension after 20 weeks' gestation without associated proteinuria or laboratory abnormalities. Women with blood pressure measurements of 140/90 mm Hg or more have mild gestational hypertension, and those with blood pressure of 160/110 mm Hg or more have severe gestational hypertension. Approximately 20% to 50% of patients with mild gestational hypertension develop preeclampsia during pregnancy.[27,28] If laboratory abnormalities arise or if the woman develops symptoms consistent with preeclampsia (headache, vision changes, right upper quadrant discomfort) without proteinuria, the diagnosis of atypical preeclampsia should be considered.[29]

Management
Blood pressure control should be initiated to prevent maternal stroke when SBPs are persistently 160 mm Hg or more and DBPs are 100 mm Hg or more. The target blood pressure is an SBP of 130 to 150 mm Hg and a DBP of 80 to 100 mm Hg. Patients with severe gestational hypertension require inpatient management.

Fetal monitoring, fetal growth assessment via US, and evaluation of umbilical artery Doppler velocimetry should be performed consistent with recommendations for evaluation and treatment of patients with preeclampsia, because the risk of adverse perinatal outcomes is similar. Patients with severe gestational hypertension (without proteinuria) have similar outcomes to patients with severe preeclampsia and worse outcomes than patients with mild preeclampsia, including increased risk of preterm delivery and fetal growth restriction (**Table 1**).[30]

Given these risks, patients with mild gestational hypertension should undergo delivery after 37 weeks' gestation or sooner if there is evidence of severe disease, fetal growth restriction, oligohydramnios, or abnormal umbilical artery Doppler results. Women with severe hypertension before 34 weeks' gestation should be offered betamethasone for fetal lung maturity and, if less than 32 weeks' gestation, magnesium sulfate for fetal neuroprotection. These patients often require hospital-based blood pressure management to titrate oral medications for adequate control. If blood pressure persists in the severe range despite maximization of oral medications, delivery is recommended. Otherwise patients with severe gestational hypertension should undergo delivery after 34 weeks, similar to management recommendations for severe preeclampsia.

Gestational hypertension is not a contraindication for vaginal delivery, and cesarean delivery should be reserved for maternal or fetal indications. Intrapartum blood

Table 1
Relative risk of adverse outcomes (severe gestational hypertension vs severe preeclampsia)

Outcome	Relative Risk	95% CI
Delivery at <37 wk	0.81	0.53–1.24
Delivery at <35 wk	0.70	0.32–1.56
SGA infant	1.83	0.56–5.71
Abruptio placentae	0.63	0.07–5.69
LGA infant	1.87	0.28–12.49
NICU admission	0.55	0.23–1.31
Respiratory distress syndrome	0.75	0.21–2.63

The severe gestational hypertension group is the reference group.
Abbreviations: CI, confidence interval; LGA, large for gestational age; NICU, neonatal intensive care unit; SGA, small for gestational age.
Data from Buchbinder A, Sibai BM, Caritis S, et al. National Institute of Child Health and Human Development Network of Maternal-Fetal Medicine Units. Adverse perinatal outcomes are significantly higher in severe gestational hypertension than in mild preeclampsia. Am J Obstet Gynecol 2002;186(1):66–71.

pressure control should follow the same recommendations as for patients with severe preeclampsia. There is no consensus as to whether patients with severe gestational hypertension require magnesium sulfate intrapartum for seizure prophylaxis.

If the hypertension resolves within 3 months postpartum, the patient retains the diagnosis of gestational hypertension. If her hypertension persists after the postpartum period, the patient is assigned the diagnosis of chronic hypertension.

THIRD-TRIMESTER VAGINAL BLEEDING

The differential diagnosis of vaginal bleeding in the third trimester includes labor (preterm and term), placenta previa, vasa previa, abruptio placentae, uterine rupture, and vaginal or cervical trauma. Given the significant consequences of each of these problems, patients should be encouraged to present for care for any sign of vaginal bleeding and should be assessed immediately by a physician.

The workup is as follows.

1. Determination of gestational age and prior obstetric history (ie, prior cesarean delivery or uterine surgery, history of abruption).
2. Vital signs (maternal and fetal). Hypertensive disorders are associated with abruptio placentae. Maternal hypotension and tachycardia may represent significant blood loss. Fetal bradycardia is concerning for abruptio placentae or uterine rupture, and frequent contractile activity is associated with both abruptio placentae and labor.
3. History. Traumatic injury in pregnancy, including minor falls or motor vehicle accidents, can provoke placental abruption. Patients with suspicious falls or injuries should be screened for intimate partner violence. Any signs or symptoms of the past several days that may reflect labor or preeclampsia should be reviewed. A history of prior uterine surgery conveys an increased risk of placenta previa.
4. Placental location. Review prior US records and perform bedside US to confirm placental location and assess for abruption.
5. Physical examination. If placenta previa suspected, do not perform vaginal examination. If there is no evidence of placenta previa, sterile speculum examination is

performed to determine the source of bleeding. Fetal fibronectin testing is invalid if a significant amount of blood is present or if the patient has had recent sexual intercourse. Evaluation for possible rupture of membranes is done; PPROM can provoke abruptio placentae. Speculum examination followed by sterile vaginal examination is done to examine for cervical changes consistent with labor.

6. Laboratory tests. Confirm maternal blood type and administer RhoGam, 300 µg for Rh-negative patients; Rh-negative women should also undergo Kleihauer-Betke testing to determine the degree of transplacental hemorrhage. CBC, blood type and screening, and coagulation studies should be collected if there is concern for significant blood loss. Tests for evaluation of severe preeclampsia are necessary if the patient is hypertensive. Anyone with new-onset hypertension and possible abruptio placentae should receive urine toxicology screening, to reveal any association with cocaine and amphetamine use.

Labor

Preterm labor with bleeding may represent abruptio placentae or a bloody show with cervical change. Cervical blood vessels may also become exposed and lacerated during labor. Patients with a cerclage in place who present with vaginal bleeding and suspicion of preterm labor may require removal of cerclage to prevent cervical injury from continued dilation. If preterm labor is complicated by extensive bleeding, forestalling labor with tocolytics to allow steroid administration may not be possible. Assessment of quantity and quality of vaginal bleeding every hour is recommended.

Placenta Previa

Placenta previa, commonly diagnosed during routine US in the second trimester, refers to a placenta that completely or partially obstructs the internal cervical os, and complicates approximately 0.5% of all pregnancies. Transvaginal US is superior to abdominal US in characterizing the position of the placenta in relation to the cervix, and transvaginal US does not increase the risk for vaginal bleeding.[31] Risk factors for placenta previa include prior uterine surgery (including termination of pregnancy and myomectomy), smoking, cocaine, and advanced maternal age. The frequency of placenta previa increases with each subsequent cesarean delivery; the relative risk of previa is 4.5 with 1 prior cesarean delivery and increases to 45% with 4 prior cesarean deliveries. The risk of abnormal placental invasion (accreta, increta, percreta) increases dramatically with the presence of previa and increasing number of prior cesarean deliveries; 11% of patients with placenta previa and 1 prior cesarean delivery have placenta accreta, whereas 61% of patients with placenta previa and 3 prior cesarean deliveries have placenta accreta.[31] US is the best way to determine the presence of accreta in patients with placenta previa.

The classic presentation of placenta previa is painless vaginal bleeding, but patients may develop painful contractions or experience no bleeding for the entire pregnancy. Patients with placenta previa and acute bleeding should be hospitalized and observed; it is reasonable to place 1 to 2 large-bore IV catheters and obtain CBC, and blood type and screen. Women between 24 and 34 weeks' gestation with bleeding should receive betamethasone to promote fetal lung maturity. Uterine contractions in patients with placenta previa can provoke continued bleeding, and several studies suggest that tocolytics may be of benefit in prolonging pregnancy in preterm patients.[30] If bleeding ceases, outpatient management may be acceptable if the patient has excellent family support and transportation and lives close to the hospital. If these things cannot be assured, the patient is best served by inpatient management for the remainder of the pregnancy. In patients with placenta previa, transvaginal sonogram is repeated in the third trimester; cesarean delivery is recommended for all patients if the placental edge is less than 2 cm from the internal os.[31] Cesarean delivery under regional anesthesia is typically scheduled at 37 weeks' gestation. Delivery may be complicated by excessive bleeding, and 2 units of packed red blood cells should be available at the time of surgery.

Patients with known placenta accreta have the same risks of bleeding in the third trimester but require cesarean hysterectomy at the time of delivery. Thus, obstetric care should be managed in a hospital with appropriate surgical and pediatric staff and in a facility with a blood bank that can manage large volume resuscitation.[32] Patients with placenta accreta may have evidence of placenta percreta at the time of delivery; the most commonly affected organ is the bladder, and patients may require partial bladder resection at the time of hysterectomy. Surgical planning with a multidisciplinary team, including the surgical staff of obstetrics and gynecology, urology, and vascular surgery, as well as the staff from anesthesia, neonatology, interventional radiology, and the blood bank, is recommended.

Vasa Previa

Vasa previa is a condition that occurs when the fetal vessels course through the amniotic sac and over the cervix, without the protection of the placenta. Vasa previa can result from a velamentous cord insertion or from vessels traversing separate placental lobes. Vasa previa is seen in approximately 1 in 2500 deliveries. Risk factors include multiple pregnancies and resolved low-lying placentas, as well as pregnancies known to have multiple placental lobes. Diagnosis of vasa previa can be made antepartum by identifying the placental cord insertion. Significant consequences can result following amniotomy, including heavy vaginal bleeding and fetal distress. Emergent delivery is often necessary. Because of the risk of fetal exsanguination following rupture of membranes, many patients with vasa previa are monitored as inpatients through the 35th week and delivered by cesarean delivery at 36 weeks without preoperative amniocentesis (to avoid provoking spontaneous rupture of membranes).[31]

Abruptio Placentae

Placental abruption is the premature separation of the placenta from the uterus and complicates 1% of all deliveries. The consequences of abruption can be severe; complete abruption can result in massive obstetric hemorrhage with DIC and renal failure. Large placental separation deprives the fetus of adequate oxygenation and can result in fetal injury or death. This is a particularly severe problem in preterm gestations. Risk factors for abruption include prior pregnancy complicated by abruption, hypertensive disorders, trauma, cocaine and methamphetamine use, and premature rupture of membranes. Fetal growth restriction and oligohydramnios also pose a risk of abruption.

Clinical presentation of abruption ranges from absence of signs or symptoms to complete hypovolemic shock with DIC and fetal death. Patients may have severe preeclampsia, which is masked because of hypotension and volume depletion and only identified after resuscitation. Management depends on gestational age and maternal/fetal well-being. If fetal death has occurred, patients can be offered vaginal delivery with intensive monitoring for evidence of hemorrhage or oliguria. Cesarean delivery may be considered if maternal condition worsens or if labor arrests, but any coagulopathy should be corrected before surgery to minimize further blood loss. Women with live fetuses greater than 34 weeks' gestation should be delivered immediately, and if less than 34 weeks' gestation and maternal/fetal well-being has been established, patients may receive steroids and tocolytics and be expectantly managed.[33] Women who have experienced trauma and are at greater than 24 weeks' gestation should be monitored for 8 hours; if there are persistent contractions on tocometry or if vaginal bleeding is evident, continued monitoring should be performed. If fetal well-being cannot be assured, patients should be delivered.

Cervical/Vaginal Trauma

Patients may present with cervical bleeding following intercourse; evaluation for cervicitis or a cervical lesion is important. Although cervical cancer is the most commonly identified gynecologic cancer in pregnancy, it remains a rare finding, with an incidence of 1 in 1200 to 10,000 pregnancies.[34] Sexual trauma may result in vaginal lacerations; all patients with evidence of vaginal or vulvar trauma should be screened for intimate partner violence. Effective evaluation and repair of any traumatic injury may require examination under anesthesia.

REFERENCES

1. Behrman RE, Stith A, editors. Committee on Understanding Premature Birth and Assuring Healthy Outcomes. Preterm birth: causes, consequences, and prevention. Washington, DC: National Academy Press; 2006.
2. Martin JA, Hamilton BE, Sutton PD, et al. Births: final data for 2007. Natl Vital Stat Rep 2010;58(24):1–85.
3. Petrini JR, Callaghan WM, Klebanoff M, et al. Estimated effect of 17 alpha-hydroxyprogesterone caproate on preterm birth in the United States. Obstet Gynecol 2005;105(2):267–72.
4. Iams JD, Berghella V. Care for women with prior preterm birth. Am J Obstet Gynecol 2010;203(2):89–100.
5. Fonseca EB, Celic E, Parra M, et al. Progesterone and the risk of preterm birth among women with a short cervix. N Engl J Med 2007;357:462–9.
6. Meis PJ, Klebanoff M, Thom E, et al. Prevention of recurrent preterm delivery by 17 alpha-hydroxyprogesterone caproate. N Engl J Med 2003;348(24):2379–85.
7. Rouse DJ, Caritis SN, Peaceman AM, et al. A trial of 17 alpha-hydroxyprogesterone caproate to prevent prematurity in twins. N Engl J Med 2007;357(5):454–61.
8. Norwitz ER, Caughey AB. Progesterone supplementation and the prevention of preterm birth. Rev Obstet Gynecol 2011;4(2):60–72.
9. American College of Obstetricians and Gynecologists. Management of Preterm Labor. ACOG practice bulletin no. 43. Obstet Gynecol 2003;101(5 Pt 1):1039–47.
10. Doyle LW, Crowther CA, Middleton P, et al. Magnesium sulphate for women at risk of preterm birth for neuroprotection of the fetus. Cochrane Database Syst Rev 2009;1:CD004661.
11. Crowther CA, Hiller JE, Doyle LW, et al. Australasian Collaborative Trial of Magnesium Sulphate (ACTOMg SO4) Collaborative Group. JAMA 2003;290(20):2669.
12. Högberg U, Holmgren PA. Infant mortality of very preterm infants by mode of delivery, institutional policies and maternal diagnosis. Acta Obstet Gynecol Scand 2007;86(6):693–700.
13. Sholapurkar SL. Is there an ideal interpregnancy interval after a live birth, miscarriage or other adverse pregnancy outcomes? J Obstet Gynaecol 2010;30(2):107–10.
14. Anonymous. Report of the National High Blood Pressure Education Program Working Group on High Blood Pressure and Pregnancy. Am J Obstet 2000;183(1):S1–22.

15. American College of Obstetricians and Gynecologists. Chronic hypertension in pregnancy. ACOG practice bulletin No. 29. Obstet Gynecol 2001;98:177–85.
16. Seely EW, Ecker J. Chronic hypertension in pregnancy. N Engl J Med 2011; 365(5):439–46.
17. Podymow T, August P, Akbari A. Management of renal disease in pregnancy. Obstet Gynecol Clin North Am 2010;37(2):195–210.
18. Sethuram R, Kiran TS, Weerakkody AN. Is the urine spot protein/creatinine ratio a valid diagnostic test for pre-eclampsia? J Obstet Gynaecol 2011;31(2):128–30.
19. Wheeler TL 2nd, Blackhurst DW, Dellinger EH, et al. Usage of spot urine protein to creatinine ratios in the evaluation of preeclampsia. Am J Obstet Gynecol 2007; 196(5):465.e1–4.
20. Sibai BM, Ramadan MK, Usta I, et al. Maternal morbidity and mortality in 442 pregnancies with hemolysis, elevated liver enzymes, and low platelets (HELLP syndrome). Am J Obstet Gynecol 1993;169(4):1000–6.
21. Belfort M, Allred J, Dildy G. Magnesium sulfate decreases cerebral perfusion pressure in preeclampsia. Hypertens Pregnancy 2008;27(4):315–27.
22. Sibai BM. Magnesium sulfate prophylaxis in preeclampsia: lessons learned from recent trials. Am J Obstet Gynecol 2004;190(6):1520–6.
23. Brown MA, Mackenzie C, Dunsmuir W, et al. Can we predict recurrence of pre-eclampsia or gestational hypertension? BJOG 2007;114(8):984–93.
24. Hernandez-Diaz S, Toh S, Cnattingius S. Risk of pre-eclampsia in first and subsequent pregnancies: prospective cohort study. BMJ 2009;338:b2255.
25. Vikse BE, Irgens LM, Leivestad T, et al. Preeclampsia and the risk of end-stage renal disease. N Engl J Med 2008;359(8):800–9.
26. Sibai BM, el-Nazer A, Gonzalez-Ruiz A. Severe preeclampsia-eclampsia in young primigravid women: subsequent pregnancy outcome and remote prognosis. Am J Obstet Gynecol 1986;155(5):1011–6.
27. Barton JR, Stamsno GJ, Sibai BM. Monitored outpatient management of mild gestational hypertension remote from term. Am J Obstet Gynecol 1994;170: 765–9.
28. Saudan P, Brown MA, Buddle ML, et al. Does gestational hypertension become pre-eclampsia? BJOG 1998;105(11):1177–84.
29. Sibai BM, Stella CL. Diagnosis and management of atypical preeclampsia-eclampsia. Am J Obstet Gynecol 2009;200(5):481.e1–7.
30. Buchbinder A, Sibai BM, Caritis S, et al. Adverse perinatal outcomes are significantly higher in severe gestational hypertension than in mild preeclampsia. Am J Obstet Gynecol 2002;186(1):66–71.
31. Oyelese Y, Smulian JC. Placenta previa, placenta accreta, and vasa previa. Obstet Gynecol 2006;107(4):927–41.
32. Publications Committee, Society for Maternal-Fetal Medicine, Belfort MA. Placenta accreta. Am J Obstet Gynecol 2010;203(5):430–9.
33. Oyelese Y, Ananth C. Placental abruption. Obstet Gynecol 2006;108(4):1005–16.
34. Nguyen C, Montz FJ, Bristow RE. Management of stage I cervical cancer in pregnancy. Obstet Gynecol Surv 2000;55(10):633–43.

Electronic Fetal Monitoring: Family Medicine Obstetrics

John R.M. Rodney, MD[a],*, Benjamin J.F. Huntley, MD[a],
Wm MacMillan Rodney, MD[b]

KEYWORDS

- Prenatal care • Labor and delivery • Intrapartum care
- Fetal monitor • Cardiotocography • Obstetrics

Continuous electronic fetal monitoring (EFM), introduced during the 1960s, was expected to provide clinicians with more accurate diagnostic information regarding maternal-fetal status that would allow for earlier intervention when necessary. Although EFM's superiority over older modalities, such as Doppler ultrasound and intermittent auscultation, was largely speculative, the ability to detect beat-to-beat variability, a major predictor of fetal distress, enabled EFM to become the United States' most common obstetric procedure.

Unfortunately, this technology and principles of interpretation are not consistently available in international and rural settings where resource restrictions and psychosocial barriers are common. Nevertheless, where the technology is available, there is a developing universal EFM language.

For both inpatient and outpatient settings, Family Medicine Obstetrics recommends that doctors, nurses, and midwives should record their findings with 9 sequential steps:

1. Clinical context
   a. Estimated gestational age
   b. Gravida and para
   c. Obstetric, gynecologic, surgical, and medical history
   d. Comorbidities—diabetes, hypertension, etc.
   e. Setting and resource limitations
2. Validity of data
   a. Legibility
   b. Labeling

The authors have nothing to disclose.
[a] Department of Family Medicine, John Peter Smith Hospital, 1500 South Main Street, Fort Worth, TX 76104, USA
[b] Medicos para la Familia, 6575 Black Thorne, Memphis, TN 38119, USA
* Corresponding author.
E-mail address: roccorodney@gmail.com

Prim Care Clin Office Pract 39 (2012) 115–133
doi:10.1016/j.pop.2011.11.006   **primarycare.theclinics.com**

  c. Technical limitations
  d. Artifacts
3. Presence of maternal contractions
4. Baseline fetal heart rate (FHR)
5. Beat-to-beat variability of the FHR
6. Presence of accelerations
7. Presence and type of decelerations
8. Interpretation – Designating FHR tracings as:
  a. Category 1, meaning reassuring or not concerning
  b. Category 2, suggesting further observation
  c. Category 3, requiring action
9. Plan – articulate a management plan, using the above steps

  The remainder of this article briefly reviews the history and standardization of EFM terminology, comments on current technologies, defines present-day parlance, highlights practice management guidelines, and discusses controversial areas within the field before concluding with future considerations.

HISTORICAL DEVELOPMENT OF STANDARDIZED TERMS AND TECHNIQUES

Although fetal heart tones were first auscultated in the early 1800s, it took nearly 150 years for FHR patterns to be scientifically defined. In 1853, William Little wrote, "...I have seen so many cases of [mental and physical] deformity traceable to causes operative at birth...[some of which are] traced to asphyxia neonatorum and mechanical injury to the foetus immediately before or during parturition."[1] These observations were supported by Sir William Osler and also Sigmund Freud who, before his famous career in psychiatry, was considered an authority on children's paralytic conditions. Subsequently, EFM has been increasingly used as a surrogate for detecting intrapartum hypoxia, a presumed predictor of fetal acidemia, morbidity, and mortality.

  Although only 45% of all American labors in 1980 used FHR monitoring, the usage rate grew steadily to 85% in 2002.[2] Despite increasing use of EFM, however, the field lacked both standard definitions and diagnostic categories that would allow researchers and clinicians to quantify FHR patterns consistently.

  In 1997, a consensus panel of physicians and nurse researchers, under the auspices of the National Institute of Child Health and Human Development (NICHD), published standard electronic FHR (EFHR) terminology.[3] A decade later the committee joined the American College of Obstetricians and Gynecologists (ACOG) and the Society for Maternal-Fetal Medicine to amend EFHR terminology and create a 3-tiered scheme for broad categorization of EFHR patterns in the United States.[4]

  This article offered basic management recommendations for normal, indeterminate, and abnormal FHR patterns. These definitions were primarily created for visual interpretation of intrapartum tracings, but they can also be applied to antepartum patterns and may be adaptable to computerized interpretation.

TECHNIQUES AND INSTRUMENTS RECOMMENDED FOR MONITORING FETAL HEART RATES
Intermittent Auscultation

FHRs fluctuate in response to changes in the uterine environment. Cardiac auscultation can be used to evaluate maternal and fetal health. Before EFM, direct intermittent auscultation assessed fetal-maternal well-being. It could not, however, reveal important dynamic characteristics of the fetal heart rate, such as beat-to-beat variability, accelerations, and decelerations. Although intermittent auscultation has largely been replaced by EFM, the American Academy of Family Physicians *Advanced Life Support in Obstetrics* text supports its limited use, stating,

> Intermittent auscultation is appropriate for healthy women with uncomplicated pregnancy. In the active stage of labor, intermittent auscultation should occur after a contraction, for a minimum of 60 seconds, and at least every 15 minutes in the first stage and every 5 minutes in the second stage. Continuous electronic monitoring is recommended if there is evidence on auscultation of a baseline less than 110 bpm or greater than 160 bpm or if there is evidence on auscultation of any decelerations or if any intrapartum risk factors develop.[5]

Electronic Fetal Monitoring

The FHR monitor is a 2-component device that graphs FHR against uterine tone. Traditional methods of sensing uterine contractions can be subdivided into (1) indirect measurements using an external tocodynamometer and (2) direct measurements using a pressure transducer inserted transcervically.

The tocodynamometer rests on the mother's abdomen and measures relative displacement of 2 sensors during abdominal contractions, serving as a surrogate for uterine tone. Although this technique is noninvasive, by virtue of recording relative physical displacement, the tocodynamometer cannot quantify intrauterine pressure. The transcervical insertion of a soft plastic catheter into the uterine cavity provides quantifiable data. This device is usually placed opposite the placental location with a sterile rigid plastic introducer. Ultrasonography is an important tool to determine placental location.

Evaluation of FHR can be subdivided into external and internal measurements. External devices include Doppler ultrasound and abdominal ECG. Internal devices have historically been restricted to the fetal electrode. For both internal and external methods, the FHR is computed based on the interval between heartbeats and is displayed on a timescale that advances at a standard speed. Beat-to-beat variability is calculated by evaluating the fluctuations in the FHR pattern.

Doppler Ultrasound

Doppler ultrasound works by transmitting sound waves into a medium and measuring the frequency of the sound waves that reflect back. The method is minimally invasive and can be used to detect FHR. Due to maternal and fetal movements during the course of gestation, these measurements often cannot reliably measure beat-to-beat variability, especially when used on morbidly obese mothers.

The Internal Fetal Electrode

The internal fetal electrode, often called a scalp lead, provides consistently valid FHR and variability recordings. This instrument detects the FHR by direct measurements through a small, typically stainless steel, corkscrew-shaped electrode placed directly into the fetal scalp. The use of scalp monitors is decreasing owing to improvements in external monitors and the complications associated with placement.

When inserting a fetal electrode, care should be taken to ensure that the spiral device is placed over a bony prominence and not over a fontanelle or suture line where cerebrum lies unprotected. The electrode can also be placed in the fetal gluteus but for cosmetic and safety reasons should never be placed on the face or on any unidentified presenting part. Other complications that may arise include rupture of placental vessels, cord compression due to catheter entanglement, placental penetration and hemorrhage, and both fetal and maternal infections.

DEFINITIONS OF 6 CRITICAL TERMS
Term 1: Uterine Contractions

The strength of uterine contractions is quantified in Montevideo units (MVU), which represent the product of the peak contraction intensity in millimeters of mercury and the number of contractions in a 10-minute window (see **Table 1** for details). These measurements are clinically relevant for their use in distinguishing Braxton Hicks contractions (typically less than 20 mm Hg) from the onset of true labor.

The first stage of labor is associated with contraction pressures of 25 to 50 mm Hg, with a frequency of 3 to 5 contractions per 10-minute window, lasting between 60 and 80 seconds before returning to a uterine basal tone of between 8 and 12 mm Hg.

The second stage of labor is associated with contraction pressures of 80 to 100 mm Hg, with a frequency of 5 contractions per 10-minute window, lasting 60 to 80 seconds.

When oxytocin is used to induce or augment labor, it is titrated to cause uterine contractions above 180 MVU. Care is taken to avoid contraction strengths above 300 MVU. It is reasonable to achieve these levels of uterine activity before considering surgical delivery.

Term 2: Baseline Fetal Heart Rate and Variability

Bradycardic fetal rhythms occur in 2% of all labors in the United States and are usually associated with fetal head compressions during uterine contractions (see **Table 2** for details). Clinicians can be more confident in this diagnosis when the heart rate is between 110 and 119 beats per minute (bpm) and it is the only abnormal parameter displayed on the EFM.[6] Furthermore, FHR between 80 and 120 bpm with good variability is reassuring.[7]

The differential diagnosis also includes placental abruption, maternal hypothermia, maternal opioid administration, fetal sleep, and fetal acidemia. Maternal hypothermia should be considered in the setting of maternal infections and intraoperative fetal bradycardia.

Tachycardic fetal rhythms raise concern of sepsis. FHRs above 160 usually arise in the context of maternal fever. In the setting of chorioamnionitis, fetal tachycardia usually precedes maternal fever.[8]

The differential diagnosis also includes both benign causes, such as prolonged accelerations in an otherwise healthy fetus, and more dangerous underlying pathologies, such as fetal compromise, cardiac arrhythmias, placental abruption, and maternal administration of either anti-parasympathetics (eg, atropine) or sympathomimetics (eg, terbutaline).

Term 3: Accelerations

Accelerations and decelerations are quantified by their zenith or nadir in beats per minute and by their duration in minutes or seconds (see **Table 3** for details). According to a study of 2000 fetal electric heart tracings, accelerations are most likely caused by fetal movements and are present in 99.8% of EFHR tracings. Presence of accelerations during the first or last 30 minutes of labor correlates with a favorable prognosis. The absence of accelerations during these periods, as an isolated finding, however, does not bear any clinical or prognostic significance.[9]

Table 1
Modified electronic fetal monitoring definitions—uterine contractions

Pattern	Definition	Tracing

Uterine contractions	• The number of contractions in a 10-minute window averaged over a 30-minute segment
	  ○ Normal: ≤5 contractions in a 10-minute period
	  ○ Tachysystole: >5 contractions in a 10-minute period; must be qualified by the presence or absence of concomitant FHR decelerations; applies to both spontaneous and stimulated FHR patterns
	  ○ Hyperstimulation and hypercontractility are not defined and should be abandoned
	• Frequency: the time interval between the start of two consecutive contractions
	• Duration: the time interval between the beginning and end of the same contraction
	• Interval: the time interval between the end of one contraction and the beginning of the next contraction
	• Intensity: the pressure of the uterus during contractions
	• Resting tone: the pressure of the uterus in between contractions
		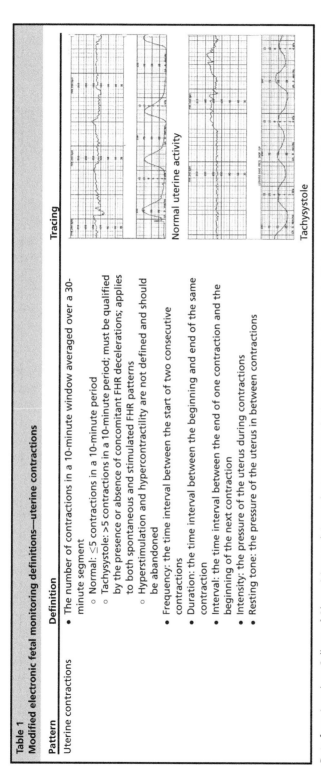
		Normal uterine activity
		
		Tachysystole

Data from American College of Obstetricians and Gynecologists. Practice bulletin no. 116: management of intrapartum fetal heart rate tracings. Obstet Gynecol 2010;116(5):1232–40. Available at: http://www.ncbi.nlm.nih.gov/pubmed/20966730. Accessed January 16, 2011; *images courtesy of* David McRay, MD, John Peter Smith Hospital.

Table 2
Modified electronic fetal monitoring definitions—baseline fetal heart rate and variability

Baseline FHR	• The mean EFHR rounded to increments of 5 bpm during a 10-minute segment, excluding
	  ○ Periodic or episodic changes
	  ○ Periods of marked FHR variability
	  ○ Segments of baseline that differ by >25 bpm
	• The baseline must be for a minimum of 2 minutes in any 10-minute segment, or the baseline for that time period is considered indeterminate. In this case, one may refer to the prior 10-minute window for determination of baseline.
	• Normal EFHR baseline: 110–160 bpm
	• Tachycardia: EFHR baseline is greater than 160 bpm
	• Bradycardia: EFHR baseline is less than 110 bpm

Variability	• Fluctuations in the baseline EFHR that are irregular in amplitude and frequency
	• Variability is visually quantified as the amplitude of peak-to-trough in bpm
	  ○ Absent: amplitude range undetectable
	  ○ Minimal: amplitude range detectable but 5 bpm or fewer
	  ○ Moderate (normal): amplitude range 6–25 bpm
	  ○ Marked: amplitude range greater than 25 bpm

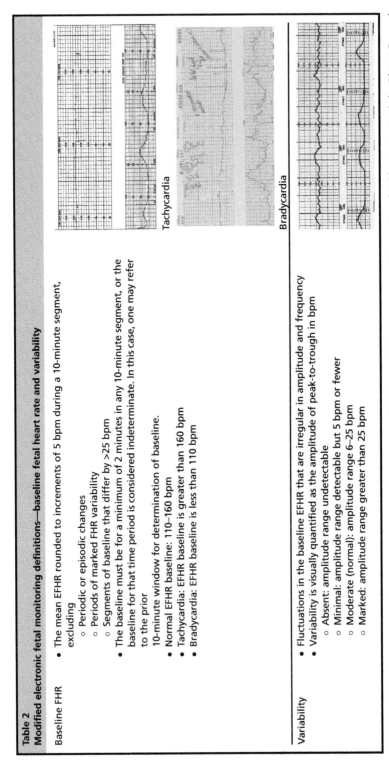

Tachycardia

Bradycardia

Data from American College of Obstetricians and Gynecologists. Practice bulletin no. 116: management of intrapartum fetal heart rate tracings. Obstet Gynecol 2010;116(5):1232–40. Available at: http://www.ncbi.nlm.nih.gov/pubmed/20966730. Accessed January 16, 2011; *images courtesy of David McRay, MD, John Peter Smith Hospital.*

Table 3
Modified electronic fetal monitoring definitions—accelerations

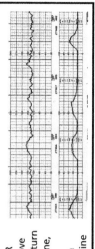

Accelerations	• A visually apparent abrupt increase (onset to peak in less than 30 seconds) in the EFHR
	• At 32 weeks of gestation and beyond, acceleration has a peak of 15 bpm or more above baseline, with duration of at least 15 seconds but less than 2 minutes from onset to return
	• Before 32 weeks of gestation, acceleration has a peak of at least 10 bpm above baseline, with duration of 10 seconds or more but less than 2 minutes from onset to return
	• A prolonged acceleration lasts 2 minutes or more but less than 10 minutes in duration
	• An acceleration that exists for more than 10 minutes constitutes a change in the baseline

Data from American College of Obstetricians and Gynecologists. Practice bulletin no. 116: management of intrapartum fetal heart rate tracings. Obstet Gynecol 2010;116(5):1232–40. Available at: http://www.ncbi.nlm.nih.gov/pubmed/20966730. Accessed January 16, 2011; *images courtesy of* David McRay, MD, John Peter Smith Hospital.

When accelerations are absent, clinicians can consider vibroacoustic stimulation to induce accelerations, thereby increasing certainty of a favorable prognosis. When attempts to stimulate the heart rate fail in the setting of fetal distress, doctors should expect a 50% risk of academia.[10,11] Other causes of accelerated FHRs include fetal stimulation from uterine contractions or maternal pelvic examinations, umbilical occlusion, and fetal scalp blood draws.

Term 4: Decelerations

Decelerations are occur frequently during the second stage of labor and can be subcategorized as either periodic (associated with contractions) or episodic (not associated with contractions) (see **Table 4** for details). Early decelerations indicate fetal head compression and usually occur during active labor between 4 and 7 cm dilation. Early decelerations are proportional to contraction strength. They rarely drop more than 20 bpm under the EFHR baseline and are not associated with poor outcomes. Early decelerations can be explained by dural stimulation during fetal head compression, which induces vagus nerve activation that causes the transient bradycardic response.[12]

Late decelerations are attributed to uteroplacental insufficiency. The first sign of uteroplacental hypoxia is late decelerations, followed by acidemia, followed by diminishing variability. The differential diagnosis for late decelerations also includes maternal hypotension (induced by epidural analgesia), iatrogenic uterine hyperactivity due to oxytocin, and placental dysfunction. Less likely etiologies include maternal hypertension, diabetes, and collagen-vascular disorders.

Variable decelerations indicate cord compression and can occur frequently, especially at the end of the first stage of labor. Tachycardic portions are attributed to partial occlusion of the umbilical vein, which decreases the amount of blood returning to the heart and elevates FHR. Bradycardic portions are attributed to complete umbilical cord occlusion (ie, occlusion of the vein and arteries), which causes systemic hypertension leading to decreased heart rate.

Fetal bradycardia may also be due to the detection of depressed arterial oxygen concentration by chemoreceptors that induce a parasympathetic response. To help providers distinguish normal from pathologic decelerations, ACOG has defined significant variable decelerations as those that drop below 70 bpm for greater than 60 seconds.[13]

Prolonged decelerations are defined as visually apparent decreases below baseline in EFHR of at least 15 bpm for 2 to 10 minutes. The differential diagnosis for prolonged decelerations includes cord entanglement, maternal hypoperfusion, maternal hypoxia, placental abruption, umbilical cord knots, umbilical cord prolapse, eclamptic or epileptic seizures, application of fetal scalp electrode, impending birth, maternal valsalva, and administration of epidural, spinal, or paracervical analgesia. Prolonged decelerations occur in 4% of pregnant women who receive epidural or intrathecal analgesia. The cumulative exposure to variable decelerations is predictive of and inversely proportional to the Apgar score.[14]

Term 5: Sinusoidal Patterns

Sinusoidal patterns strongly suggest fetal anemia stemming from Rh isoimmunization due to fetomaternal hemorrhage, but the differential diagnosis also includes vasa previa, severe fetal asphyxia, chorioamnionitis, maternal narcotic use, umbilical cord occlusion, and, less commonly, twin-to-twin transfusion syndrome (see **Table 5** for details).

Term 6: Fetal Heart Rate Variability

Baseline EFHR variability hinges on autonomic nervous system tone (see **Table 6** for details). Short-term variability is defined as true beat-to-beat variability: the difference in rate between two adjacent homologous intervals of the fetal ECG (ie, rates projected from consecutive R-R or p-p segments). In fetuses, short-term variability is associated with body movements. Long-term variability, alternatively, describes broader oscillations seen in an EFHR tracing over many heartbeats and is usually present at 3 to 5 hertz.

Because EFHR patterns are interpreted visually, short-term and long-term variability are interpreted as one, the individual parts of which should not be quantified. Variability is unaffected by gender, is inversely proportional to rate, and increases proportionately with gestational age beyond 30 weeks. Although decreased baseline EFHR variability is generally considered the most reliable sign of fetal compromise, by itself variability cannot be used as a prognostic indicator. Furthermore, good variability must be interpreted within the context of the entire tracing and a patient's comorbidities.

PROFESSIONAL MANAGEMENT GUIDELINES

As discussed previously, professional guidelines regarding the interpretation and management of EFHR patterns have been slow in coming and fraught with considerable controversy. To date no clinically adequate algorithm has been unanimously accepted by the medical community. A 2008 NICHD consensus panel, however, moved obstetricians in the direction of consistent interpretation first by defining 3 categories of EFHR patterns and second by advising basic management principles for each diagnostic tier (as shown in **Table 7**).

Category I tracings strongly predict normal fetal acid-base status and should be continued with routine management using either continuous or intermittent monitoring.

Category II tracings cover a vast range of patterns that do not necessarily predict abnormal acid-base status but should be carefully evaluated and continuously monitored. Fetal heart rate tracings that triage into category II may include but are not limited to deviations in baseline rate, such as bradycardia in the absence of variability or any form of tachycardia. Perturbations in EFHR variability also fall under category II, including minimal or marked variability or absent variability without recurrent decelerations. Absence of accelerations even after fetal stimulation is also a foreboding yet indeterminate sign that does not necessarily indicate fetal metabolic acidemia and thus is not considered a category III pattern. Lastly, prolonged decelerations, recurrent late decelerations with moderate variability, and recurrent variable decelerations accompanied by minimal or moderate variability are also categorized into the indeterminate tier.

Category III tracings, however, predict fetal acidemia and warrant prompt intervention to resolve the abnormal EFHR pattern. Maternal-fetal pairs with category III patterns should quickly be evaluated for maternal hypotension, maternal hypoxia, and umbilical cord occlusion.

Thus, practitioners are able to determine that EFHR patterns are either clearly normal, clearly abnormal, or clearly something in-between whose interpretation and management is poorly understood. One useful strategy for interpreting category II FHR patterns is to look for moderate variability and/or accelerations (either spontaneous or induced), which are highly predictive of normal fetal acid-base status and should guide clinical management. Absent variability, that is not accompanied by

Table 4
Modified electronic fetal monitoring definitions—decelerations

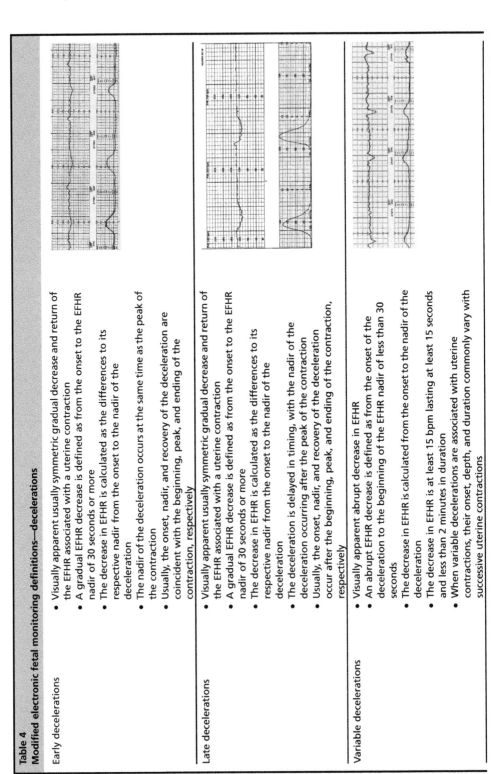

Early decelerations	• Visually apparent usually symmetric gradual decrease and return of the EFHR associated with a uterine contraction • A gradual EFHR decrease is defined as from the onset to the EFHR nadir of 30 seconds or more • The decrease in EFHR is calculated as the differences to its respective nadir from the onset to the nadir of the deceleration • The nadir of the deceleration occurs at the same time as the peak of the contraction • Usually, the onset, nadir, and recovery of the deceleration are coincident with the beginning, peak, and ending of the contraction, respectively
Late decelerations	• Visually apparent usually symmetric gradual decrease and return of the EFHR associated with a uterine contraction • A gradual EFHR decrease is defined as from the onset to the EFHR nadir of 30 seconds or more • The decrease in EFHR is calculated as the differences to its respective nadir from the onset to the nadir of the deceleration • The deceleration is delayed in timing, with the nadir of the deceleration occurring after the peak of the contraction • Usually, the onset, nadir, and recovery of the deceleration occur after the beginning, peak, and ending of the contraction, respectively
Variable decelerations	• Visually apparent abrupt decrease in EFHR • An abrupt EFHR decrease is defined as from the onset of the deceleration to the beginning of the EFHR nadir of less than 30 seconds • The decrease in EFHR is calculated from the onset to the nadir of the deceleration • The decrease in EFHR is at least 15 bpm lasting at least 15 seconds and less than 2 minutes in duration • When variable decelerations are associated with uterine contractions, their onset, depth, and duration commonly vary with successive uterine contractions

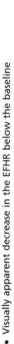

Prolonged decelerations	• Visually apparent decrease in the EFHR below the baseline • Decrease in EFHR from the baseline that is 15 bpm or more, lasting 2 minutes or more but less than 10 minutes in duration • If a deceleration lasts 10 minutes or longer, it is a baseline change

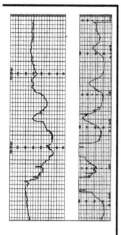

Data from American College of Obstetricians and Gynecologists. Practice bulletin no. 116: management of intrapartum fetal heart rate tracings. Obstet Gynecol 2010;116(5):1232–40. Available at: http://www.ncbi.nlm.nih.gov/pubmed/20966730. Accessed January 16, 2011; *images courtesy of David McRay, MD, John Peter Smith Hospital.*

Table 5
Modified electronic fetal monitoring definitions—sinusoidal patterns

Sinusoidal pattern	• Visually apparent, smooth, sine wave-like undulating pattern in EFHR baseline with a cycle frequency of 3–5 per minute, which persists for 20 minutes or more

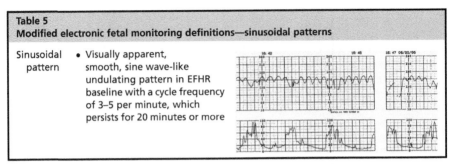

Data from American College of Obstetricians and Gynecologists. Practice bulletin no. 116: management of intrapartum fetal heart rate tracings. Obstet Gynecol 2010;116(5):1232–40. Available at: http://www.ncbi.nlm.nih.gov/pubmed/20966730. Accessed January 16, 2011; *image adapted from* Yeo L, Ananth CV, Vintzileos AM. Placental abruption. The global library of women's medicine. 2009. Available at: http://www.glowm.com/index.html?p=glowm.cml/section_view&articleid=122. Accessed May 23, 2011.

any other tracing abnormalities, does not reliably predict fetal metabolic acidemia. This is better demonstrated visually in the diagram from an ACOG practice bulletin (**Fig. 1**).

Although the significance of marked variability is unknown, decreased variability may be caused by the fetal sleep cycle, maternal medications, fetal hypoxic bradycardia, or fetal acidemia. Analgesic narcotics, barbiturates, phenothiazines,

Table 6
Modified electronic fetal monitoring definitions—fetal heart rate variability

Pattern	EFHR Tracing
Absent EFHR variability: undetectable	
Minimal EFHR variability: > undectable but ≤5 bpm	
Moderate EFHR variability: 6–25 bpm	
Marked EFHR variability: >25 bpm	

Data from American College of Obstetricians and Gynecologists. Practice bulletin no. 116: management of intrapartum fetal heart rate tracings. Obstet Gynecol 2010;116(5):1232–40. Available at: http://www.ncbi.nlm.nih.gov/pubmed/20966730. Accessed January 16, 2011; *images courtesy of* David McRay, MD, John Peter Smith Hospital.

Table 7	
Three-tiered EFHR categorical system	
Modified Three-Tiered EFHR Interpretation System	**Management**

Category I (Normal)
• Must include all of the following:
   ◦ Baseline rate: 110–160 bpm
   ◦ Baseline EFHR variability: moderate
   ◦ Late or variable decelerations: absent
   ◦ Early decelerations and accelerations may or may not be present
	Routine management

Category II (Indeterminant) • Includes all EFHR tracings not defined elsewhere	Evaluation and continued surveillance and reevaluations

Category III (Abnormal)
• Must include either
   ◦ Sinusoidal pattern OR
   ◦ Absent baseline FHR variability AND either bradycardia, recurrent late decelerations, or recurrent variable decelerations
	Expeditious evaluation and intervention
	• Repositioning
	• Supplemental oxygen
	• Fluid bolus
	• Cessation of labor induction agents

Adapted from Macones GA, Hankins GD, Spong CY, et al. The 2008 National Institute of Child Health and Human Development workshop report on electronic fetal monitoring: update on definitions, interpretation, and research guidelines. Obstet Gynecol 2008;112:661–6; *data from* Macones GA, Hankins GD, Spong CY, et al. The 2008 National Institute of Child Health and Human Development workshop report on electronic fetal monitoring: update on definitions, interpretation, and research guidelines. J Obstet Gynecol Neonatal Nurs 2008;37(5):510–5. Available at: http://www.ncbi.nlm.nih.gov/pubmed/18761565. Accessed May 23, 2011.

tranquilizers, and general anesthetics also decrease variability. Minimal variability due to opioid use should resolve within 1 to 2 hours. Magnesium sulfate does not significantly decrease variability.

Intermittent variable decelerations are the most common EFHR abnormality during labor, are associated with normal fetal outcomes, and do not ordinarily necessitate further intervention.

Recurrent variable decelerations are usually caused by umbilical cord compression. First attempts to relieve recurrent variable decelerations should include lateral maternal repositioning, which takes the weight of the fetus off the maternal great vessels posteriorly. Amnioinfusion of 250-mL to 500-mL warm saline via an intrauterine pressure catheter followed by a 50-mL to 60-mL per hour drip can also be considered and has been shown to decrease recurrence of variable decelerations and cesarean delivery rates; however, outcome data supporting this practice are limited. Other appropriate interventions may include fluid bolus for treatment of maternal hypotension, supplemental oxygen, and cessation of labor stimulants, such as oxytocin.

Recurrent late decelerations are associated with uteroplacental insufficiency and commonly form as manifestations of postepidural maternal hypotension, maternal hypoxia, and uterine tachysystole. They confer a low predictive value for fetal metabolic acidemia, however, and have a high false-positive rate for neurologic damage. Management recommendations are the same for recurrent variable decelerations.

Uterine tachysystole with recurrent decelerations should be treated with decreased dosing of oxytocin. Tachysystole is less concerning when associated with

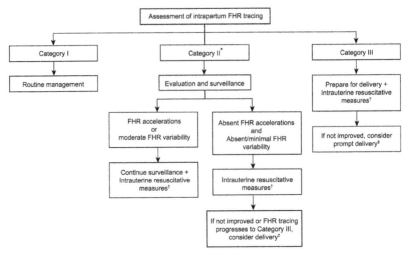

*Given the wide variation of FHR tracings in Category II, this algorithm is not meant to represent assessment and management of all potential FHR tracings, but provide an action template for common clinical situations.

†See Table 2 for list of various intrauterine resuscitative measures.

‡Timing and mode of delivery based on feasibility and maternal-fetal status.

Goal	Associated Fetal Heart Rate Abnormality*	Potential Intervention (S)†
Promote fetal oxygenation and improve uteroplacental blood flow	Recurrent late decelerations Prolonged decelerations or bradycardia Minimal or absent fetal heart rate variability	Initiate lateral positioning (either left or right) Administer maternal oxygen administration Administer intravenous fluid bolus Reduce uterine contraction frequency
Reduce uterine activity	Tachysystole with Category II or III tracing	Discontinue oxytocin or cervical ripening agents Administer tocolytic medication (eg, terbutaline)
Alleviate umbilical cord compression	Recurrent variable decelerations Prolonged decelerations or bradycardia	Initiate maternal repositioning Initiate amnioinfusion If prolapsed umbilical cord is noted, elevate the presenting fetal part while preparations are underway for operative delivery

*Evaluation for the underlying suspected cause(s) is also an important step in management of abnormal FHR tracings.

Fig. 1. ACOG management algorithm of intrapartum fetal heart rate tracings based on the NIHCD 3-tiered category system. (*Data from* American College of Obstetricians and Gynecologists. Practice bulletin no. 116: management of intrapartum fetal heart rate tracings. Obstet Gynecol 2010;116(5):1232–40. Available at: http://www.ncbi.nlm.nih.gov/pubmed/20966730. Accessed January 16, 2011.)

accelerations or moderate EFHR variability. An ACOG flowchart for the management of uterine tachysystole is displayed in **Fig. 2.**

If all reasonable clinical interventions are exhausted and the category III pattern persists, definitive treatment is emergent delivery.

When interpreting EFHR tracings, bear in mind that patterns are dynamic and should be interpreted in the context of their clinical development. Therefore, multiple management strategies may exist for equivalent EFHR findings arising in different contexts. Furthermore, EFHR tracings commonly switch categories over time and thus should be evaluated frequently. Unfortunately, no evidence-based medicine is available to establish what constitutes an appropriate time interval between EFHR pattern assessments. An ACOG 2010 practice bulletin, however, recommends reviewing the EFHR tracings of uncomplicated patients every 30 minutes during the first

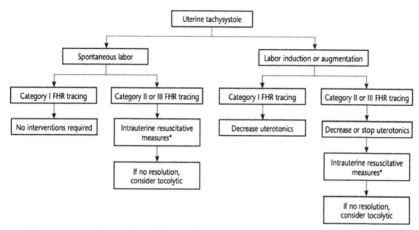

Fig. 2. Management of uterine tachysystole. (*Data from* American College of Obstetricians and Gynecologists. Practice bulletin no. 116: management of intrapartum fetal heart rate tracings. Obstet Gynecol 2010;116(5):1232–40. Available at: http://www.ncbi.nlm.nih.gov/ pubmed/20966730. Accessed January 16, 2011.)

stage of labor and every 15 minutes throughout the second stage; complicated patients should be evaluated every 15 minutes during the first stage of labor and every 5 minutes after that.[15]

Although the current 3-tiered EFHR pattern schematic is useful for its ease of comprehension, many clinicians feel that it falls short of providing a thorough construct to interpret accurately and respond reliably to the large majority of indeterminate patterns. Organizations, such as the Society of Obstetricians and Gynaecologists of Canada and the Royal College of Obstetricians and Gynaecologists, have posited their own versions of the 3-tiered system that incorporate more specific recommendations for intrapartum EFHR pattern interpretation and management.

Systematic Management

When describing an EFM tracing, the mnemonic, "Dr C. Bravado," from the American Academy of Family Physicians ALSO, provides a systematic method of incorporating the information into a decision algorithm with the intention of optimizing managements and outcomes.

DR	Define Risk—low or high
C	Contractions—comment on frequency, etc.
BRa	Baseline Rate—bradycardia, normal, tachycardia
V	Variability—at least 10–15 bpm (persistent, reduced variability is ominous)
A	Accelerations—present or absent
D	Decelerations—early, variable, or late
O	Overall—assessment (category I/II/III) and plan of management

Discussion and Controversy

The benefit of EFM is controversial. It is not a good universal screening tool. When used to predict neurologic injury, EFHR's positive predictive value is only 0.14% in singleton newborns with birth weights greater than 2500 g, and it confers an overall false-positive rate of 99%.[16] To its credit, the presence of accelerations does have an acceptable negative predictive value for metabolic acidemia, with sensitivity and specificity of 57% and 69%, respectively.[17]

Some clinicians maintain that there is no evidence to indicate that EFHR confers any advantage over intermittent auscultation in otherwise healthy singleton pregnancies. A 2006 Cochrane review comparing EFHR monitoring with intermittent auscultation showed no significant change in perinatal mortality or cerebral palsy between the two methods but documented an increase in the rate of operative obstetric interventions with EFM.[18] In essence, EFM has become universal even though fetal outcome data is lacking and its use puts mothers at undue risk of surgical complications.

Not everyone agrees with the standard terminology put forth by the NICHD. Although ACOG has adopted the NICHD definitions into their practice bulletins, some groups do not consider these recommendations to constitute standard of care. Those in opposition cite that the time frames for intervention are logistically impossible. Recommendations for timely resolution of abnormal patterns by means of emergent operative delivery lack evidence. Emergent procedures for category 3 patterns may only increase maternal health risk without providing an outcomes benefit to fetuses that have already developed irreversible brain damage. This is supported by a study of 2808 emergent cesarean sections in which, although greater than 30% of deliveries were delayed by more than half an hour after the decision was made to operate, no adverse neonatal outcomes differences resulted between the two groups.[19]

In spite of standard definitions for interpreting EFHR patterns, reliance on human assessment causes the current diagnostic system to have exceedingly poor interobserver and intraobserver reliability. But recent improvements in EFHR analysis and better risk stratification will change this. Algorithms and resource realities will allow low-tech deliveries with limited EFHR in community settings. Science will recommend early transfer to high-tech birth centers for those with elevated risk and the financial resources to support this expensive service. As usual, errors of omission and commission will persist.

Complications and Considerations

Beyond increasing operative delivery rates, EFM is not a completely benign clinical assessment tool. Insertion of catheters and pressure transducers has been documented to cause physical complications, such as uterine perforation, hemorrhage, chorioamnionitis, and fetal scalp osteomyelitis. Its use also medicalizes an otherwise natural birthing process. Thus, although ACOG guidelines leave the decision to use EFM or intermittent auscultation up to individual clinicians, the efficacy of this decision and its risk-benefit profile should not be taken lightly.

Medicolegal

EFHR tracings provide information on the current acid-base status of the fetus. Although they have been associated with cerebral palsy and fetal acidemia, their poor positive predictive value limits the prognostic value for neurologic outcomes.

Future Considerations

Since recommendations for further evaluation of the effectiveness of computer interpretation systems were made by the 2008 NICHD report, much research has accumulated. Recent advancements in computerized ST-segment and EFHR analysis look promising for reliably streamlining a more reliable EFHR pattern interpretation system.

Although these technologies have become standard in other parts of the world, ST analysis remains on the horizon of mainstream American obstetric practice.

SUMMARY

In summary, this article reviews the history and standardization of EFM terminology, citing publications from both the NICHD and the ACOG that led to the 3-tiered scheme for broad categorization of EFHR patterns in the United States. The article comments on current technologies, such as intermittent auscultation, EFM, tocodynamometry, abdominal ECG, Doppler ultrasound, and internal fetal electrodes. After defining these 6 terms—uterine contractions, baseline FHR and variability, accelerations, decelerations, sinusoidal patterns, and FHR variability—practice management guidelines are highlighted, which included a description of the 3-tiered system of FHR pattern categorization. Lastly, controversial areas within the field are discussed before briefly concluding with future considerations.

REFERENCES

1. Raju TN. Historical perspectives on the etiology of cerebral palsy. Clin Perinatol 2006;33(2):233–50. Available at: http://www.ncbi.nlm.nih.gov/pubmed/16765722. Accessed May 23, 2011.
2. Martin JA, Hamilton BE, Sutton PD, et al. Births: final data for 2002. Natl Vital Stat Rep 2003;52(10):1–113. Available at: http://www.ncbi.nlm.nih.gov/pubmed/14717305. Accessed May 23, 2011.
3. Electronic fetal heart rate monitoring: research guidelines for interpretation. National Institute of Child Health and Human Development Research Planning Workshop. Am J Obstet Gynecol 1997;177(6):1385–90. Available at: http://www.ncbi.nlm.nih.gov/pubmed/9423739. Accessed May 23, 2011.
4. Macones GA, Hankins GD, Spong CY, et al. The 2008 National Institute of Child Health and Human Development workshop report on electronic fetal monitoring: update on definitions, interpretation, and research guidelines. J Obstet Gynecol Neonatal Nurs 2008;37(5):510–5. Available at: http://www.ncbi.nlm.nih.gov/pubmed/18761565. Accessed May 23, 2011.
5. Cline MK, Taylor H, BE, editors. ALSO syllabus. American Academy of Family Physicians. Available at: http://www.aafp.org/online/en/home/cme/aafpcourses/clinicalcourses/also/syllabus.html. Accessed May 23, 2011.
6. Young BK, Weinstein HM. Moderate fetal bradycardia. Am J Obstet Gynecol 1976;126(2):271–5. Available at: http://www.ncbi.nlm.nih.gov/pubmed/961768. Accessed May 23, 2011.
7. Freeman RK. The evolution of antepartum fetal testing methods. Am J Obstet Gynecol 2003;189(1):310. Available at: http://www.ncbi.nlm.nih.gov/pubmed/12861191. Accessed May 23, 2011.
8. Gilstrap LC, Hauth JC, Hankins GD, et al. Second-stage fetal heart rate abnormalities and type of neonatal acidemia. Obstet Gynecol 1987;70(2):191–5. Available at: http://www.ncbi.nlm.nih.gov/pubmed/3601281. Accessed May 23, 2011.
9. Krebs HB, Petres RE, Dunn LJ, et al. Intrapartum fetal heart rate monitoring. VI. Prognostic significance of accelerations. Am J Obstet Gynecol 1982;142(3):297–305. Available at: http://www.ncbi.nlm.nih.gov/pubmed/7065019. Accessed May 23, 2011.
10. Clark SL, Gimovsky ML, Miller FC. The scalp stimulation test: a clinical alternative to fetal scalp blood sampling. Am J Obstet Gynecol 1984;148(3):274–7. Available at: http://www.ncbi.nlm.nih.gov/pubmed/6695974. Accessed May 23, 2011.

11. Smith CV, Nguyen HN, Phelan JP, et al. Intrapartum assessment of fetal well-being: a comparison of fetal acoustic stimulation with acid-base determinations. Am J Obstet Gynecol 1986;155(4):726–8. Available at: http://www.ncbi.nlm.nih.gov/pubmed/3766625. Accessed May 23, 2011.

12. Paul JD, Gahres EE, Rhoads JC, et al. CR51 placenta localization and blood loss determinations in placenta previa accreta: report of a case. Obstet Gynecol 1964;23:259–61. Available at: http://www.ncbi.nlm.nih.gov/pubmed/14117337. Accessed May 23, 2011.

13. ACOG technical bulletin. Fetal heart rate patterns: monitoring, interpretation, and management. Number 207–July 1995 (replaces No. 132, September 1989). Int J Gynaecol Obstet 1995;51(1):65–74. Available at: http://www.ncbi.nlm.nih.gov/pubmed/8582524. Accessed May 23, 2011.

14. Spong CY, Rasul C, Collea JV, et al. Characterization and prognostic significance of variable decelerations in the second stage of labor. Am J Perinatol 1998;15(6):369–74. Available at: http://www.ncbi.nlm.nih.gov/pubmed/9722057. Accessed May 23, 2011.

15. American College of Obstetricians and Gynecologists. Practice bulletin no. 116: management of intrapartum fetal heart rate tracings. Obstet Gynecol 2010; 116(5):1232–40. Available at: http://www.ncbi.nlm.nih.gov/pubmed/20966730. Accessed January 16, 2011.

16. ACOG Practice Bulletin No. 106: intrapartum fetal heart rate monitoring: nomenclature, interpretation, and general management principles. Obstet Gynecol 2009; 114(1):192–202. Available at: http://www.ncbi.nlm.nih.gov/pubmed/19546798. Accessed April 26, 2011.

17. Larma JD, Silva AM, Holcroft CJ, et al. Intrapartum electronic fetal heart rate monitoring and the identification of metabolic acidosis and hypoxic-ischemic encephalopathy. Am J Obstet Gynecol 2007;197(3):301.e1–8. Available at: http://www.ncbi.nlm.nih.gov/pubmed/17826429. Accessed May 23, 2011.

18. Alfirevic Z, Devane D, Gyte GM. Continuous cardiotocography (CTG) as a form of electronic fetal monitoring (EFM) for fetal assessment during labour. Cochrane Database Syst Rev 2006;3:CD006066. Available at: http://www.ncbi.nlm.nih.gov/pubmed/16856111. Accessed April 20, 2011.

19. Bloom SL, Leveno KJ, Spong CY, et al. Decision-to-incision times and maternal and infant outcomes. Obstet Gynecol 2006;108(1):6–11. Available at: http://www.ncbi.nlm.nih.gov/pubmed/16816049. Accessed May 23, 2011.

FURTHER READINGS

Coonrod A, Kelly BF, Ellert W, et al. Tiered maternity care training in family medicine: a consensus statement. Fam Med 2011;43(9):631–7.

Dresang LT, Rodney WM, Dees J. Teaching prenatal ultrasound to family medicine residents. Fam Med 2004;36:98–107.

Dresang LT, Rodney WM, Leeman L, et al. ALSO in Ecuador: teaching the teachers. J Am Board Fam Pract 2004;17(4):276–82. Available at: http://www.jabfp.org/cgi/content/full/17/4/276. Accessed May 23, 2011.

Rodney WM, Rodney JR. Family Medicine-OB 1989-2009: Applications for Developing Countries. Scientific Assembly [abstract]. New York: American Institute for Ultrasound in Medicine; 2009.

Rodney WM, Rodney JR. Medicos para la Familia: a successful model for service through procedurally enriched family medicine obstetrics. Rockford (IL): University of Illinois; Department of Family Medicine. May 5, 2010, and the World Organization of Family Doctors in Cancun, Mexico May 25, 2010.

Rodney WM, Hardison RD, McKenzie LM, et al. The impact of deliveries on office hours and physician sleep. J Natl Med Assoc 2006;98:1685–90.

Rodney WM, Martinez C, Chiu KW, et al. Prenatal patients not delivered: unplanned events, uncounted services, risks. Am J Clin Med 2009;6(2):31–6.

Rodney WM, Martinez C, Collins MC, et al. The obstetrics fellowship 1992-2010: where do they go, what do they do, and how many stop doing OB? Fam Med 2010;42:712–5.

Complications of Labor and Delivery: Shoulder Dystocia

Jane E. Anderson, MD, MS

KEYWORDS

- Shoulder dystocia • Macrosomia • Brachial plexus injury
- McRoberts maneuver

There is no such thing as routine labor and delivery until after the fact, when a healthy live infant is born. Even in uncomplicated pregnancies, situations may arise during parturition that turn an unremarkable labor or delivery into an obstetric emergency with increased risk or morbidity and mortality for mother and infant. One of the less common but most dreaded complications of labor and deliver, shoulder dystocia, is reviewed.

SHOULDER DYSTOCIA

Shoulder dystocia is an infrequent but potentially devastating event that results from impaction of the fetal shoulders in the maternal pelvis. Although maternal, fetal, and intrapartum risk factors are identified, they have poor predictive value. Shoulder dystocia occurs most commonly in patients without identified risk factors, and can result in both maternal and fetal morbidity. Prophylactic measures including intrapartum maneuvers and cesarean section have not been shown to be effective at preventing the incidence of dystocia except in select populations (maternal diabetes and macrosomia). A series of maternal and clinician maneuvers may be effective in reducing the dystocia. Because the vast majority of cases of shoulder dystocia are unpredictable, obstetric care providers must be prepared to recognize dystocia and respond appropriately in every delivery. Detailed documentation is essential after any delivery complicated by shoulder dystocia.

Definition

Shoulder dystocia has a somewhat subjective definition that is not universally agreed on by delivering providers. Based on physical presentation, shoulder dystocia may be

This work received no grant funding.
The author has nothing to disclose.
Department of Family Medicine, University of Wisconsin School of Medicine and Public Health, 1100 Deleplaine Ct. Madison, WI 53715-1896, USA
E-mail address: jane.anderson@fammed.wisc.edu

Prim Care Clin Office Pract 39 (2012) 135–144
doi:10.1016/j.pop.2011.12.002   primarycare.theclinics.com
0095-4543/12/$ – see front matter Published by Elsevier Inc.

defined as impaction of the anterior shoulder against the maternal symphysis pubis, the posterior shoulder against the maternal sacral promontory, or both.[1] The American College of Obstetrics and Gynecologists Practice Bulletin defines shoulder dystocia as "a delivery that requires additional obstetric maneuvers following failure of gentle downward traction on the fetal head to effect delivery of the shoulders."[1] In an effort to create a more objective definition, Spong and colleagues[2] proposed a prolonged head-to-body delivery time of more than 60 seconds or the need for ancillary obstetric maneuvers (McRoberts, suprapubic pressure, rotational maneuvers, or hands' and knees' positioning). This proposal is based on a prospective study in which patients who did not require obstetric maneuvers had an average head-to-body delivery time of 24.2 seconds, with 2 standard deviations above the mean being 60 seconds.

Incidence

Rates of shoulder dystocia vary because of differences in diagnostic criteria, and range in various reports from 0.3% to 3% of vaginal deliveries of term vertex infants.[3] The incidence of shoulder dystocia increases correspondingly with increasing fetal weight and with maternal diabetes. Nesbitt and colleagues[4] conducted a retrospective study of 175,886 infants weighing greater than 3500 g. Among nondiabetic patients, rates of shoulder dystocia increased in spontaneous vaginal deliveries from 5.2% for infants weighing 4000 to 4250 g up to 21.1% for those weighing 4750 to 5000 g. Vacuum or forceps-assisted deliveries are associated with even higher rates of dystocia. Incidence of shoulder dystocia in diabetic patients with assisted births (vacuum or forceps) increased to a dramatic 34.8% for infants weighing 4750 to 5000 g.

Risk Factors

Maternal, fetal, and intrapartum variables can contribute to increased risk of shoulder dystocia. Risk factors alone or in combination, however, have a poor positive predictive value for any individual delivery.[3] Many cases of shoulder dystocia have no identifiable risk factors,[5] and the vast majority of deliveries, even in patients with multiple risk factors, are uneventful.

Maternal risk factors include maternal diabetes, maternal obesity, postdates pregnancy, advanced maternal age, increased parity, and history of a previous shoulder dystocia.[6-9] These risk factors have increased likelihood of a macrosomic infant as the common element. Additional risk factors include maternal short stature and abnormal pelvic anatomy.[8]

The primary fetal factor is suspected macrosomia, defined as weight greater than 4500 g by the American College of Obstetricians and Gynecologists (ACOG).[1] Frustratingly, efforts to predict fetal weight antenatally have proved to be inaccurate. There are multiple formulas that try to predict fetal weight based on ultrasonography during the third trimester, but these formulas have been found to have an error rate that results in lower accuracy by ultrasound than clinician estimates based on Leopold maneuvers or maternal estimates.[9,10] The larger the fetus, the less accurate the estimate. An additional fetal risk factor is male gender.

Intrapartum risk factors include induction of labor, prolonged first or second stage of labor, and operative vaginal delivery (vacuum having greater risk than forceps).[11,12] Precipitous delivery is also a risk factor. Although this seems counterintuitive, the proposed mechanism is insufficient time for the fetus to rotate into an oblique position in the maternal pelvis. Use of epidural anesthesia is not associated with an increased risk of shoulder dystocia.[13]

Maternal diabetes and fetal macrosomia have the strongest evidence as independent risk factors, which may be related to the pattern of weight gain in infants of diabetic mothers who demonstrate a larger head, trunk and chest circumference, and increased bisacromial diameter.[6] This pattern of weight gain may hamper the ability of the fetal shoulders to rotate during the second stage, further complicating the birth of an already large fetus.

Despite multiple analyses of risk factors in the literature, shoulder dystocia cannot be predicted or prevented because accurate methods for identifying which fetuses will experience this complication do not exist.[1]

Complications

Maternal complications after a shoulder dystocia may include postpartum hemorrhage, uterine rupture, and a third-degree or fourth-degree tear with risk of increased pain, rectovaginal fistula, and incontinence of stool.[1,7,8,10]

Fetal complications include brachial plexus injury leading to temporary or permanent palsy, fracture of the clavicle or humerus, hypoxia with potential neurologic sequela, and even fetal demise.[1,7]

The most frequent fetal complication is brachial plexus injury. Erb-Duchenne palsy affects nerve roots C5 to C6. This palsy is the most common and has a high likelihood of resolution within 1 year. The injury persists in 5% to 8% of cases. Klumpke palsy affects C8 to T1 and is less common, but up to 40% of cases persist beyond 1 year.[14] Despite the uncertain etiology of the brachial plexus injury (maternal vs iatrogenic), brachial plexus injuries are a frequent source of litigation.[15] Until the past decade, it has been presumed that brachial plexus injuries were caused by excessive or inappropriate lateral traction on the fetal head and neck by the delivering physician, causing stretch on the fetal brachial plexus.[16] Data suggest that this injury is multifactorial, however. Brachial plexus injury has been documented in anterior and posterior shoulders of uncomplicated vaginal deliveries without shoulder dystocia and in cesarean section deliveries. The rate of brachial plexus injury has been static for decades despite increasing rates of cesarean section.[17,18] The proposed mechanisms for brachial plexus injuries in deliveries without shoulder dystocia include in utero malpositioning (uterine septum, bicornuate uterus, and uterine fibroid) and endogenous maternal forces during the second stage of labor, which can generate greater pressure than exogenous forces applied by delivering providers.[19-21]

Hypoxic-ischemic encephalopathy and death are the most devastating outcomes of a shoulder dystocia. The proposed pathology includes compression of the umbilical cord, compression of fetal carotid arteries, and premature placental separation in prolonged dystocia. A retrospective review of 200 shoulder dystocias documented a gradual linear decline in cord arterial pH with increasing time interval to delivery. The overall incidence of acidosis, hypoxic-ischemic encephalopathy, and death after shoulder dystocia is low when the head-to-body delivery interval is less than 5 minutes, suggesting a target delivery of the trunk by 5 minutes.[22]

Prevention

Prevention of macrosomia

Because increasing fetal weight is strongly correlated with increased risk of shoulder dystocia, treatment of gestational diabetes has been considered a means to prevent shoulder dystocia. However, this perception has not been convincingly demonstrated in the literature. Crowther and colleagues[23] conducted a randomized controlled trial of patients in Australia and the United Kingdom (ACHOIS Trial) who had moderately increased glucose on gestational screening tests. Women were randomized to usual care versus intervention with dietary advice, glucose monitoring, and insulin. Although there was an overall significant decrease in serious perinatal outcomes among infants in the intervention group ($P = 0.01$), there was not a significant difference in rates of shoulder dystocia per se ($P = 0.08$). A subsequent article with a secondary analysis of the ACHOIS data concludes that there is a positive relationship between the severity of maternal hyperglycemia and the risk of shoulder dystocia with macrosomic and large for gestational age infants, having an increased relative risk of 6.72 and 4.57, respectively, for shoulder dystocia.[24] This trend is supported by retrospective analysis of birth weight and perinatal morbidity.[4]

Prophylactic intrapartum maneuvers

There are several maneuvers that are used to facilitate delivery in a shoulder dystocia (see sections on Management and Maneuvers for full description). The McRoberts maneuver is commonly used as the initial response, accompanied by suprapubic pressure. These maneuvers alone will lead to resolution of half of all dystocias.[25] The McRoberts maneuver consists of flexing the maternal hips to effectively increase the diameter of the maternal pelvis. Suprapubic pressure is applied by a second provider in an attempt to disimpact the shoulder from behind the maternal pubis. Beall and colleagues[26] completed a prospective study to evaluate whether prophylactic use of the McRoberts maneuver and suprapubic pressure before delivery of the fetal head would decrease head-to-body time interval in a group of patients with estimated fetal weight of more than 3800 g. Prophylactic maneuvers were associated with reduction in therapeutic maneuvers after delivery of the fetal head, thus reducing the rate of recognized dystocia. However, there was no decrease in delivery time in the intervention group. Because there is a small risk for maternal morbidity with the McRoberts maneuver and suprapubic pressure, the investigators concluded that those measures should not be used prophylactically but should be reserved for therapeutic use in evident cases of shoulder dystocia.

A Cochrane review concluded that there was not enough data to support or refute the use of prophylactic maneuvers, and recommended additional data with larger sample sizes.[27]

Induction of labor in select populations

It may seem intuitive that the risk of shoulder dystocia could be reduced by inducing patients with suspected macrosomia at an earlier gestational age when the fetus is smaller. However, although multiple studies have been conducted, none have shown evidence of improved outcomes.[24] The investigators of a Cochrane review concluded that compared with expectant management, induction of labor for suspected fetal macrosomia in nondiabetic women did not reduce perinatal morbidity, including shoulder dystocia (relative risk 1.06, 95% confidence interval 0.44–2.56).[28]

Elective induction versus expectant management for women with insulin-requiring diabetes reduced macrosomia without increasing the rates of cesarean section. However, this observation was based on one trial and the overall rate of shoulder dystocia was low; therefore, there is no evidence to support early induction. The ACOG Practice Bulletin for Shoulder Dystocia concurs that labor induction in nondiabetic women with suspected macrosomia has not been effective at decreasing shoulder dystocia.[1]

Cesarean section in select populations

Studies have evaluated whether prophylactic cesarean delivery in pregnancies with suspected macrosomic fetuses (>4000 g) would reduce rates of shoulder dystocia. One study used a decision-analysis model to evaluate the effect of performing cesarean sections on all fetuses suspected of weighing 4000 g or more. They estimated that the cost of the additional cesarean sections would be $4.9 million annually to prevent one permanent injury from shoulder dystocia.[29] Based on the same study, ACOG recommends that prophylactic cesarean section may be considered for suspected macrosomia greater than 4500 g for women with gestation diabetes and greater than 5000 g for women without.[1]

Recurrent dystocia

Although primary shoulder dystocia is difficult to predict, patients with a history of dystocia may have a uniquely increased risk for recurrence. In an effort to provide evidence-based counseling to women with a history of shoulder dystocia, Bingham and colleagues[30] conducted a review of pregnancies resulting in recurrent shoulder dystocia, and found that patients with a history of shoulder dystocia in one pregnancy (1.6% of pregnancies) have a 12% risk of a recurrent shoulder dystocia in subsequent pregnancies (odds ratio [OR] 8.25). The risk factors for recurrent dystocia were similar to those identified for primary dystocia (macrosomia, gestational diabetes, induction of labor, and operative delivery). The investigators acknowledge that risk factors continue to be poor predictors of which specific deliveries will be complicated by dystocia.

The risk of brachial plexus injury was increased from 19/1000 per first episode of dystocia to 45/1000 in recurrent dystocia. This figure represents a significant increase from 1% to 4% of births (OR 3.59). Brachial plexus injury occurred in 13 of 1000 subsequent deliveries without documented dystocia. These data are consistent with contemporary data suggesting multiple causes for brachial plexus injury in addition to shoulder dystocia.

Additional studies support prior shoulder dystocia as a risk factor for subsequent shoulder dystocia. Fetal size in the subsequent pregnancy is consistently identified as the primary risk factor.[31,32]

The ACOG guideline recommends evaluating risk factors (estimated fetal weight of current pregnancy compared with prior pregnancy, gestational age, maternal glucose status, and prior neonatal injury) and discussing the risks and benefits of cesarean delivery for patients with a previous shoulder dystocia.[1]

MANAGEMENT

Because shoulder dystocia cannot be predicted, it should be anticipated in every delivery, particularly in patients with one or more risk factors. It is important to recognize shoulder dystocia when it occurs: this is often described as the turtle sign, whereby the head delivers but does not undergo external rotation and the neonatal cheeks and chin recoil tightly against the perineum. Gentle downward traction fails to deliver the anterior shoulder.[7] After confirming the shoulder dystocia, the patient and nursing staff should be informed and the physician should call for help. Most institutions have a protocol to summon additional obstetric, neonatal, anesthesia, and nursing staff. One staff member should be dedicated to recording the order and duration of events and monitoring time intervals for the delivering clinician.

Maneuvers

There are several maneuvers that may be attempted to reduce a dystocia. In general, there has not been strong evidence that any one maneuver is superior to another in releasing an impacted shoulder or reducing the risk of injury to the fetus. The American Academy of Family Physicians (through ALSO [the Advanced Life Support in Obstetrics program]), the ACOG, and the Royal College of Obstetricians and Gynecologists

(RCOG) support following a systematic sequence of maneuvers starting with the simplest and least invasive.[1,33,34]

To assess comparative efficacy of maneuvers at reducing dystocia and minimizing neonatal injury, 2 retrospective reviews were recently conducted. Hoffman and colleagues[35] found that McRoberts and suprapubic pressure were widely practiced and were associated with low rates of neonatal injury. However, in terms of efficacy, delivery of the posterior shoulder had the highest overall rate of success when compared with all other maneuvers, without increasing injury to the neonate. Leung and colleagues[36] found that rotational maneuvers and posterior arm delivery had similar success rates after a failed McRoberts maneuver. Rotational maneuvers were associated with lower rates of fetal injury.

In practice, the order of maneuvers is flexible depending on the experience of the delivering clinician and the position and mobility of the mother. If one maneuver is not successful after 20 to 30 seconds, it is important to move on to another maneuver until delivery is accomplished.

There are additional maneuvers of last resort (deliberate clavicle fracture, cephalic replacement and cesarean section, symphysiotomy, abdominal surgery, and hysterotomy), but these maneuvers are not within the scope of this article.

McRoberts maneuver

The ACOG Bulletin states that McRoberts is a reasonable initial maneuver.[1] This maneuver consists of abducting, externally rotating, and hyperflexing the maternal hips, typically with an assistant supporting each maternal leg. This procedure causes superior rotation of the symphysis pubis and straightening of the lumbosacral angle, which effectively helps rotate the pubis over the impacted anterior shoulder and creates a large pelvic diameter.[11] The McRoberts maneuver alone is successful at reducing the dystocia 42% of the time. The addition of suprapubic pressure increases the success rate to 54%.[3] By contrast, a 15-year retrospective review found no improvement in reducing rates of shoulder dystocia and brachial plexus injury despite the introduction and near universal adoption of the McRoberts maneuver.[37] Although this maneuver is generally safe, there have been reports in the literature of damage to the symphysis pubis cartilage and transient femoral neuropathy. Common sense would dictate avoiding overaggressive or prolonged flexion, particularly in patients with epidural anesthesia.

Suprapubic pressure

It is important that suprapubic pressure not be confused with fundal pressure, which would add to the shoulder impaction and increased risk of uterine rupture. Suprapubic pressure is applied by an assistant (usually standing on a stool for better leverage) to the posterior aspect of the anterior shoulder just proximal to the symphysis pubis. This pressure adducts the fetal shoulder and helps disimpact the shoulder from the symphysis pubis, pushing the fetal shoulders into the oblique diameter. Pressure is applied continuously or a rocking, "CPR-like," motion may be used.[11,33] Suprapubic pressure is also known as the Rubin maneuver or Rubin I maneuver.

Rotational maneuvers

The Rubin II and the Woods screw are maneuvers that both entail entering the vagina and manually attempting to rotate the fetal shoulder girdle. The Rubin II maneuver consists of applying pressure to the posterior aspect of the anterior shoulder to adduct/flex the anterior shoulder. The Woods screw maneuver involves applying pressure to the anterior aspect of the posterior shoulder to abduct/extend the posterior shoulder. Both Rubin II and Woods screw may be attempted at the same time to facilitate corkscrewing the fetal shoulder through the maternal pelvis. These maneuvers may also be done concurrently with the McRoberts maneuver. An episiotomy may be required to allow room for the clinician's hand to enter the vaginal canal, particularly for the maneuvers involving the posterior shoulder.

If these maneuvers are not successful in dislodging the fetus, the Reverse Woods screw may be attempted. The entering hand is placed behind the posterior shoulder to adduct/flex the posterior shoulder, which essentially attempts to rotate the fetus in the opposite direction to that used in the Rubin II and Woods screw maneuvers.

Delivery of the posterior arm

The clinician inserts a hand into the vagina (again, this may require episiotomy) and locates the posterior fetal forearm, which is swept across the chest and delivered hand-first. Care should be taken to avoid direct pressure on the upper arm, which could fracture the midshaft of the humerus. Delivery of the posterior arm results in a reduction in shoulder diameter and allows the anterior shoulder to drop below the symphysis pubis.

Gaskin maneuver

This maneuver is probably the oldest technique, although it may be the least familiar to physicians. The Gaskin or "all-fours" involves assisting the patient into a hands' and knees' position, which changes the dimensions of the pelvic diameter, and the process of maternal repositioning and gravity may aid in disimpacting the shoulders. This position may be difficult for a patient who is limited in mobility by exhaustion or epidural anesthesia, but is possible even then with sufficient assistance. The hands' and knees' position may be somewhat disorienting to the delivering provider, because the posterior shoulder is delivered first. The rotational maneuvers may be repeated with the patient in this position.

SIMULATION AND SKILLS TRAINING

The Joint Commission on the Accreditation of Healthcare Organizations issued a Sentinel Event Alert in 2004 recommending clinical drills for shoulder dystocia to prepare staff, evaluate team performance, and identify areas for improvement.[38] Observations of shoulder dystocia simulations have found common management errors, including ambiguity in diagnosing dystocia, failure to call for help, excessive traction on the fetal head, failure to execute appropriate maneuvers, poor communication among team members, and poor documentation.[39,40]

Improved management and clinical outcomes have been documented after mandatory multiprofessional shoulder dystocia simulation training. Recommended maneuvers were used more frequently and there was a reduction in excessive traction. Clinical outcomes were improved, with a significant reduction in the number of brachial palsies recorded at birth.[41] The improvement in management of dystocia persisted up to 1 year after training in a simulation setting.[42]

DOCUMENTATION

It is imperative that documentation be accurate and comprehensive, to demonstrate standard of care management in the event of litigation.[43,44] A review of documentation after both simulated and actual deliveries complicated by shoulder dystocia indicated that crucial elements of documentation are often missing.[40,43,44] Simulations may help raise awareness, and standardized forms (rather than free text narrative) provide more complete and consistent documentation. This documentation can be in the form of an electronic template or preformatted checklist that is scanned into the electronic record.

Documentation should include who was present, the time interval between delivery of the head and the body, fetal position, sequence of maneuvers, time spent on each maneuver, whether cord gas was sent, and condition of the infant including arm motion after delivery. Implementation of a checklist significantly improves documentation for almost all key components.[44]

Even before the delivery, documentation should reflect consideration for possible dystocia in the setting of known risk factors (gestational diabetes, anticipated macrosomia, and so forth). Estimated fetal weight at the time of presentation in labor should be recorded even with the understanding that it may be inaccurate, which can help both the patient and provider to be prepared for maneuvers that may be needed at the time of delivery.

SUMMARY POINTS

Shoulder dystocia occurs in about 1.6% of all births.
Be mindful of risk factors but recognize there is no way to predict a shoulder dystocia in a given delivery.
Think about dystocia before every delivery. Practice simulation with team to improve skills and confidence.
Recognize dystocia. Communicate this diagnosis to delivery team. Call for help as soon as dystocia is recognized.
Proceed in systematic fashion. Avoid excess traction on the fetal head.
After resolution, document comprehensively.

REFERENCES

1. ACOG Committee on Practice Bulletins—Gynecology, The American College of Obstetrician and Gynecologists. ACOG practice bulletin clinical management guidelines for obstetrician-gynecologists. Number 40, November 2002. Obstet Gynecol 2002;100(5 Pt 1):1045–50.
2. Spong CY, Beall M, Rodriques D, et al. An objective definition of shoulder dystocia: prolonged head-to-body delivery intervals and/or the use of ancillary obstetric maneuvers. Obstet Gynecol 1995;86(3):433–6.
3. Gherman RB. Shoulder dystocia: an evidence-based evaluation of the obstetric nightmare. Clin Obstet Gynecol 2002;45(2):345–62.
4. Nesbitt TS, Gilbert WM, Harrchen B. Shoulder dystocia and associated risk factors with macrosomic infants born in California. Am J Obstet Gynecol 1998;179(2):476–80.
5. Lewis DF, Edwards MF, Asrat T, et al. Can shoulder dystocia be predicted? Preconceptive and prenatal factors. J Reprod Med 1998;43(8):654–8.
6. Gherman RB, Chauhan S, Ouzounian JG, et al. Shoulder dystocia: the unpreventable obstetric emergency with empiric management guidelines. Am J Obstet Gynecol 2006;195(3):657–72.
7. Baskett TF. Shoulder dystocia. Best Pract Res Clin Obstet Gynecol 2002;16(1):57–68.
8. Baxley EG, Gobbo RW. Shoulder dystocia. Am Fam Physician 2004;69(7):1707–14.

9. Gottlieb AG, Galan HL. Shoulder dystocia: an update. Obstet Gynecol Clin North Am 2007;34(3):501–31, xii.
10. Wagner RK, Nielsen PE, Gonik B. Shoulder dystocia. Obstet Gynecol Clin North Am 1999;26(2):371–83.
11. Neill AM, Thornton S. The Obstetrician & Gynaecologist [letter]. Obstet Gynecol 2000;2(4):45–7.
12. Gherman RB, Goodwin TM, Souter I, et al. The McRoberts' maneuver for the alleviation of shoulder dystocia: how successful is it? Am J Obstet Gynecol 1997; 176(3):656–61.
13. Nocon JJ, McKenzie DK, Thomas LJ, et al. Shoulder dystocia: an analysis of risks and obstetric manuevers. Am J Obstet Gynecol 1993;168:1732–9.
14. Doumouchtsis SK, Arulkumaran S. Is it possible to reduce obstetrical brachial plexus palsy by optimal management of shoulder dystocia? Ann N Y Acad Sci 2010;1205:135–43.
15. Gilbert WM, Nesbitt TS, Danielsen B. Associated factores in 1611 cases of brachial plexus injury. Obstet Gynecol 1999;93(4):536–40.
16. Sandmire HF, DeMott RK. Erb's palsy causation: a historical perspective. Birth 2002;29(1):52–4.
17. Sandmire HF, Demott RK. Controversies surrounding the causes of brachial plexus injury. Int J Gynaecol Obstet 2009;104(1):9–13.
18. Walsh JM, Kandamany N, Ni Shuibhne N, et al. Neonatal brachial plexus injury: comparison of incidence and antecedents between 2 decades. Am J Obstet Gynecol 2011;204(4):324.e1–6.
19. Sandmire HF, DeMott RK. Erb's palsy without shoulder dystocia. Int J Gynaecol Obstet 2002;78(3):253–6.
20. Allen RH. On the mechanical aspects of shoulder dystocia and birth injury. Clin Obstet Gynecol 2007;50(3):607–23.
21. Doumouchtsis SK, Arulkumaran S. Are all brachial plexus injuries caused by shoulder dystocia? Obstet Gynecol Surv 2009;64(9):615–23.
22. Leung TY, Stuart O, Sahota DS, et al. Head-to-body delivery interval and risk of fetal acidosis and hypoxic ischaemic encephalopathy in shoulder dystocia: a retrospective review. BJOG 2011;118(4):474–9.
23. Crowther CA, Hiller JE, Moss JR, et al. Effect of treatment of gestational diabetes mellitus on pregnancy outcomes. N Engl J Med 2005;352(24):2477–86.
24. Athukorala C, Crowther CA, Willson K, et al. Women with gestational diabetes mellitus in the ACHOIS trial: risk factors for shoulder dystocia. Aust N Z J Obstet Gynecol 2007;47:37–41.
25. Romoff A. Shoulder dystocia: lessons from the past and emerging concepts. Clin Obstet Gynecol 2000;43(2):226–35.
26. Beall MH, Spong CY, Ross MG. A randomized controlled trial of prophylactic maneuvers to reduce head-to-body delivery time in patients at risk for shoulder dystocia. Obstet Gynecol 2003;102(1):31–5.
27. Athukorala C, Middleton P, Crowther CA. Intrapartum interventions for preventing shoulder dystocia. Cochrane Database Syst Rev 2009;4:CD005543.
28. Irion O, Boulvain M. Induction of labour for suspected fetal macrosomia. Cochrane Database Syst Rev 2000;2:CD000938.
29. Rouse DJ, Owen J, Goldenberg RL, et al. The effectiveness and costs of elective cesarean delivery for fetal macrosomia diagnosed by ultrasound. JAMA 1996; 276(18):1480–6.
30. Bingham J, Chauhan SP, Hayes E, et al. Recurrent shoulder dystocia: a review. Obstet Gynecol Surv 2010;65(3):183–8.

31. Usta IM, Heyek S, Yahya F, et al. Shoulder dystocia: what is the risk of recurrence? Acta Obstet Gynecol Scand 2008;87:992–7.
32. Overland EA, Spydslaug A, Nielsen CS, et al. Risk of shoulder dystocia in second delivery: does a history of shoulder dystocia matter? Am J Obstet Gynecol 2009; 200(5):506.e1–6.
33. Gobbo R, Baxley EG. Shoulder dystocia. In: Leeman L, editor. ALSO: advance life support in obstetrics provider course syllabus. Leawood (KS): American Academy of Family Physicians; 2000. p. 5. Chapter 1.
34. Chauhan SP, Gherman R, Hendrix NW, et al. Shoulder dystocia: comparison of the ACOG practice bulletin with another national guideline. Am J Perinatol 2010;27(2):129–36.
35. Hoffman MK, Bailit JL, Branch DW, et al. A comparison of obstetric maneuvers for the acute management of shoulder dystocia. Obstet Gynecol 2011;117(6):1–7.
36. Leung T, Stuart O, Suen S, et al. Comparison of perinatal outcomes of shoulder dystocia alleviated by different type and sequence of manoeuvres: a retrospective review. BJOG 2011;118(8):985–90.
37. MacKenzie IZ, Mutayyab S, Lean K, et al. Management of shoulder dystocia: trends in incidence and maternal and neonatal morbidity. Obstet Gynecol 2011;110(5):1059–68.
38. Joint Commission on Accreditation of Healthcare Organizations. Preventing infant death and injury during delivery. Sentinel Event Alert 2004;(30):180–1.
39. Grobman WA, Hornbogen A, Burke C, et al. Development and implementation of a team-centered shoulder dystocia protocol. Simul Healthc 2010;5(4):199–203.
40. Maslovitz S, Barkai G, Lessing JB, et al. Recurrent obstetric management mistakes identified by simulation. Obstet Gynecol 2007;109(6):1295–300.
41. Draycott TJ, Crofts JF, Ash JP, et al. Improving neonatal outcome through practical shoulder dystocia training. Obstet Gynecol 2008;112(1):14–20.
42. Crofts JF, Fox R, Ellis D, et al. Observations from 450 shoulder dystocia simulations: lessons for skills training. Obstet Gynecol 2008;112(4):906–12.
43. Goffman D, Heo H, Chazotte C, et al. Using simulation training to improve shoulder dystocia documentation. Obstet Gynecol 2008;112(6):1284–7.
44. Deering SH, Tobler K, Cypher R. Improvement in documentation using an electronic checklist for shoulder dystocia deliveries. Obstet Gynecol 2010;116(1): 63–6.

Cesarean Delivery

Lee T. Dresang, MD[a],*, Lawrence Leeman, MD, MPH[b]

KEYWORDS

• Cesarean section • Obstetrics • Delivery • Complications
• Obstetric labor

HISTORY

The first cesareans were perimorterm cesareans when a woman was dying in child-birth. A Babylonian cuneiform tablet contains an apparent reference to a cesarean birth in 1772 BC.[1] In the eighth century BC law, Lex Regia, stated that a baby should be taken from a mother's womb if she dies before giving birth.[2] The word cesarean is derived from the Latin verb "caedere," which means "to cut"; it is likely a myth that Julius Caesar was born by cesarean.[2] "La section Caesarienne" was described but denounced in a midwife text by Jacques Guillimeau in 1598.[2] In 1879, a British physician in Uganda described the cesarean technique of Banyoro surgeons, which included banana wine for anesthesia and antisepsis, a red hot iron for thermocautery, suture of the abdominal wall and root paste for wound care.[3] Aseptic technique was an important development in the safety of both vaginal and cesarean delivery. In 1882, Max Sanger emphasized the importance of suturing the uterus and introduced a silver suture which did not cause tissue reaction.[1] The Pfannenstiel transverse skin incision was described in the early 1900s and first made popular when described by Monro Kerr in 1926.[4] The Joel-Cohen modification of the Misgav-Ladach technique of using primarily blunt dissection for cesarean was first introduced in 1983 based on the Joel-Cohen technique for hysterectomy.[5,6] This article will describe the evidence behind various details of current cesarean technique.

EPIDEMIOLOGY

Cesarean delivery is the most frequent major surgery performed in the United States with approximately 2 cesareans started every minute.[7] The US cesarean delivery rate for 2009 hit an all-time high of 32.9%.[8–10] The rate increased every year from 1996

The authors have nothing to disclose.
[a] Department of Family Medicine, University of Wisconsin School of Medicine and Public Health, 1100 Delaplaine Ct, Madison, WI 53715, USA
[b] Departments of Family and Community Medicine, and Obstetrics and Gynecology, University of New Mexico School of Medicine, 2400 Tucker Avenue Northeast, Albuquerque, NM 87131, USA
* Corresponding author.
E-mail address: lee.dresang@fammed.wisc.edu

Prim Care Clin Office Pract 39 (2012) 145–165
doi:10.1016/j.pop.2011.11.007
0095-4543/12/$ – see front matter © 2012 Elsevier Inc. All rights reserved.

when the rate was 20.7%[9] to 2009, however the preliminary 2010 cesarean rate demonstrated a slight decrease to 32.8%.[11] The World Health Organization recommended 15% as an ideal cesarean rate and US Healthy People 2020 goals have recommended decreasing the primary cesarean rate to 23.9% and increasing the vaginal birth after cesarean (VBAC) rate to 18.3%, although there is limited evidence to support specific goals.[12–14]

A 2011 study extrapolating the effect of recent cesarean trends to the future found that "if primary and secondary cesarean rates continue to rise as they have in recent years, by 2020 the cesarean delivery rate will be 56.2%, and there will be an additional 6236 placenta previas, 4504 placenta accretas, and 130 maternal deaths annually. The rise in these complications will lag behind the rise in cesareans by approximately 6 years."[15]

The likelihood of a woman in the United States having a cesarean delivery is affected by her age, ethnicity, gestational age at delivery, body mass index (BMI; calculated as the weight in kilograms divided by height in meters squared, ie, kg/m^2), and state in which she gives birth. Cesarean rate increases with age: the 2007 rate for women younger than 20 years is 22.7% compared with 47.7% for women older than 40.[9] Cesarean rates increased for all age groups from 1996 to 2007.[8] The 2007 cesarean rates are highest among African Americans (34%), and lowest among American Indian and Alaskan Natives (28%) and Hispanics (30%).[8] Cesarean rates increased for all racial and ethnic groups from 1996 to 2007.[8] Cesarean rates are consistently higher for early preterm deliveries (<34 weeks) and late preterm deliveries (34–36 weeks) than for term deliveries. Cesarean rates increased for all gestational ages from 1996 to 2007.[8] BMI is strongly associated with cesarean rate in nulliparous women, with an 11.1% rate in women with a BMI less than 25 compared with 33% when BMI was between 35 and 39.9.[16] Each increase of 1 kg/m^2 in BMI increased the risk for cesarean in nulliparous women by 5%.[16] Cesarean rates in the United States vary widely between different regions and states, as illustrated by New Jersey's rate of 38.3%, which is 42% greater than Utah's 22.2% rate in 2007. The regional variations suggest differences in maternity care provider practices and thresholds for operative intervention as well as variations in the paitent populations.[9]

There are potential adverse consequences to having delays in initiating necessary operative delivery, this being particularly an issue in rural areas.[17–20] Rural hospitals often rely on family physicians for maternity care and operative delivery services.[21] In Colorado, 92% of counties have family physicians and only 36% have obstetricians.[22] In 77% of rural Washington hospitals, family physicians performed the majority of cesareans and in the other 23%, family physicians performed 28% of cesareans.[23] The American Academy of Family Physicians has a position paper on Cesarean Delivery in Family Medicine that addresses issues of training and credentialing.[24] The development of fellowships in Family Medicine Obstetrics over the past 20 years has expanded opportunities for advanced training in operative and high-risk obstetrics.[25] Since 2009, the American Board of Physician Specialties has offered certification in Family Medicine Obstetrics for physicians trained in operative obstetrics by fellowship or practice track.[26]

INDICATIONS
Overall

In 1994, indications for cesareans in the United States were labor dystocia (40.3%), elective repeat (21.2%), breech (13.4%), fetal distress (9.8%), and other (15.4%) (**Table 1**).[27]

Table 1	
Indications for cesarean delivery	
Indication	**Percentage**
Labor dystocia	40.3
Elective repeat	21.2
Breech	13.4
Fetal distress	9.8
Other:	15.4
Herpes	
Human immunodeficiency virus with viral load greater than 1000 counts/mL	
Maternal request	
Placenta previa	
Previous cesarean with vertical uterine scar	
Previous uterine surgery	
Gestational diabetes with estimated fetal weight of 4500 g or more	
Worsening severe preeclampsia distant from delivery	
Perimortem cesarean	

A study of more than 200,000 deliveries at 19 hospitals in the United States from 2002 to 2008 revealed that 47.1% of intrapartum cesarean deliveries were for labor dystocia, 27.1% for nonreassuring fetal heart tones, and 7.5% for malpresentation.[28] Forty-five percent of cesareans that occurred before labor were for a prior uterine scar and 17.1% were for malpresentation.[28]

Labor Dystocia

Labor dystocia includes cesareans for failure to progress (in active labor) and arrest of descent (in the second stage of labor). A study of 542 women found that cesarean delivery for failure to progress can be decreased without adverse maternal or perinatal outcomes if women are given at least four hours with adequate contractions (>200 Montevideo Units) in active phase labor before proceeding to cesarean delivery instead of the traditional 2 hours.[29] In an observational study of women who remain in latent labor after 12 hours of induction with oxytocin and rupture of membranes, 40% still had a vaginal delivery.[30] A 2010 analysis of first-stage labor demonstrated a wider variation in labor progress compared with previous observations, suggesting that a proportion of the cesareans for failure to progress at 5 cm or less may be avoidable.[31] The need for cesarean delivery for second stage arrest of descent can be decreased without adverse maternal or perinatal outcomes if women are allowed to continue pushing beyond the traditional definition of prolonged second stage as long as there is progress and maternal vital signs and fetal heart tones are reassuring.[32] The Zuni-Ramah maternity service achieved a cesarean delivery rate of 7.3% in a higher-risk population with perinatal outcomes similar to national statistics; 46% of the lower cesarean rate was attributed to lower cesarean rates for labor dystocia.[33]

Repeat Elective Cesarean

While cesarean rates have increased from 1996 to 2007, vaginal births after cesarean (VBAC) rates have decreased. The VBAC rate reached a high of 28.3% in 1996[34] compared with 8.5% in 2006.[35] Many attribute the decrease in support for VBAC to a 1999 American College of Obstetricians and Gynecologists (ACOG) statement that "VBAC should be attempted in institutions equipped to respond to emergencies with physicians immediately available to respond to provide emergency care."[36] A 2003-2005 study of 312 hospitals in 4 states found that 30.6% of hospitals that offered trial of labor after cesarean (TOLAC) in 1999 no longer offered this option.[37] A 2008 ACOG and American Society of Anesthesiologists statement reinforced the 1999 ACOG recommendation calling for "immediate availability of appropriate facilities and personnel, including obstetric anesthesia, nursing personnel, and a physician capable of monitoring labor and performing cesarean delivery, including an emergency cesarean delivery in cases of vaginal birth after cesarean delivery."[38]

A 2010 National Institutes of Health (NIH) VBAC consensus conference called for increased support for TOLAC. The conference highlighted that high-grade evidence suggests that maternal mortality risk is decreased by a TOLAC in comparison with a repeat cesarean (3.8/100,000 vs 13.4/100,000).[38] The committee recommended: "Given the level of evidence for the requirement for 'immediately available' surgical and anesthesia personnel in current guidelines, we recommend that the ACOG and the American Society of Anesthesiologists reassess this requirement relative to other obstetric complications of comparable risk, risk stratification, and in light of limited physician and nursing resources."[38]

In 2011, the ACOG updated its Practice Bulletin on VBAC. Though it did not reverse its call for "immediately available" surgical and anesthesia personnel, it did support consideration of TOLAC in settings that did not meet this standard: "When resources for immediate cesarean are not available, the College recommends that health care providers and patients considering TOLAC discuss the hospital's resources and availability of obstetric, pediatric, anesthetic and operating room staffs ... After counseling, the ultimate decision to undergo TOLAC or a repeat cesarean delivery should be made by the patient in consultation with her health care provider."[35]

The 2011 ACOG Practice Bulletin also expanded eligibility criteria for TOLAC to include women with 2 prior cesarean deliveries or an undocumented uterine scar. Whereas the 2004 ACOG Practice Bulletin on VBAC recommended "for women with 2 prior cesarean deliveries, only those with a prior vaginal delivery should be considered candidates for a spontaneous trial of labor,"[39] the 2010 update recommends "women with 2 previous low transverse cesarean deliveries may be considered candidates for TOLAC."[35] In a study of 975 women with multiple prior cesareans and 16,915 women with a single prior cesarean undergoing TOLAC, multiple prior cesareans were not associated with an increased risk of uterine rupture,[40] although there was an increased risk of hysterectomy (0.6 vs 0.2%, $P = .023$) and transfusion (3.2 vs 1.6%, $P<.001$).[40]

The 2004 ACOG Practice Bulletin on VBAC stated that with undocumented uterine scar "many authorities question the safety of offering VBAC under these circumstances; others suggest that the uterine scar type usually can be inferred based on the indication for the prior cesarean delivery."[39] The 2010 ACOG Practice Bulletin update states "TOLAC is not contraindicated for women with previous cesarean delivery with an unknown uterine scar type unless there is high clinical suspicion of previous classical uterine incision."[35] The risk of uterine rupture in labor is 0.2% to 1.5% after a cesarean with a low transverse uterine incision and 4% to 9% with a classical vertical uterine incision.[41] A review of TOLAC for 300 women with an undocumented uterine incision and 88 with a documented low transverse uterine incision did not find a difference in vaginal delivery rate, maternal morbidity, or neonatal morbidity.[42] In a review of TOLAC for 97 women with an undocumented uterine incision and 204 with a documented low transverse uterine incision, there was no statistically significant difference in estimated blood loss (EBL) greater than 1000 mL, maternal fever, uterine scar separation, perinatal mortality associated with a TOLAC, and 5-minute Apgar score of less than 7.[43]

Malpresentation/Breech

Approximately 3% to 4% of pregnancies at term are breech.[44] In 2002, 86.9% of women with breech presentation in labor had a cesarean.[45] Cesarean rates for breech can be decreased by diagnosis prior to labor and offering the option of external cephalic version (ECV). Although uncommon in the United States, recent studies[46,47] suggest that vaginal breech delivery is a reasonable option for selected women using appropriate hospital-based guidelines. As many as 92.8% of births with nonvertex presentation occur by cesarean delivery and most of these women will have elective repeat cesarean births in future pregnancies, indicating that failure to diagnose and/or successfully perform ECV for breech presentation may be responsible for a substantial overall proportion of cesarean deliveries.[28]

ECV has a low complication rate, with emergency cesarean being needed after approximately 1 in 200 procedures.[48] A 2011 Cochrane review found that attempted ECV was not associated with Apgar score ratings of less than 7 at 1 minute (2 trials, 108 women; relative risk [RR] 0.95, 95% confidence interval [CI] 0.47–1.89) or 5 minutes (4 trials, 368 women; RR 0.76, 95% CI 0.32–1.77), low umbilical artery pH levels (1 trial, 52 women; RR 0.65, 95% CI 0.17–2.44), neonatal admission (1 trial, 52 women; RR 0.36, 95% CI 0.04–3.24), perinatal death (6 trials, 1053 women; RR 0.34, 95% CI 0.05–2.12), or time from enrollment to delivery (2 trials, 256 women; weighted mean difference [WMD] −0.25 days, 95% CI −2.81 to 2.31).[49] ECV is not contraindicated for women with a prior cesarean with a low transverse uterine incision.[35]

Success rates vary widely from 35–85% with most studies showing increased success rates with transverse and oblique lie and increasing parity; studies are conflicting regarding the effect of amniotic fluid, maternal weight and placental position.[44] Attempted ECV results in a lower risk of noncephalic birth (7 trials, 1245 women; RR 0.46, 95% CI 0.31–0.66) and caesarean section (7 trials, 1245 women; RR 0.63, 95% CI 0.44–0.90).[49]

Tocolysis increases the likelihood of successful version. A 2010 Cochrane review showed that a β-mimetic before attempted ECV resulted in fewer unsuccessful versions (6 trials, 617 women; RR 0.74, 95% CI 0.64–0.87) and fewer cesareans (3 trials, 444 women; RR 0.85, 95% CI 0.72–0.99).[50] One study found a decreased ECV failure rate when acoustic stimulation was used when the fetal spine was midline (1 trial, 26 women; RR 0.17, 95% CI 0.05–0.60).[50] A 2011 meta-analysis of 6 RCTs found that regional anesthesia was connected with a higher ECV success rate than intravenous or no anesthesia (59.7% vs 37.6%; pooled RR 1.58; 95% CI 1.29–1.93).[51] There was no significant difference in cesarean or other adverse outcomes.[51]

Vaginal breech delivery is another means of decreasing cesarean rates for malpresentation. Planned vaginal breech delivery in the United States became uncommon after the 2000 Term Breech Trial study of short term outcomes found higher neonatal morbidity and mortality after vaginal breech delivery compared with cesarean.[52] The same authors two year follow-up study found that vaginal breech delivery was no longer associated with adverse perinatal outcomes.[46,47] An ACOG Committee Opinion supports vaginal birth delivery for appropriate candidates with hospital specific guidelines for patient selection and labor management but recognizes that few people have the skills to attend vaginal breech delivery now that cesarean has been the standard for the last decade.[53] In Canada the Society of Obstetricians and Gynecologists is now encouraging women to consider the option of vaginal breech delivery under specific guidelines, and encourages the retraining of physicians to offer this option.[54] The PRMODA study of 5579 cesarean and 2526 attempted vaginal deliveries for breech in Belgium and France found that 71% of attempted vaginal breech deliveries were successful with no worsening of neonatal outcomes.[55]

The maneuvers for delivering breech at cesarean are similar to those for vaginal breech delivery. First, the feet or the buttocks and then the feet are delivered with the baby rotated back-up. When the scapula is visible, the baby is rotated away from each arm and the arm swept in front of the baby and delivered; the oropharynx can be bulb suctioned when visible, and finally the head is delivered with flexion using the modified Mauriceau-Smellie-Veit maneuver whereby the operator's second and third fingers are placed on maxillary prominence and the other hand applies pressure to the occiput.

Human Immunodeficiency Virus with Viral Load of More Than 1000 Copies/mL

A 2000 ACOG Committee Opinion recommends that elective cesarean be offered to women with a viral load of greater than 1000 copies/mL.[56] A 2009 Cochrane review of one RCT and 5 observational studies concluded that while cesarean is recommended for women with higher viral loads, it is not clear that there is a benefit with cesarean delivery for women receiving antiretroviral therapy in pregnancy and with low viral loads and cesarean delivery is not routinely recommended for this group.[57,58]

Diabetes in Pregnancy with Estimated Fetal Weight 4500 g or Greater

Cesarean delivery may be considered in the setting of suspected macrosomia and a pregnancy complicated by diabetes to prevent shoulder dystocia and its consequences. With the recognition that ultrasound estimation of fetal weight is imprecise, ACOG recommends that cesarean only be considered for women with diabetes in pregnancy when the estimated fetal weight is greater than 4500 g.[59] A study of 2604 women with diabetes in pregnancy were followed after instituting a protocol whereby women with an ultrasound estimated fetal weight of 4250 g or more were delivered by cesarean and those with a lower estimated fetal weight were given a trial of labor. Using this protocol, the rate of shoulder dystocia decreased from 2.4% to 1.1% (odds ratio [OR] 2.2).[60] However, the cesarean rate increased from 21.7% to 25.1% (P<.04).[60] Ultrasonography correctly identified the presence or absence of macrosomia in 87% of women.[60] Shoulder dystocia was 7.4% for women who delivered vaginally.[60] In women without diabetes in pregnancy, offering elective cesarean for macrosomia is only recommended when the ultrasound EFW is greater than 5000 g.[59]

Maternal Request for Cesarean

Maternal-request cesarean may account for 4% to 18% of cesareans in the United States, and the incidence appears to be increasing although reliable statistics are not available.[61] The reasons women request primary elective cesarean delivery include concerns about the effect of vaginal birth on future pelvic floor function, a fear of labor, and unfounded concerns for the risk to the fetus of vaginal delivery. Cesarean delivery will not prevent anal and urinary incontinence. A 2010 Cochrane review of 21 nonrandomized trials involving 6028 cesarean deliveries and 25,170 vaginal deliveries did not find enough evidence to support cesarean delivery for prevention of anal incontinence.[62] Cesarean delivery does initially decrease the incidence of urinary incontinence; however, by age 50 years the predominant risk factor is age and there is no evidence of an effect from mode of delivery.[63] Fear of childbirth was a common reason for maternal-request cesarean in several European studies, and when women were offered and received counseling, 86% chose vaginal delivery.[64,65]

A 2006 NIH consensus conference concluded that not enough information is available on the risks and benefits of maternal-request cesarean.[61] The panel recommended: "Until quality evidence becomes available, any decision to perform a cesarean delivery on maternal request should be carefully individualized and consistent with ethical principles."[61] Because of increasing morbidity including invasive placenta with the increasing number of deliveries, maternal-request cesarean should be discouraged for women wishing to have several children.[61]

INFORMED CONSENT

Before cesarean, as before any procedure, risks should be discussed and questions answered. Counseling should be well documented and written consent obtained. Risks of cesarean include bleeding, infection, anesthesia reaction, organ damage (bowel or bladder injury), maternal death, fetal death, and fetal morbidity. Compared with vaginal birth, cesarean birth has an increased risk of overall severe morbidity (OR 3.1; 95% CI 3.0–3.3), hemorrhage requiring hysterectomy (OR 2.1; 95% CI 1.2–3.8), hysterectomy (OR 3.2; 95% CI 2.2–4.8), anesthetic complication (OR 2.3; 95% CI 2.0–2.6), cardiac arrest (OR 5.1; 95% CI 4.1–6.3), venous thromboembolism (OR 2.2; 95% CI 1.5–3.2), major puerperal infection (OR 3.0; 95% CI 2.7–3.4), and obstetric wound hematoma (OR 5.1; 95% CI 4.6–5.5).[66]

Cesarean counseling should explain that cesarean complication risk increases when a woman has had a greater number of prior cesarean deliveries. Risk for invasive placenta, transfusion, hysterectomy, bowel or bladder injury, and intensive care unit (ICU) admission increases with the increasing number of cesareans.[67–69] In a study of 30,132 women with prior cesarean, hysterectomy was required in 40 (0.65%) first, 67 (0.42%) second, 57 (0.90%) third, 35 (2.41%) fourth, 9 (3.49%) fifth, and 8 (8.99%) sixth or more cesarean deliveries.[68]

Fig. 1 is a model cesarean consent form.

TIMING

Once viability is reached, cesarean may be indicated regardless of fetal maturity for certain indications such as category 3 fetal heart rate monitoring unresponsive to conservative measures or complications of severe pre-eclampsia such as pulmonary edema remote from vaginal delivery. When timing is elective as occurs with repeat cesarean delivery or malpresentation, delivery should not take place until 39 weeks estimated gestational age, with dating determined by (1) ultrasonography before 20 weeks, (2) fetal heart tones documented by Doppler for 30 weeks, or (3) 36 weeks since a positive pregnancy test.[70] Fetal lung maturity can be confirmed by amniocentesis prior to elective cesarean when the aforementioned criteria are not met. In a study of 24,077 elective repeat cesareans in the United States between 1999 and 2002, 6.3% were performed at 37 weeks and 29.5% at 38 weeks.[71] The rates of adverse respiratory outcomes, mechanical ventilation, newborn sepsis, hypoglycemia, admission to the neonatal ICU, and hospitalization for 5 days or more were increased by a factor of 1.8 to 4.2 for births at 37 weeks and 1.3 to 2.1 for births at 38 weeks.[71] A study of 2687 infants delivered by term elective cesarean found the risk of respiratory morbidity (compared with vaginal delivery) to increase with decreasing gestational age (37 weeks: OR 3.9, 95% CI 2.4–6.5; 38 weeks: OR 3.0, 95% CI 2.1–4.3; 39 weeks: OR 1.9, 95% CI 1.2–3.0).[72] Even comparing the last 3 days before 39 weeks with 39 weeks, there is a significant increased risk of a composite of neonatal death and any of

Patient:

Medical record number: **Birth date:**

Indication:

Surgeon:

Risks reviewed including:

____   Bleeding

____   Infection

____   Anesthesia reaction

____   Organ damage (bladder or intestinal injury)

____   Maternal mortality

____   Poor fetal outcome (laceration, morbidity, mortality)

____   Increasing risk of placenta acreta, organ damage, hysterectomy, transfusion with increasing

number of cesareans

Signature: _____   **Date:** _____

Fig. 1. Consent form for cesarean delivery.

several adverse events, including respiratory complications, treated hypoglycemia, newborn sepsis, and admission to the neonatal ICU (RR 1.21, 95% CI 1.04–1.40; $P = .01$).[71]

Cesarean as soon as lung maturity can be confirmed by amniocentesis may be considered for women with a previous cesarean with a vertical uterine incision,[73] other surgery involving the more muscular portion of the uterus, or placenta previa. In the setting of a prior vertical uterine incision or placenta previa, it is appropriate to schedule a cesarean before 39 weeks to prevent the risks of uterine rupture or hemorrhage when labor occurs; however, the specific timing remains controversial, with recommendations varying between 36 and 38 weeks.[74,75]

Cesarean for women with human immunodeficiency virus and a viral load of greater than 1000 copies/mL is recommended at 38 weeks.[56] Amniocentesis is not recommended, as it may increase the risk of mother-to-child transmission. Scheduled delivery at 38 weeks rather than 39 weeks is recommended to decrease the probability of rupture of membranes before cesarean.[56]

TECHNIQUE
Skin Incision

Transverse skin incision results in less postoperative pain and a better cosmetic result than a vertical skin incision.[7] A 2009 Cochrane review of 2 studies involving 411 women comparing Pfannenstiel (2 fingerbreadths above the pubic symphysis) and Joel-Cohen (3 cm below the line between the anterior-superior iliac spines) skin incision found that the Joel-Cohen incision was preferable because it reduced postoperative morbidity (RR 0.35; 95% CI 0.14–0.87).[76] A 2010 Cochrane review comparing Pfannenstiel with Joel-Cohen techniques found that the latter resulted in less blood loss

(5 trials, 481 women; WMD −64.45 mL, 95% CI −91.34 to −37.56 mL); shorter operating time (5 trials, 581 women; WMD −18.65 minutes, 95% CI −24.84 to −12.45 minutes); postoperatively, reduced time to oral intake (5 trials, 481 women; WMD −3.92 hours, 95% CI −7.13 to −0.71 hours); less fever (8 trials, 1412 women; RR 0.47, 95% CI 0.28–0.81); shorter duration of postoperative pain (2 comparisons from 1 trial, 172 women; WMD −14.18 hours, 95% CI −18.31 to −10.04 hours); fewer analgesic injections (2 trials, 151 women; WMD −0.92, 95% CI −1.20 to −0.63); and shorter time from skin incision to birth of the baby (5 trials, 575 women; WMD −3.84 minutes, 95% CI −5.41 to −2.27 minutes).[77] Use of chlorhexidine solution for skin washing[78] and using clippers rather than a razor when removal of hair is needed at the surgical site decreases the incidence of postcesarean surgical site infections.[79]

Dissection of Rectus Muscle from Fascia

There have not been any well-designed trials to compare blunt with sharp dissection of the rectus muscle from the fascia. Some have questioned whether this step is even necessary.[7]

Uterine Incision

Low transverse uterine incision is recommended over vertical incision because of a lower rate of rupture in subsequent pregnancies, less blood loss, and a lower risk of bladder laceration. A 2008 Cochrane review of 2 RCTs involving 1241 women looked at blunt versus sharp dissection of the uterine incision. Blunt dissection resulted in less blood loss (1 study, 945 women; mean difference −43.00, 95% CI −66.12 to −19.88).[80] There was no statistically significant difference in blood transfusion rates (1 study, 945 women; RR 0.22, 95% CI 0.05–1.01).[80]

Antibiotic Prophylaxis

Antibiotic prophylaxis with ampicillin or a first-generation cephalosporin is recommended for cesarean delivery. A 2010 Cochrane review comparing antibiotic prophylaxis with no prophylaxis found that antibiotic prophylaxis resulted in lower febrile morbidity (50 studies, 8141 women; average RR 0.45, 95% CI 0.39–0.51), wound infection (77 studies, 11,961 women; average RR 0.39, 95% CI 0.32–0.48), endometritis (79 studies, 12,142 women; RR 0.38, 95% CI 0.34–0.42), and serious maternal infectious complications (31 studies, 5047 women; RR 0.31, 95% CI 0.19–0.48).[81] A 2010 Cochrane review of 51 RCTs found no difference between ampicillin and first-generation cephalosporins for preventing endometritis.[82] A separate 2010 Cochrane review of 29 trials including 6367 women reached the same conclusion.[83] The first Cochrane review also noted no benefit from using multidrug regimens.[82] A 2010 ACOG Committee Opinion recommends preoperative antibiotics (within 60 minutes of skin incision) over antibiotics at cord clamping, based on evidence emanating from studies including 2 RCTs.[84–86]

Delivery of Placenta

Delivery of the placenta by cord traction and uterine fundal massage rather than entering the uterus for manual placental extraction is recommended. A 2008 Cochrane review of 15 studies involving 4694 women comparing manual extraction with cord traction plus massage found that manual extraction resulted in: more endometritis (4134 women, 13 trials; RR 1.64, 95% CI 1.42–1.90); more blood loss above 1000 mL (872 women, 2 trials; RR 1.81, 95% CI 1.44–2.28); lower hematocrit after delivery (384 women, 2 trials; WMD −1.55%, 95% CI −3.09% to −0.01%); greater hematocrit decrease after delivery (1777 women, 5 trials; WMD 0.39%, 95% CI 0.00% to 0.78%);

and longer duration of hospital stay (546 women, 3 trials; WMD 0.39 days, 95% CI 0.17–0.61 days).[87]

Exteriorization

A 2011 Cochrane review of 6 studies including 1221 women did not find strong evidence for or against exteriorization of the uterus for repair.[88] The only statistically significant findings were that exteriorization of the uterus resulted in lower risk of febrile morbidity (RR 0.41, 95% CI 0.17–0.97), but a longer hospital stay (WMD 0.24 days, 95% CI 0.08–0.39 days).[88]

Uterine Closure

Double-layer closure is preferred over single-layer closure because of a lower risk of uterine rupture. An observational cohort study of 2142 women found a fourfold risk of uterine rupture with labor after a single-layer closure (OR 3.95, 95% CI 1.35–11.49).[80,89] In a study of 948 women (35 with single-layer closure and 913 with double-layer closure), the uterine rupture rate was higher with single-layer closure (8.6% vs 1.3%; $P = .015$).[90]

Bladder Flap Closure

An RCT of 102 women suggests that nonclosure of the bladder flap results in decreased median skin incision to delivery interval (5 vs 7 minutes, $P<.001$), median total operating time (35 vs 40 minutes, $P<.004$), median blood loss (hemoglobin 0.5 vs 1 g/dL, $P<.009$), median need for analgesics (diclofenac 75.0 vs 150.0 mg, $P<.001$), and percentage of patients receiving analgesics 2 or more days after cesarean (26.4% vs 55.1%, $P<.006$). The study was not powered to look at bladder injuries or long term effects.[91]

Peritoneal Closure

A 2003 Cochrane review of 14 RCTs involving 2908 women found that nonclosure of the peritoneum was associated with shorter operating time (6.05 minutes, 95% CI −6.74 to −5.37) and reduced dose of postoperative analgesic (WMD −0.20, 95% CI −0.33 to −0.08).[92] There was also a statistically significant decrease in postoperative fever and postoperative stay in the hospital.[92] A study of repeat cesareans in women prospectively randomized to closure versus, nonclosure of the parietal peritoneum failed to demonstrate a significant difference in the presence of adhesions or time to delivery.[93]

Intra-Abdominal Irrigation

An RCT of 97 women looking at 500 to 1000 mL of intra-abdominal normal saline irrigation versus no irrigation found no statistically significant differences in EBL, operating time, incidence of intrapartum complications, hospital stay, return of gastrointestinal function, incidence of infectious complications, or neonatal outcomes.[94]

Closure of Fascia

Closure of the fascia has not been well studied. Most experts support nonlocking continuous closure with delayed absorbable suture (0 Vicryl).[7]

Subcutaneous Tissue Closure

A 2008 Cochrane review of 7 trials involving 2056 women found that closure of the subcutaneous tissue resulted in a lower risk of hematoma or seroma (RR 0.52, 95% CI 0.33–0.82) and a lower risk of wound complication (hematoma, seroma, wound infection, or wound separation) (RR 0.68, 95% CI 0.52–0.88).[95] Two studies found that closing the subcutaneous tissue when less than 2 cm deep did not decrease the risk of wound complication (RR 1.01, 95% CI, 0.46–2.20); therefore, subcutaneous tissue closure is only recommended when the tissue thickness is 2 cm or more in depth.[7]

Skin Closure

A 2010 Cochrane review of one RCT involving 25 cesareans with sutures in comparison with 25 with staples found that the sutures took longer to place (mean, 605 vs 47 seconds; P<.001), but women reported less pain at time of discharge (10-point pain scale 5.1 vs 6.6; P<.003) and at a postoperative visit (pain scale 0.5 vs 2.0; P<.002), and cosmetic results were preferred both by patients (rated excellent 60% vs 36%, good 40% vs 48%, fair 0% vs 4%; P = .04) and physicians (rated excellent 60% vs 24%, good 32% vs 48%, fair 8% vs 24%, poor 0% vs 4%; P = .01).[96,97] A meta-analysis demonstrated a twofold increased risk of wound infection or separation with staples, with a number needed to harm of 16.[98]

TREATMENT OF COMPLICATIONS

Cesarean complications include postpartum hemorrhage, infection, venous thromboembolism (VTE), and bladder and bowel laceration. Management of each is discussed in this section.

Postpartum Hemorrhage

Average EBL at vaginal delivery is 500 mL and at cesarean delivery 1000 mL.[99] A study comparing visual with calculated blood loss for primary and repeat cesareans with a calculated blood loss of more than 1000 mL and 1500 mL found a statistically significant underestimation of blood loss in each case.[99] Of 149 primary cesareans, only 8% were estimated to have an EBL greater than 1000 mL whereas 46% had a calculated EBL greater than 1000 mL (P = .0002).[99] Of 149 primary cesareans, only 1% were estimated to have an EBL greater than 1500 mL whereas 18% had a calculated EBL greater than 1500 mL (P<.0001).[99] Of 82 repeat cesareans, only 5% were estimated to have an EBL of more than 1000 mL whereas 27% had a calculated EBL of more than 1000 mL (P = .0001).[99] Of 82 repeat cesareans, none were estimated to have an EBL greater than 1500 mL whereas 10% had a calculated EBL greater than 1500 mL.[99] Accurate estimation of blood loss is important at cesarean because pregnant women do not develop tachycardia or hypotension as early as nonpregnant patients.

Postpartum hemorrhage at cesarean is most often attributable to atony but may also be due to other causes including uterine artery laceration, retained placental tissue, invasive placenta, and coagulopathy (most commonly disseminated intravascular coagulopathy). Atony can be controlled with uterine massage, medicines, uterine packing, and the B-Lynch suture. Retained placental tissue can be removed, sweeping inside the uterus with gauze over 2 fingers. Hysterectomy is usually needed for invasive placenta. Coagulopathy can be treated by addressing the underlying cause and replacing appropriate blood components. When bleeding is the result of uterine artery laceration or another cause, uterine artery ligation can reduce uterine blood flow and often avoids the need for hysterectomy.[100]

Packing

Bleeding can sometimes be controlled with packing or a balloon device, thus avoiding the need for hysterectomy. The only balloon made specifically for the uterus is the Bakri balloon, which has a double lumen shaft that can hold up to 800 mL, and has holes so that blood can drain and ongoing hemorrhage can be detected even after inflation. In one study, the Bakri balloon stopped bleeding in 4 of 7 women (57%) who had postpartum hemorrhage after cesarean. The other 3 cases involved either placenta previa (2) or placenta accreta (1).[101] Other balloon devices that can be used in a similar manner include the Sengstaken-Blakemore tube, the Rusch balloon, the condom catheter, and the Foley catheter.[102]

Uterine artery ligation

Uterine artery ligation is a technique that can control severe hemorrhage at cesarean while preserving the uterus. The technique is effective because the uterine arteries are responsible for 90% of uterine blood flow.[100] To ligate a uterine artery, a no. 1 chromic needle is passed through the myometrium anteriorly to posteriorly 2 to 3 cm medial to the uterine artery, then brought forward through an avascular area of the broad ligament lateral to the uterine artery.[100]

B-Lynch suture

The B-Lynch suture is another method for preserving the uterus when faced with severe hemorrhage at cesarean from atony refractory to medicines and massage.[103] The suture (2-0 chromic) is passed from 3 cm below the right lower edge of the uterine incision and 3 cm from the right lateral border of the uterus vertically, to come out 3 cm above the right upper edge of the uterine incision. The suture is passed over the fundus and a stitch is placed transversely on the back of the uterus, entering the back of the uterus at the level where the suture exited anteriorly. The entry and exit points on the back of the uterus should be 3 cm from the uterine borders. After exiting the left back of the uterus, the suture is passed over the fundus to the front of the uterus where a stitch is passed from 3 cm above the left upper edge of the uterine incision to 3 cm below the left lower edge of the uterine incision. The two ends of suture are tied while an assistant compresses the fundus. The uterine incision is now closed.[103]

Hemostatic square suturing

Another surgical technique to control bleeding at cesarean is hemostatic square suturing. A no. 7 or 8 needle is used to pass no. 1 chromic catgut in a square: (1) from the anterior uterus through the entire uterus, (2) from the back of the uterus through the anterior uterus 2 to 3 cm medial to the original pass, (3) anterior to posterior 2 to 3 cm inferior to the second suture point, and (4) posterior through anterior uterus 2 to 3 cm lateral to point 3 and inferior to point 1. The ends are tied, forming the square. In a case series, 23 of 23 women who had postpartum hemorrhage not responding to conservative measures had decreased bleeding and did not need hysterectomy following a hemostatic square suture.[104] However, cases have been reported of post-hemostatic square suture uterine cavity synechiae[105] and pyometria.[106]

Infection

Postpartum endometritis and wound infections are much more common in cesarean than in vaginal delivery. In a multicenter Latin American study, both elective (OR 4.24, 95% CI 2.78–6.46) and intrapartum (OR 5.53, 95% CI 3.77–8.10) cesarean had a substantially increased risk of postpartum infection as measured by the surrogate outcome of use of postpartum antibiotics.[107] A Cochrane review found the traditional regimen of intravenous clindamycin (900 mg IV every 8 hours) and gentamicin to be more effective than the comparison regimens, and daily dosing of gentamicin (5 mg/kg/day) superior to thrice-daily dosing.[108] There was no benefit to continuing oral antibiotics after the completion of the intravenous regimen following clinical resolution.[108] Failure of presumptive postpartum endometritis to resolve with 48 to 72 hours of intravenous antibiotics requires consideration of the possibility of an intra-abdominal abscess or septic pelvic thrombophlebitis.

Postcesarean surgical site infections are common, affecting 2% to 10% of women after cesarean and with risk factors including obesity, chorioamnionitis, and failure to administer perioperative prophylaxis prior to skin incision.[109,110] Mild cellulitic infections may respond to oral or intravenous antibiotics; however, it is common for wound separation to occur with infection, or for opening of the incision to be required to drain out purulent tissue or to debride necrotic areas. When the wound is opened the incision should be gently probed to ensure fascial integrity.

Venous Thromboembolism

A 2010 decision analysis concluded that low-molecular-weight heparin (LMWH) is the best postcesarean prophylaxis, although the benefit is minimal in women without additional risk factors.[111] Given the minimal benefit of LMWH in low-risk women, a recommended approach is to use early ambulation and sequential compression devices during cesarean delivery and the immediate postoperative period in all women, and to reserve LMWH for women with multiple risk factors.[112,113]

The Royal College of Obstetricians and Gynecologists and the American College of Chest Physicians recommend adjusting thromboprophylaxis based on level of risk. Low-risk women (women with a cesarean delivery for normal pregnancy with no other risk factors) should be encouraged to ambulate early. Moderate-risk women (age >35 years, BMI >30, parity >3, gross varicose veins, current infection, preeclampsia, immobility for >4 days before surgery, major current illness, emergency cesarean during labor) should receive LMWH or compression stockings. High-risk women (presence of more than 2 risk factors from moderate risk list, cesarean hysterectomy, previous deep vein thrombosis, or known thrombophilia) should receive LMWH and compression stockings.[112]

With one or more of the risk factors of an emergency procedure, a BMI greater than 25, or tobacco smoking, reductions in VTE greatly outnumbered the increase in major hemorrhages, with a modest benefit on mortality.[111] In women with a history of thromboembolism or thrombophilia, LMWH may be recommended for 6 weeks postpartum or for a longer period.[114] For women on LMWH in pregnancy needing a scheduled cesarean, the LMWH should be stopped 24 hours before the procedure and a prophylactic dose given no sooner than 3 hours after the operation, with therapeutic LMWH resumed that evening.[115]

Diagnosis and Treatment of Bladder Laceration

Bladder injury occurs in 1 to 3 per 1000 cesarean deliveries.[7] It occurs most commonly when trying to develop a bladder flap and when there is scarring from a previous cesarean.[116] Seventy-five percent occur during emergency cesareans.[117] When bladder injury is suspected, 200 mL of 5% methylene blue or sterile milk can be infused into the bladder through a Foley catheter.[116,118] The Foley is then clamped, and the leaking of methylene blue or sterile milk intra-abdominally is diagnostic of bladder laceration.[116] Identified defects can be repaired with two layers of 2-0 or 3-0 chromic suture.[116] A Foley catheter is left in place until hematuria resolves (7–14 days).[116,119] In many centers, urological consultation is available and indicated. When bladder laceration is recognized and repaired intraoperatively, complications are rare.[119]

Diagnosis and Treatment of Bowel Laceration

Bowel laceration occurs in approximately 0.08% of cesarean deliveries.[120] As with bladder laceration, bowel laceration is most likely to occur when there are adhesions from previous surgery and with emergency cesareans.[118] If bowel injury is noticed before delivery of the baby, it can be marked with a stitch and covered with a warm laparotomy pack.[118] Small serosal injuries do not need repair.[118] The repair will depend on whether the injury is to the small or large intestine, the size of the laceration, whether it compromises the blood supply, and whether there are multiple injuries.[118] Compromising the lumen is more of a concern with small intestine repair; the suture line should be perpendicular to the axis of the bowel.[118] Antibiotics are generally not necessary after small intestine repair, but are indicated intraoperatively and postoperatively with large intestine repair.[118] Early clear liquids but no regular diet for 3 to 4 days is recommended.[118] In many centers, general surgery consultation is available and indicated.

PERIMORTEM CESAREAN

A 1986 study indicated that for optimal fetal survival, perimortem cesarean should be performed within 4 minutes of maternal cardiac arrest.[121] A review of 38 perimortem cesareans from 1985 to 2004 supported the 4-minute rule.[122] With perimortem cesarean, time is of the essence: vertical skin and vertical uterine incisions are indicated. In some cases the maternal condition improves after delivery of the fetus.[121]

POSTCESAREAN CARE

Women should be encouraged to ambulate as soon after surgery as their clinical condition and pain control permits, to decrease the risk of venous thromboembolism and pulmonary complications (atelectasis and pneumonia) from immobility. The Foley catheter can be removed as soon as the patient can ambulate. The patient may start on clear liquids in the recovery room if there are no concerns regarding nausea or postoperative bleeding requiring additional surgery. Once clear liquids are tolerated, the diet may be advanced to a regular diet on the day of the surgery. Immediate postoperative analgesia varies in different maternity units, and options include injection of long-acting opioids at the time of regional anesthesia to provide 12 to 18 hours of pain relief, patient-controlled analgesia with parenteral opioids, or intermittent use of parenteral opioids. Most women can transition to oral opioids, acetaminophen, and nonsteroidal anti-inflammatory agents within 24 hours of their cesarean delivery. It is typical for postcesarean patients to be discharged home within 2 to 4 days of their surgery. Timing of the removal of surgical skin staples will vary based on habitus, concerns for tension at the skin site, timing of discharge, and local practices.

After cesarean delivery women were traditionally discharged home with a list of limitations regarding lifting, walking up stairs, bathing, driving, and the resumption of sexual intercourse. These limitations were not evidence based, and frequently unduly restricted the resumption of postoperative activities.[123] Patients may be permitted to lift and walk up stairs on hospital discharge, and both Valsalva with bowel movement and arising from a supine position increase intra-abdominal pressure more than these activities. Once the bandage is removed at 24 to 48 hours, tub bathing can be resumed. There are no data regarding the need to defer vaginal intercourse after cesarean delivery, and the time for initiation of sexual intercourse should be based on the patient's comfort because minimal risk for ascending infection should exist after 2 weeks postpartum.[123] Positions that allow her to control the depth of vaginal penetration and the use of lubricants can facilitate comfort at the time of resumption of vaginal intercourse.

TEAMWORK

Patient outcomes with cesarean delivery depend not only on medical decision making and technical skills of individuals, but also on communication and functioning of systems and teams. The Joint Commission determined that 72% of perinatal sentinel events in the United States have communication errors as a cause.[124] Many tools used to promote communication and patient safety in medicine are derived from successes in the aviation industry.[125] One example is the "two-challenge rule," which empowers all team members to speak up when they feel uncomfortable with a situation. If a person's concern is not addressed the first time, they issue a second challenge and the procedure is halted until the problem is addressed.[126] Time-outs before procedures make sure everyone is on the same page. Call-outs during procedures notify all of significant events. Debriefings after procedures allow teams to identify what went well, what did not go well, and what could be done better in the future. Debriefings often identify systems issues to be addressed. For example, a debriefing may identify that someone needs to be designated in emergencies to address the needs of a significant other. CareTeam OB (TM) is a patient safety curriculum which helps hospitals teach and monitor teamwork for cesareans and other aspects of maternity care.[127]

SUMMARY

Cesarean delivery can be life-saving for a woman and her baby. The cesarean rate in the United States is at an all-time high. The incidence of placenta previa and placenta accreta, hysterectomy, urological injury, blood transfusion, and other operative complications increases in relation to the number of prior cesarean deliveries that the patient has undergone.[68,128] Decreasing the number of cesareans for labor dystocia and malpresentation as well as encouraging TOLAC can decrease cesarean rates without compromising outcomes. Evidence-based medicine can guide indications for cesarean, surgical technique, and effective team function.

REFERENCES

1. Lurie S, Glezerman M. The history of cesarean technique. Am J Obstet Gynecol 2003;189:1803–6.
2. Todman D. A history of caesarean section: from ancient world to the modern era. Aust N Z J Obstet Gynaecol 2007;47:357–61.
3. Wilson C, Felkin R. Uganda and Egyptian Sudan. London: Low; 1882.
4. Kerr J. The technique of cesarean section, with special reference to the lower uterine segment incision. Am J Obstet Gynecol 1926;12:729–34.
5. Joel-Cohen S. Abdominal and vaginal hysterectomy: new techniques based on time and motion studies. London: William Heinemann; 1972.
6. Holmgren G, Sjöholm L, Stark M. The Misgav Ladach method for cesarean section: method description. Acta Obstet Gynecol Scand 1999;78:615–21.
7. Berghella V, Baxter J, Chauhan S. Evidence-based surgery for cesarean delivery. Am J Obstet Gynecol 2005;193:1607–17.
8. Menacker F, Hamilton B. Recent trends in cesarean delivery in the United States. NCHS Data Brief 2010;35:1–8.

9. Martin J, Hamilton B, Sutton P, et al. Births: final data for 2007. Natl Vital Stat Rep 2010;58:1–85.
10. Hamilton B, Martin J, Ventura S. Births: preliminary data for 2009. National vital statistics reports, vol. 59. Hyattsville (MD): National Center for Health Statistics; 2010.
11. Hamilton B, Martin J, Ventura S. Births: Preliminary data for 2010. National vital statistics reports web release, vol 60. Issue 2. Hyattsville (MD): National Center for Health Statistics; 2011.
12. Appropriate technology for birth. Lancet 1985;2:436–7.
13. Greer I. The special case of venous thromboembolism in pregnancy. Haemostasis 1998;28:22–34.
14. Maternal, infant and child health. Healthy People 2020 Summary of Objectives. Available at: http://healthypeople.gov/2020/topicsobjectives2020/pdfs/MaternalChildHealth.pdf. Accessed November 19, 2011.
15. Solheim K, Esakoff T, Little S, et al. The effect of cesarean delivery rates on the future incidence of placenta previa, placenta accreta, and maternal mortality. J Matern Fetal Neonatal Med 2011;24(11):1341–6.
16. Kominiarek M, Vanveldhuisen P, Hibbard J, et al. The maternal body mass index: a strong association with delivery route. Am J Obstet Gynecol 2010; 203:e1–7.
17. Nesbitt T, Connell F, Hart L, et al. Access to obstetric care in rural areas: effect on birth outcomes. Am J Public Health 1990;80:814–8.
18. Larimore W, Davis A. Relation of infant mortality to the availability of maternity care in rural Florida. J Am Board Fam Pract 1995;8:392–9.
19. Allen D, Kamradt J. Relationship of infant mortality to the availability of obstetrical care in Indiana. Fam Pract 1991;33:609–13.
20. Lynch N, Thommasen H, Anderson N, et al. Does having cesarean section capability make a difference to a small rural maternity service? Can Fam Physician 2005;51:1238–9.
21. Dresang L, Koch P. The need for rural family physicians who can perform cesareans. Am J Clin Med 2009;6:39–41.
22. Deutchman M. Who ever heard of family physicians performing cesarean sections? J Fam Pract 1996;43:449–53.
23. Norris T, Reese J, Pirani M, et al. Are rural family physicians comfortable performing cesarean sections? J Fam Pract 1996;43:455–60.
24. Gerhardt A, Scharf R, Beckman M, et al. Prothrombin and factor V mutations in women with a history of thrombosis during pregnancy and the puerperium. N Engl J Med 2000;342:374–80.
25. Pecci C, Leeman L, Wilkinson J. Family medicine obstetrics fellowship graduates: training and post-fellowship experience. Fam Med 2008;40:326–32.
26. Friederich P, Sanson B, Simioni P, et al. Frequency of pregnancy-related venous thromboembolism in anticoagulant factor-deficient women: implications for prophylaxis. Arch Intern Med 1996;125:955–60.
27. Gregory K, Curtin S, Taffel S, et al. Changes in indications for cesarean delivery: United States, 1985 and 1994. Am J Public Health 1998;88:1384–7.
28. Zhang J, Troendle J, Reddy U, et al. Contemporary cesarean delivery practice in the United States. Am J Obstet Gynecol 2010;203:1–10.
29. Rouse D, Owen J, Hauth J. Active-phase labor arrest: oxytocin augmentation for at least 4 hours. Obstet Gynecol 1999;93:323–8.
30. Rouse D, Weiner S, Bloom S, et al. Failed labor induction: toward an objective diagnosis. Obstet Gynecol 2011;117:267–72.

31. Zhang J, Troendle J, Mikolajczyk R, et al. The natural history of the normal first stage of labor. Obstet Gynecol 2010;115:705–10.
32. Shields S, Ratcliffe S, Fontaine P, et al. Dystocia in nulliparous women. Am Fam Physician 2007;75:1671–8.
33. Leeman L, Leeman R. A Native American community with a 7% cesarean delivery rate: does case mix, ethnicity, or labor management explain the low rate? Ann Fam Med 2003;1:36–43.
34. Wall E, Roberts R, Deutchman M, et al. Trial of Labor After Cesarean (TOLAC), formerly trial of labor versus elective repeat cesarean section for the woman with a previous cesarean section. Leawood (KS): American Academy of Family Physicians; 2005.
35. American College of Obstetricians and Gynecologists. ACOG Practice bulletin no. 115: vaginal birth after previous cesarean delivery. Obstet Gynecol 2010; 116:450–63.
36. American College of Obstetricians and Gynecologists. Vaginal birth after previous cesarean delivery. ACOG Practice Bulletin No. 5. 1999.
37. Roberts R, Deutchman M, King V, et al. Changing policies on vaginal birth after cesarean: impact on access. Birth 2007;34:316–22.
38. National Institutes of Health Consensus Development Conference Panel. National Institutes of Health Consensus Development conference statement: vaginal birth after cesarean: new insights March 8-10, 2010. Obstet Gynecol 2010;115:1279–95.
39. American College of Obstetricians and Gynecologists. Vaginal birth after previous cesarean delivery. Obstet Gynecol 2004;104:203–12.
40. Landon M, Spong C, Thom E, et al. Risk of uterine rupture with a trial of labor in women with multiple and single prior cesarean delivery. Obstet Gynecol 2006; 108:12–20.
41. Society of Obstetricians and Gynaecologists of Canada. SOGC clinical practice guidelines. Guidelines for vaginal birth after previous caesarean birth. Number 155. Int J Gynaecol Obstet 2005;89(3):319–31.
42. Pruett K, Kirshon B, Cotton D. Unknown uterine scar and trial of labor. Am J Obstet Gynecol 1988;159(4):807–10.
43. Beall M, Eglinton G, Clark S, et al. Vaginal delivery after cesarean section in women with unknown types of uterine scar. J Reprod Med 1984;29(1):31–5.
44. American College of Obstetricians and Gynecologists. ACOG practice bulletin, number 13. External cephalic version. Obstet Gynecol 2000. p. 1–7. Available at: http://www.acog.org/publications/pdfs/pb013.pdf. Accessed November 2, 2011.
45. American College of Obstetricians and Gynecologists. Committee on Obstetric Practice. ACOG committee opinion. Mode of term singleton breech delivery. Number 265, December 2001. Int J Gynaecol Obstet 2002;77(1):65–6.
46. Whyte H, Hannah M, Saigal S, et al. Outcomes of children at 2 years after planned cesarean birth versus planned vaginal birth for breech presentation at term: the International Randomized Term Breech Trial. Am J Obstet Gynecol 2004;191(3):864–71.
47. Hannah M, Whyte H, Hannah W, et al. Maternal outcomes at 2 years after planned cesarean section versus planned vaginal birth for breech presentation at term: the international randomized Term Breech Trial. Am J Obstet Gynecol 2004;191(3):917–27.
48. Collins S, Ellaway P, Harrington D, et al. The complications of external cephalic version: results from 805 consecutive attempts. BJOG 2007;114:636–8.

49. Hofmeyr G, Kulier R. External cephalic version for breech presentation at term. Cochrane Database Syst Rev 2011;1:CD000083.
50. Hofmeyr G, Gyte G. Interventions to help external cephalic version for breech presentation at term. Cochrane Database Syst Rev 2010;1:CD000184.
51. Goetzinger K, Harper L, Tuuli M, et al. Effect of regional anesthesia on the success rate of external cephalic version: a systematic review and meta-analysis. Obstet Gynecol 2011;118:1137–44.
52. Hannah M, Harrah W, Hewson S, et al. Planned caesarean section versus planned vaginal birth for breech presentation at term: a randomized multicentre trial. Lancet 2000;356(9239):1375–83.
53. ACOG Committee Opinion: mode of term singleton breech delivery. Obstet Gynecol 2006;108:235–7.
54. Kotaska A, Menticoglou S, Gagnon R, et al. SOGC clinical practice guideline: vaginal delivery of breech presentation. Int J Gynaecol Obstet 2009;107: 169–76.
55. Goffinet F, Carayol M, Foidart J, et al. Is planned vaginal delivery for breech presentation at term still an option? Results of an observational prospective survey in France and Belgium. Am J Obstet Gynecol 2006;194:1002–11.
56. American College of Obstetricians and Gynecologists. ACOG committee opinion scheduled Cesarean delivery and the prevention of vertical transmission of HIV infection. Number 234, May 2000 (replaces number 219, August 1999). Committee on Obstetric Practice. Int J Gynaecol Obstet 2001;73:279–81.
57. Read J, Newell M. Efficacy and safety of cesarean delivery for prevention of mother-to-child transmission of HIV-1. Cochrane Database Syst Rev 2009;1: CD000102.
58. Panel on Treatment of HIV-Infected Pregnant Women and Prevention of Perinatal Transmission. Recommendations for Use of Antiretroviral Drugs in Pregnant HIV-1-Infected Women for Maternal Health and Interventions to Reduce Perinatal HIV Transmission in the United States. 2011. p. 1–207. Available at: http://aidsinfo.nih.gov/contentfiles/PerinatalGL.pdf. Accessed November 19, 2011.
59. ACOG practice bulletin no. 22: fetal macrosomia. 2000.
60. Conway D, Langer O. Elective delivery of infants with macrosomia in diabetic women: reduced shoulder dystocia versus increased cesarean deliveries. Am J Obstet Gynecol 1998;178:922–5.
61. National Institutes of Health state-of-the-science conference statement. Cesarean delivery on maternal request. March 27-29, 2006. Obstet Gynecol 2006;107:1386–97.
62. Nelson R, Furner S, Westercamp M, et al. Cesarean delivery for the prevention of anal incontinence. Cochrane Database Syst Rev 2010;2:CD006756.
63. Rortveit G, Daltveit A, Hannestad Y, et al. Norwegian EPINCONT Study. Urinary incontinence after vaginal delivery or cesarean section. N Engl J Med 2003;348: 900–7.
64. Nerum H, Halvorsen L, Sørlie T, et al. Maternal request for cesarean section due to fear of birth: can it be changed through crisis-oriented counseling? Birth 2006;33:221–8.
65. Rouhe H, Salmela-Aro K, Halmesmäki E, et al. Fear of childbirth according to parity, gestational age, and obstetric history. BJOG 2009;116:67–73.
66. Leeman L. Prenatal counseling regarding cesarean delivery. Obstet Gynecol Clin North Am 2008;35:473–95.
67. Nisenblat V, Barak S, Griness O, et al. Maternal complications associated with multiple cesarean deliveries. Obstet Gynecol 2006;108:21–6.

68. Silver R, Landon M, Rouse D, et al. Maternal morbidity associated with multiple repeat cesarean deliveries. Obstet Gynecol 2006;107:1226–32.
69. Ananth C, Smulian J, Vintzileos A. The association of placenta previa with history of cesarean delivery and abortion: a metaanalysis. Am J Obstet Gynecol 1997; 177:1071–8.
70. American College of Obstetricians and Gynecologists. ACOG practice bulletin no. 97: fetal lung maturity. Obstet Gynecol 2008;112:717–26.
71. Tita A, Landon M, Spong C, et al. Timing of elective repeat cesarean delivery at term and neonatal outcomes. N Engl J Med 2009;360:111–20.
72. Hansen A, Wisborg K, Uldbjerg N, et al. Risk of respiratory morbidity in term infants delivered by elective caesarean section: cohort study. BMJ 2008;336:85–7.
73. Stotland N, Lipschitz L, Caughey A. Delivery strategies for women with a previous classic cesarean delivery: a decision analysis. Am J Obstet Gynecol 2002;187:1203–8.
74. Royal College of Obstetricians and Gynaecologists. Placenta praevia, placenta praevia accreta and vasa praevia: diagnosis and management. Green-top Guideline No. 27. London: Royal College of Obstetricians and Gynaecologists; 2011. Available at: http://www.rcog.org.uk/files/rcog-corp/GTG27PlacentaPraevia January2011.pdf. Accessed November 2, 2011.
75. Zlatnik M, Little S, Kohli P, et al. When should women with placenta previa be delivered? A decision analysis. J Reprod Med 2010;55:373–81.
76. Mathai M, Hofmeyr G. Abdominal surgical incisions for caesarean section. Cochrane Database Syst Rev 2009;1:CD004453.
77. Hofmeyr G, Mathai M, Shah A, et al. Techniques for caesarean section. Cochrane Database Syst Rev 2010;1:CD004662.
78. Darouiche R, Wall MJ, Itani K, et al. Chlorhexidine-alcohol versus povidone-iodine for surgical-site antisepsis. N Engl J Med 2010;362:18–26.
79. Duff P. A simple checklist for preventing major complications associated with cesarean delivery. Obstet Gynecol 2010;116:1393–6.
80. Dodd J, Anderson E, Gates S. Surgical techniques for uterine incision and uterine closure at the time of caesarean section. Cochrane Database Syst Rev 2008;3:CD004732.
81. Smaill F, Gyte G. Antibiotic prophylaxis versus no prophylaxis for preventing infection after cesarean section. Cochrane Database Syst Rev 2010;1:CD007482.
82. Hopkins L, Smaill F. Antibiotic prophylaxis regimens and drugs for cesarean section. Cochrane Database Syst Rev 2010;2:CD001136.
83. Alfirevic Z, Gyte G, Dou L. Different classes of antibiotics given to women routinely for preventing infection at caesarean section. Cochrane Database Syst Rev 2010;10:CD008726.
84. Sullivan S, Smith T, Chang E, et al. Administration of cefazolin prior to skin incision is superior to cefazolin at cord clamping in preventing postcesarean infectious morbidity: a randomized, controlled trial. Am J Obstet Gynecol 2007;196: e1–5.
85. American College of Obstetricians and Gynecologists. Committee opinion no. 465: antimicrobial prophylaxis for cesarean delivery: timing of administration. Obstet Gynecol 2010;116:791–2.
86. Thigpen B, Hood W, Chauhan S, et al. Timing of prophylactic antibiotic administration in the uninfected laboring gravida: a randomized clinical trial. Am J Obstet Gynecol 2005;192:1868–71.
87. Anorlu R, Maholwana B, Hofmeyr G. Methods of delivering the placenta at caesarean section. Cochrane Database Syst Rev 2008;3:CD004737.

88. Jacobs-Jokhan D, Hofmeyr G. Extra-abdominal versus intra-abdominal repair of the uterine incision at caesarean section. Cochrane Database Syst Rev 2011;4:CD000085.

89. Bujold E, Bujold C, Hamilton E, et al. The impact of a single-layer or double-layer closure on uterine rupture. Am J Obstet Gynecol 2002;186:1326–30.

90. Gyamfi C, Juhasz G, Gyamfi P, et al. Single- versus double-layer uterine incision closure and uterine rupture. J Matern Fetal Neonatal Med 2006;19:639–43.

91. Hohlagschwandtner M, Ruecklinger E, Husslein P, et al. Is the formation of a bladder flap at cesarean necessary? A randomized trial. Obstet Gynecol 2001;98:1089–92.

92. Bamigboye A, Hofmeyr G. Closure versus non-closure of the peritoneum at caesarean section. Cochrane Database Syst Rev 2003;4:CD000163.

93. Kapustian V, Anteby E, Gdalevich M, et al. Effect of closure versus nonclosure of peritoneum at cesarean section on adhesions: a prospective randomized study. Am J Obstet Gynecol 2011.

94. Harrigill K, Miller H, Haynes D. The effect of intraabdominal irrigation at cesarean delivery on maternal morbidity: a randomized trial. Obstet Gynecol 2003;101:80–5.

95. Anderson E, Gates S. Techniques and materials for closure of the abdominal wall in caesarean section. Cochrane Database Syst Rev 2008;4: CD004663.

96. Alderdice F, McKenna D, Dornan J. Techniques and materials for skin closure in caesarean section. Cochrane Database Syst Rev 2010;2:CD003577.

97. Frishman G, Schwartz T, Hogan J. Closure of Pfannenstiel skin incisions. Staples vs. subcuticular suture. J Reprod Med 1997;42:627–30.

98. Tuuli M, Rampersad R, Carbone J, et al. Staples compared with subcuticular suture for skin closure after cesarean delivery: a systematic review and meta-analysis. Obstet Gynecol 2011;117:682–90.

99. Stafford I, Dildy G, Clark S, et al. Visually estimated and calculated blood loss in vaginal and cesarean delivery. Am J Obstet Gynecol 2008;199:e1–7.

100. O'Leary J. Uterine artery ligation in the control of postcesarean hemorrhage. J Reprod Med 1995;40:189–93.

101. Vitthala S, Tsoumpou I, Anjum Z, et al. Use of Bakri balloon in post-partum haemorrhage: a series of 15 cases. Aust N Z J Obstet Gynaecol 2009;49: 191–4.

102. Georgiou C. Balloon tamponade in the management of postpartum haemorrhage: a review. BJOG 2009;116:747–57.

103. B-Lynch C, Coker A, Lawal A, et al. The B-Lynch surgical technique for the control of massive postpartum haemorrhage: an alternative to hysterectomy? Five cases reported. Br J Obstet Gynaecol 1997;104:372–5.

104. Cho J, Jun H, Lee C. Hemostatic suturing technique for uterine bleeding during cesarean delivery. Obstet Gynecol 2000;96:129–31.

105. Wu H, Yeh G. Uterine cavity synechiae after hemostatic square suturing technique. Obstet Gynecol 2005;105:1176–8.

106. Ochoa M, Allaire A, Stitely M. Pyometria after hemostatic square suture technique. Obstet Gynecol 2002;99:506–9.

107. Villar J, Carroli G, Zavaleta N, et al. Maternal and neonatal individual risks and benefits associated with caesarean delivery: multicentre prospective study. BMJ 2007;335:1025.

108. French L, Smaill F. Antibiotic regimens for endometritis after delivery. Cochrane Database Syst Rev 2004;4:CD001067.

109. Kaimal A, Zlatnik M, Cheng Y, et al. Effect of a change in policy regarding the timing of prophylactic antibiotics on the rate of postcesarean delivery surgical-site infections. Am J Obstet Gynecol 2008;199:e1–5.
110. Tran T, Jamulitrat S, Chongsuvivatwong V, et al. Risk factors for postcesarean surgical site infection. Obstet Gynecol 2000;95:367–71.
111. Blondon M, Perrier A, Nendaz M, et al. Thromboprophylaxis with low-molecular-weight heparin after cesarean delivery. Thromb Haemost 2010;103:129–37.
112. Marik P, Plante L. Venous thromboembolic disease and pregnancy. N Engl J Med 2008;359:2025–33.
113. Casele H, Grobman W. Cost-effectiveness of thromboprophylaxis with intermittent pneumatic compression at cesarean delivery. Obstet Gynecol 2006; 108(3 Pt 1):535–40.
114. Dresang L, Fontaine P, Leeman L, et al. Venous thromboembolism during pregnancy. Am Fam Physician 2008;77:1709–16.
115. Greer I, Thomson A. Thromboembolic disease in pregnancy and the puerperium. Leawood (KS): Guidelines and Audit Committee of the Royal College of Obstetricians and Gynaecologists; 2001.
116. Eisenkop S, Richman R, Platt L, et al. Urinary tract injury during cesarean section. Obstet Gynecol 1982;60:591–6.
117. Rajasekar D, Hall M. Urinary tract injuries during obstetric intervention. Br J Obstet Gynaecol 1997;104:731–4.
118. Davis J. Management of injuries to the urinary and gastrointestinal tract during cesarean section. Obstet Gynecol Clin North Am 1999;26:469–80.
119. Rahman M, Gasem T, Al Suleiman S, et al. Bladder injuries during cesarean section in a University Hospital: a 25-year review. Arch Gynecol Obstet 2009; 279:349–52.
120. Nielsen T, Hökegård K. Cesarean section and intraoperative surgical complications. Acta Obstet Gynecol Scand 1984;63:103–8.
121. Katz V, Dotters D, Droegemueller W. Perimortem cesarean delivery. Obstet Gynecol 1986;68:571–6.
122. Katz V, Balderston K, DeFreest M. Perimortem cesarean delivery: were our assumptions correct? Am J Obstet Gynecol 2005;192:1916–20.
123. Minig L, Trimble E, Sarsotti C, et al. Building the evidence base for postoperative and postpartum advice. Obstet Gynecol 2009;114:892–900.
124. Pronovost P, Holzmueller C, Ennen C, et al. Overview of progress in patient safety. Am J Obstet Gynecol 2011;204:5–10.
125. Mann S, Marcus R, Sachs B. Lessons from the cockpit: how team training can reduce errors on L&D. Contemp Ob Gyn 2006;51:34–45.
126. Macready N. Two-challenge rule averts errors, improves safety. OR Manager 1999;15:12.
127. American Academy of Family Physicians (AAFP). CareTeam OB. 2010. Available at: http://www.aafp.org/online/en/home/cme/aafpcourses/clinicalcourses/also/contactus.html. Accessed August 8, 2011.
128. Guise J, Eden K, Emeis C, et al. Vaginal birth after cesarean: new insights. Evid Rep Technol Assess 2010;(191):1–397.

Postpartum Hemorrhage

Cindy W. Su, MD

KEYWORDS

- Postpartum hemorrhage • Uterine atony • Uterotonic agents
- Uterine tamponade • Perineal lacerations
- Active management of third stage of labor

Postpartum hemorrhage (PPH) is an obstetric emergency that can follow either vaginal or cesarean delivery. It is the single most significant cause of maternal mortality worldwide. Annually an estimated 140,000 women die of PPH worldwide: one every 4 minutes.[1–3] The World Health Organization (WHO) estimates that approximately one-quarter of maternal deaths worldwide are caused by PPH.[1] In addition to death, serious morbidity may follow PPH because of the complications of adult respiratory distress syndrome, coagulopathy, shock, loss of fertility, and pituitary necrosis (Sheehan syndrome).

DEFINITION

There is no consensus on the single best definition of PPH. Traditionally PPH has been defined as estimated blood loss of 500 mL or more after vaginal delivery, or 1000 mL or more after a cesarean delivery. There are, however, two problems with this definition. First, studies have shown that objectively measured average blood loss after vaginal and cesarean deliveries is about 500 mL and 1000 mL, respectively.[4,5] Second, clinicians are more likely to underestimate than overestimate the volume of blood loss.[5] Using the traditional definitions would thus inaccurately categorize at least one-half of deliveries as having PPH.

Another classic definition of PPH is a 10% decline in postpartum hemoglobin concentration from antepartum levels. The problem with this definition is that determinations of hemoglobin or hematocrit concentrations may not reflect the current hematologic status, because this change depends on the timing of the test and amount of fluid resuscitation given.[6] More importantly, the diagnosis would be retrospective, perhaps useful for research but not so in the clinical setting.

Some clinicians have suggested defining PPH as excessive bleeding that makes the patient symptomatic (eg, lightheadedness, weakness, palpitations, diaphoresis, and syncope) and/or results in signs of hypovolemia (eg, hypotension, tachycardia,

The author has nothing to disclose.
Department of Obstetrics & Gynecology, Contra Costa Regional Medical Center, 2500 Alhambra Avenue, Martinez, CA 94553, USA
E-mail address: cindy.su@hsd.cccounty.us

Prim Care Clin Office Pract 39 (2012) 167–187
doi:10.1016/j.pop.2011.11.009   **primarycare.theclinics.com**

oliguria, and low oxygen saturation [<95%]). However, this method of diagnosis also has its shortcomings. Maternal blood volume expands 40% to 50% during pregnancy because of an increase in both plasma volume and red blood cell mass. This increased blood volume, to some extent, protects the mother from the consequences of hemorrhage during and after delivery. Thus, after delivery a woman may lose up to 20% of her blood volume before clinical signs become apparent.[7] Consequently, waiting for signs of excessive bleeding may delay initiating appropriate treatment.

INCIDENCE

Because of these varied definitions, the exact incidence of PPH is difficult to ascertain. However, estimates suggest that PPH complicates 4% to 6% of all deliveries.[7]

ETIOLOGY AND RISK FACTORS

PPH generally is classified as primary or secondary, with primary (also known as early) PPH occurring within 24 h after delivery, and secondary (also known as delayed) PPH occurring between 24 h and 6 to 12 weeks postpartum. **Box 1** lists the most common causes of primary and secondary PPH. The "Four Ts" mnemonic (Tone, Tissue, Trauma, and Thrombin) is another simple and effective way to remember and detect the specific causes (**Table 1**).

Tone

The most common cause of PPH is uterine atony (ie, lack of effective contraction of the uterus after delivery), which complicates 1 in 20 births and is responsible for at least 80% of cases of PPH.[6] At term, blood flow through the placental site averages 600 mL/min. After placental delivery, the uterus contracts its myometrial fibers to occlude the spiral arterioles. If inadequate uterine contraction occurs, rapid blood loss will ensue. Risk factors for uterine atony include[6,8]:

- Uterine overdistention (multiple gestation, polyhydramnios, and fetal macrosomia)
- Prolonged oxytocin use
- Rapid or prolonged labor
- Multiparity
- Chorioamnionitis

Box 1
Etiology of PPH

Primary (early or within 24 h)

    Uterine atony

    Retained placenta, especially placenta accreta

    Defects in coagulation

    Uterine inversion

Secondary (delayed or between 24 h and 12 weeks)

    Subinvolution of placental site

    Retained products of conception

    Infection

    Inherited coagulation defects

Table 1 "Four Ts" mnemonic device for causes of postpartum hemorrhage	
Four Ts	Cause
Tone	Uterine atony
Trauma	Lacerations, hematomas, inversion, rupture
Tissue	Retained tissue, invasive placenta
Thrombin	Coagulopathies

- Preeclampsia
- Placenta previa and accreta
- Uterine-relaxing agents (tocolytic therapy, halogenated anesthetics, and nitroglycerin)
- History of uterine atony in previous pregnancy
- Uterine inversion
- Retained placenta or placental fragment
- Asian or Hispanic ethnicity.

Trauma

Trauma-related bleeding can be caused by genital tract lacerations, episiotomies, or uterine rupture. Genital tract lacerations involve the maternal soft-tissue structures, and can be associated with large hematomas and rapid blood loss if unrecognized. The most common lower genital tract lacerations include perineal, vulvar, vaginal, and cervical. Upper genital tract lacerations are typically associated with broad ligament and retroperitoneal hematomas. Although it is difficult to ascertain their exact incidence, genital tract lacerations are the second leading cause of PPH.[8] Risk factors include[8,9]:

- Operative vaginal delivery (forceps or vacuum)
- Fetal malpresentation
- Fetal macrosomia
- Episiotomy, especially mediolateral
- Precipitous delivery
- Prior cerclage placement
- Shoulder dystocia.

Tissue

Retained products of conception, namely placental tissue and amniotic membranes, can inhibit the uterus from adequate contraction and result in hemorrhage. Retained placenta (ie, failure of the placenta to deliver within 30 minutes of birth) complicates 1 in 100 to 1 in 200 deliveries.[10] Risk factors include midtrimester delivery, chorioamnionitis, and accessory placental lobes.

Invasive placenta is a cause of PPH that has significant morbidity and can also, at times, be life threatening.[10] One study reported that abnormally adherent placentation caused 65% of cases of intractable PPH requiring emergency peripartum hysterectomy at Brigham and Women's Hospital.[11] The incidence is estimated at 1 in 2500 deliveries, a tenfold rise in the last 50 years that is most likely due to the increase in cesarean section rates.[12] Classification is based on the depth of invasion and can be easily remembered through alliteration: placenta accreta adheres to the myometrium, placenta increta invades the myometrium, and placenta percreta penetrates the myometrium to or beyond the serosa.[13] The greatest risk factor is a placenta previa in the setting of a prior cesarean section (increasing to 67% with 4 or more[14]). Other risk factors include prior myomectomy, prior cesarean delivery, Asherman syndrome, submucous leiomyomata, and maternal age of 35 years or greater.[12]

Thrombin

Coagulation disorders are a rare cause of PPH, and are usually identified before delivery. These disorders include idiopathic thrombocytopenic purpura (ITP), thrombotic thrombocytopenic purpura (TTP), von Willebrand disease, and hemophilia. Disorders of coagulation should be suspected in patients with a family history of such abnormalities and in patients with a history of menorrhagia.[15] Women with von Willebrand disease are prone to postabortal bleeding, but are unlikely to experience PPH at term. On the other hand, women with factor XI deficiency or who are hemophilia carriers are at increased risk of both early and late PPH (16%–22% for early and 11%–24% for late).[16–19] However, PPH alone is not a strong indication for screening for these defects, given that bleeding disorders are rarely the cause of PPH.

Patients can also develop hemolysis, elevated liver enzyme levels, low platelets (HELLP), and disseminated intravascular coagulation (DIC). The overall incidence of DIC in the obstetric population has not been reported; however, several risk factors have been documented. These include massive antepartum hemorrhage or PPH, sepsis, severe preeclampsia, amniotic fluid embolism, tissue necrosis (eg, retained intrauterine fetal demise and trauma), placental abruption, and acute fatty liver of pregnancy.[20]

PREVENTION OF PPH

Two preventive methods that have been suggested to reduce PPH from uterine atony are active management of the third stage of labor and spontaneous delivery of the placenta after cesarean delivery. Active management of the third stage of labor involves three steps: (1) giving a prophylactic uterotonic (most commonly oxytocin), (2) early cord clamping, and (3) controlled cord traction to deliver the placenta. A Cochrane review showed that patients who were actively managed during the third stage of labor had significant reductions in mean blood loss (weighted mean difference −79.33 mL, 95% confidence interval [CI] −94.29 to −64.37), PPH of more than 500 mL (relative risk 0.38, 95% CI 0.32–0.46), and the length of third stage of labor (weighted mean difference −9.77 minutes, 95% CI −10.00 to −9.53).[21] Controversy exists regarding whether prophylactic oxytocin should be given before or after delivery of the placenta. A systematic review showed that the timing of administration of the uterotonic agent made no significant impact on the incidence of PPH, the rate of placental retention, or the length of the third stage or labor.[22] The recommended dose of oxytocin (Pitocin) is 10 to 40 units in 1 L of lactated Ringer's intravenously at a rate of 125 to 250 mL/h or 10 units intramuscularly.[7]

Spontaneous delivery of the placenta during a cesarean section (ie, delivery of the placenta with cord traction as opposed to manual removal) has also been associated with reduced blood loss. In a Cochrane review, spontaneous delivery reduced blood loss by 30% and postpartum endometritis by sevenfold when compared with manual removal.[23]

MANAGEMENT OF PPH

Prompt recognition of excessive bleeding after delivery is crucial. A healthy woman may lose 10% to 15% of her blood volume without a drop in blood pressure.[7] By the time her blood pressure drops appreciably, the patient frequently has lost at least 30% of her blood volume. Thus, relying on vital signs to initiate treatment or to assess the severity of the bleeding could be misleading and may cause an unnecessary delay in initiating appropriate treatment.

PRIMARY INTERVENTIONS FOR PPH

Because the single most common cause of hemorrhage is uterine atony, the first interventions should be directed toward ensuring that the uterus is contracted. The bladder should be emptied and a bimanual pelvic examination performed. If the uterus is soft (atonic), massage is performed by placing one hand made into a fist in the anterior fornix and pushing against the body of the uterus while the other hand compresses the fundus from above through the abdominal wall (**Fig. 1**).[24] The posterior aspect of the uterus is massaged with the abdominal hand and the anterior aspect with the vaginal hand. The fundus should be massaged vigorously for at least 15 seconds and continued until the uterus remains firm and bleeding has abated. Massage should be maintained while other interventions are being initiated. These measures may include ensuring adequate intravenous access (preferably with two large-bore 18-gauge catheters), ordering appropriate laboratory tests, and requesting uterotonic agents.

The first-line treatment for ongoing blood loss in the setting of decreased uterine tone is the administration of additional uterotonics.[7] The 3 categories of uterotonic agents include oxytocin, ergot alkaloids, and prostaglandins (**Table 2**). There is no evidence that one sequence is better than another.[25] The important point is not the sequence of drugs, but the prompt initiation of uterotonic therapy and prompt assessment of effect. The choice of the agent also depends on its side-effect profile as well as its contraindications. It should be possible to determine within 30 minutes whether

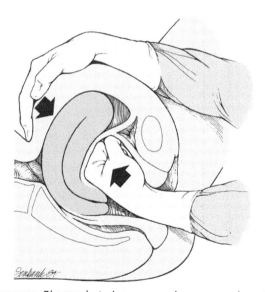

Fig. 1. Bimanual massage. Bimanual uterine compression massage is performed by placing one hand in the vagina and pushing against the body of the uterus while the other hand compresses the fundus from above through the abdominal wall. The posterior aspect of the uterus is massaged with the abdominal hand and the anterior aspect with the vaginal hand. (*From* Gabbe SG, Niebyl JR, Simpson JL. Obstetrics: normal and problem pregnancies. 4th edition. New York: Churchill Livingstone; 2002. p. 468; with permission.)

Table 2
Uterotonic agents for management of postpartum hemorrhage

Agent	Dose/Route	Frequency	Contraindications	Side Effects
Oxytocin (Pitocin)	IV: 10–40 units in 1 L normal saline or lactated Ringer's solution IM: 10 units	Continuous	None	Nausea, vomiting, water intoxication
Methylergonovine (Methergine)	IM: 0.2 mg	Every 2–4 h	Hypertension, preeclampsia	Hypertension, hypotension, nausea, vomiting
15-Methyl prostaglandin $F_{2\alpha}$ (Carboprost, Hemabate)	IM: 0.25 mg	Every 15–90 min, 8 doses maximum	Asthma	Nausea, vomiting, diarrhea, headache, flushing, fever
Prostaglandin E_2 (Dinoprostone)	Suppository: vaginal or rectal 20 mg	Every 2 h	Hypotension	Nausea, vomiting, diarrhea, fever, chills, headache
Misoprostol (Cytotec)	800–1000 µg rectally	Single dose	None	Shivering, fever, diarrhea

Abbreviations: IM, intramuscular; IV, intravenous.

pharmacologic treatment will reverse uterine atony.[26] If it does not, prompt invasive intervention is usually warranted.

Oxytocin

Oxytocin (Pitocin) is usually given as a first-line agent, and is often already administered prophylactically as part of active management of the third stage of labor.[7] The recommended dose is 10 to 40 units in 1 L of normal saline or lactated Ringer's intravenously at a rate of 125 to 250 mL/h or 10 units intramuscularly (including directly into the myometrium in the setting of a cesarean section).[7] As much as 500 mL can be infused over 10 minutes without complications.[13] Higher doses of oxytocin (up to 80 units in 1000 mL) can be infused intravenously for a short duration to manage uterine atony.[27] Oxytocin generally is well tolerated and has few side effects, but rapid intravenous push may, rarely, contribute to hypotension and lead to cardiovascular collapse.[28]

Carbetocin, a long-acting analogue of oxytocin, is available in many countries (but not the United States) for preventing uterine atony and hemorrhage. It seems to be as effective as oxytocin and shares a similar toxicity spectrum.[29] The recommended dose is 100 µg given by a single, slow intravenous injection.[29]

Ergot Alkaloids

When oxytocin fails to produce adequate uterine tone, a second-line therapy must be initiated. Ergot alkaloids such as methylergonovine (Methergine) and ergometrine (not available in the United States) cause smooth muscle contractions and thus rapidly induce strong tetanic uterine contractions. These agents may be given orally or intramuscularly, but never intravenously. In cases of PPH, the recommended dose is 0.2 mg given intramuscularly (including directly into the myometrium) and repeated at 2- to 4-hour intervals as needed.[7] These medications may cause significantly rapid increases in blood pressure and are, therefore, contraindicated in patients who have hypertension and preeclampsia. Other side effects include nausea and vomiting.[30]

Prostaglandins

Prostaglandins enhance uterine contractility and vasoconstriction.[31] Carboprost (Hemabate) is a 15-methyl prostaglandin $F_{2\alpha}$ analogue that is potent and has a long duration of action. The recommended dose is 250 µg intramuscularly (including directly into the myometrium) every 15 to 90 minutes, as needed, to a total cumulative dose of 2 mg (8 doses).[7] Carboprost has been proved to control hemorrhage in up to 87% of patients.[32,33] In cases where it is not effective, chorioamnionitis or other risk factors for hemorrhage often are present.[31] Asthma is a strong contraindication to its use because it has bronchoconstrictive properties. Other side effects include diarrhea, nausea, vomiting, headache, flushing, and pyrexia.[31]

Misoprostol (Cytotec), a synthetic prostaglandin E_1 analogue, has also been shown to increase uterine tone and decrease PPH.[33,34] Extremely inexpensive, misoprostol is especially useful for reducing blood loss in resource-poor settings where injectable uterotonics and/or refrigeration are unavailable. It can be administered sublingually, orally, vaginally, and rectally. Doses range from 200 to 1000 µg; the dose recommended by the American College of Obstetricians and Gynecologists (ACOG) is 800 to 1000 µg administered rectally.[2,7,34,35] There are no contraindications to misoprostol, although common side effects include shivering, pyrexia, and diarrhea.[36] Although misoprostol is widely used in the treatment of PPH, it is not approved by the US Food and Drug Administration (FDA) for this indication.

Dinoprostone is a prostaglandin E_2 that is not as commonly used but has also been shown to be effective in treating PPH.[37] The recommended dose is a 20 mg suppository administered either vaginally or rectally and repeated every 2 hours as necessary.[7] It is not to be given in the setting of hypotension and has known side effects of nausea, vomiting, diarrhea, fever, chills, and headache.[7]

SECONDARY INTERVENTIONS FOR PPH

If bleeding persists despite the initial interventions described earlier, other etiological factors besides atony must be considered. Even if atony is present, there may also be other contributing factors.

Genital Tract Lacerations

Even if inspection for lacerations has been already performed at delivery, a thorough examination should be repeated, as it is possible that a bleeding site was missed. The lower genital tract (cervix and vagina) should be examined carefully starting superiorly at the cervix and progressing inferiorly to the vagina, perineum, and vulva. This examination requires proper patient positioning, adequate operative assistance, good lighting, appropriate instrumentation (eg, Simpson or Heaney retractors), and adequate anesthesia. If necessary, performing the laceration repair in a well-equipped operating room should be considered.

Sutures should be placed if direct pressure does not stop the bleeding. Episiotomy increases blood loss as well as the risk of anal sphincter tears (third-degree lacerations) and rectal mucosa tears (fourth-degree lacerations).[6,38] Consequently, this procedure should be avoided unless urgent delivery is necessary, and the perineum is thought to be a limiting factor.[39]

Figs. 2–4 illustrate second-, third-, and fourth-degree lacerations of the perineum and the techniques for their repair. For third- and fourth-degree lacerations, a prophylactic dose of a second-generation cephalosporin (cefotetan or cefoxitin) or of clindamycin, if the patient is allergic to penicillin at the time of repair, has been shown to decrease perineal wound complications at 2 weeks postpartum.[40]

In repairing cervical lacerations it is important to secure the apex of the laceration, which is often a major source of bleeding. However, this area is frequently the most

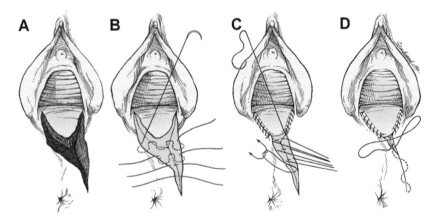

Fig. 2. (*A–D*) Second-degree laceration repair. A first-degree laceration involves the four-chet, the perineal skin, and the vaginal mucous membrane. A second-decree laceration also includes the muscles of the perineal body. The rectal sphincter remains intact. (*From* Gabbe SG, Niebyl JR, Simpson JL. Obstetrics: normal and problem pregnancies. 4th edition. New York: Churchill Livingstone; 2002. p. 472; with permission.)

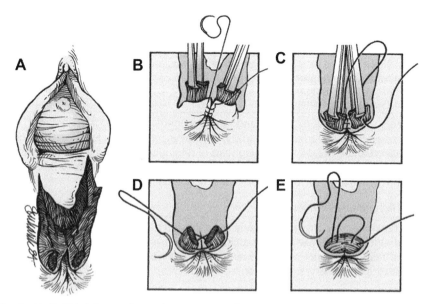

Fig. 3. (*A–E*) Third-degree laceration repair. A third-degree laceration not only extends through the skin, mucous membrane, and perineal body, but includes the anal sphincter. Interrupted figure-of-eight sutures should be placed in the capsule of the sphincter muscle. (*From* Gabbe SG, Niebyl JR, Simpson JL. Obstetrics: normal and problem pregnancies. 4th edition. New York: Churchill Livingstone; 2002. p. 473; with permission.)

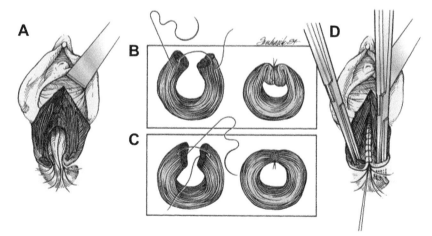

Fig. 4. Fourth-degree laceration repair. This laceration extends through the rectal mucosa. (*A*) The extent of the laceration is shown, with a segment of the rectum exposed. (*B*) Approximation of the rectal submucosa. This is the most commonly recommended method for repair. (*C*) Alternative method of approximating the rectal mucosa in which the knots are actually buried inside the rectal lumen. (*D*) After closure of the rectal submucosa, an additional layer of running sutures may be placed. The rectal sphincter is then repaired. (*From* Gabbe SG, Niebyl JR, Simpson JL. Obstetrics: normal and problem pregnancies. 4th edition. New York: Churchill Livingstone; 2002. p. 473; with permission.)

difficult to visualize, especially in the setting of an active bleed. A helpful technique to use in these cases is to start to suture the laceration at its proximal end, using the suture for traction to expose the more distal portion of the cervix until the apex is in view (**Fig. 5**).[13] Risk factors for cervical lacerations associated with excessive bleeding or requiring repair include precipitous labor, operative vaginal delivery, and cerclage.[41]

Retained Products of Conception

The uterus should be explored and any retained placental fragments of fetal membranes should be removed manually, if possible, or with ring forceps. Ultrasound examination can be helpful for the diagnosis of retained tissue and to guide removal.[7] Curettage with a 16-mm suction catheter or a large blunt curette (banjo curette) is performed if manual removal is unsuccessful in controlling hemorrhage.[26]

Uterine Tamponade Techniques

Uterine tamponade is effective in many patients with atony or lower uterine segment bleeding. Such approaches can be particularly useful as a temporizing measure, but if a prompt response is not seen, preparations should be made for exploratory laparotomy and, if necessary, hysterectomy.

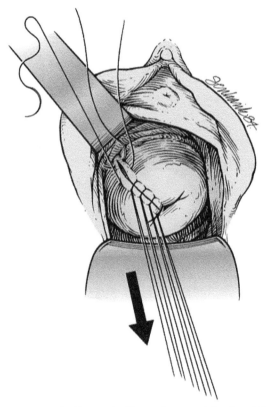

Fig. 5. Cervical laceration repair. The cervical laceration repair begins at the proximal part of the laceration, using traction on the previous sutures to aid in exposing the distal portion of the defect. (*From* Gabbe SG, Niebyl JR, Simpson JL. Obstetrics: normal and problem pregnancies. 4th edition. New York: Churchill Livingstone; 2002. p. 474; with permission.)

Either a balloon or a pack can be used for tamponade. Packing with gauze requires careful layering of the material, such as Kerlix, back and forth from one cornu to the other using a sponge stick and ending with extension of the gauze through the cervical os.[7] The gauze can be impregnated with 5000 units thrombin in 5 mL sterile saline to enhance clotting. Often, broad-spectrum antibiotics (such as gentamicin, 1.5 mg/kg every 8 hours and clindamycin 300 mg every 6 hours) are administered while the pack is in place.[26] If packing does not control hemorrhage, repacking is not advised.[42]

The same effect often can be derived more easily using a balloon device such as a Foley catheter, Rusch catheter, condom catheter, Sengstaken-Blakemore tube or, more recently, the Surgical Obstetric Silicone (SOS) Bakri tamponade balloon.[43] The advantages of such devices are that they allow some assessment of ongoing hemorrhage, are easy to place, and are effective.[44] A success rate of 84% has been reported.[45] The SOS Bakri balloon was specifically designed for placement in the uterus for control of PPH, and is one of two such devices approved by the US FDA for this application. It consists of a silicone balloon connected to a 24F, 54-cm long silicone catheter. The balloon provides a tamponade to the uterine surface while the catheter allows drainage of blood from the uterine cavity. **Fig. 6** shows its proper placement.

Regardless of the method used, hemoglobin and urine output should be closely monitored. Such monitoring is especially important when a gauze pack is used because a large amount of blood can collect behind the pack.[26] The balloon or pack should be removed by 12 to 24 hours.[43,44]

Arterial Embolization

A patient who has persistent bleeding despite all the aforementioned measures but is hemodynamically stable may be a candidate for arterial embolization.[7] The technique involves pelvic angiography to visualize the bleeding vessels and placement of Gelfoam (gelatin) pledgets, coils, or glue into the vessels for occlusion. Balloon occlusion is also a technique used in such circumstances. A cumulative success rate of 95% has been reported.[46]

Arterial embolization has several advantages over surgical intervention. First, it allows for selective occlusion of bleeding vessels, which can be extremely valuable in patients with aberrant pelvic vasculature (eg, uterine arteriovenous malformations).[47–49] Second, the uterus and potential future fertility are preserved as long as the uterus and ovaries are intact.[50–55] Finally, the procedure has minimal morbidity, enables the physician to avoid or delay surgical intervention, and can be performed in coagulopathic patients, allowing more time for blood and clotting factor replacement.[13] Serious complications are unusual, and the procedure-related morbidity of 3% to 6% is much

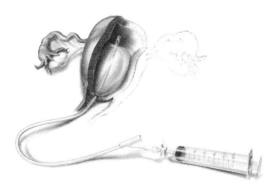

Fig. 6. SOS Bakri balloon. (© Lisa Clark, *courtesy of* Cook Medical Inc.)

less than with laparotomy.[46,56] Postembolization fever is the most common complication; other less common complications include buttock ischemia, vascular perforation, and infection.

Surgical Interventions

When uterine atony is unresponsive to conservative management, surgical intervention through laparotomy is necessary. Possible interventions include (1) those that decrease blood supply to the uterus (arterial ligation), (2) those aimed at causing uterine contraction or compression (B-Lynch), and (3) those that remove the uterus (hysterectomy).

Arterial ligation techniques

The goal of arterial ligation is to decrease uterine perfusion and subsequent bleeding. Success rates have varied from 40% to 95% in the literature, depending on which vessels are ligated.[56] Described by O'Leary nearly 40 years ago, uterine artery ligation is one of the easiest and most effective techniques, and is the recommended initial step in surgical intervention for refractory PPH.[57] To perform the procedure, a large curved needle with an absorbable suture is passed anterior to posterior through the uterine myometrium at the level of the lower uterine segment, approximately 1 to 2 cm medial to the broad ligament. The suture then is directed posterior to anterior through a cleared avascular space in the broad ligament close to the lateral border of the uterus. The suture is then tied to compress the vessels (**Fig. 7**). Unilateral artery ligation will control hemorrhage in 10% to 15% of cases, whereas bilateral ligation will control an additional 75%.[58]

If bleeding persists despite bilateral uterine artery ligations, the utero-ovarian vessels can be ligated in a similar fashion. Alternatively, the ovarian artery can be ligated directly between the medial margin of the ovary and the lateral aspect of the fundus in the area of the utero-ovarian ligament (also known as infundibulopelvic vessels). A stepwise combination of unilateral and then bilateral ligatures starting with the uterine artery and working toward the ovarian vessels is the recommended strategy.[58]

Hypogastric (internal iliac) artery ligation can be technically challenging and time consuming, and should really be performed only by an experienced surgeon who is familiar with pelvic anatomy. If this procedure fails, it is important to proceed quickly to more definitive therapy (ie, hysterectomy).[59]

Uterine suturing techniques

Two uterine suturing techniques that have been described for atony control include placement of a B-Lynch compression suture and multiple square sutures.[60,61] The

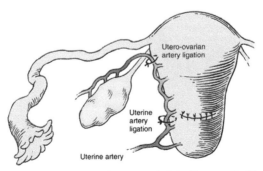

Fig. 7. Uterine artery ligation. (*From* Gabbe SG, Niebyl JR, Simpson JL. Obstetrics: normal and problem pregnancies. 4th edition. New York: Churchill Livingstone; 2002. p. 470; with permission.)

B-Lynch compression suture technique involves anchoring a large absorbable suture within the uterine myometrium, both anteriorly and posteriorly.[62] It is then passed in a continuous fashion around the external surface of the uterus and tied firmly so that adequate uterine compression occurs (**Fig. 8**). Numerous case reports have demonstrated the efficacy of B-Lynch compression sutures in resolving PPH due to uterine atony.[63,64] Furthermore, successful term pregnancies after the B-Lynch technique have been reported.[65,66]

A recent report demonstrated efficacy of multiple square sutures within the uterine wall to control PPH caused by uterine atony, placenta previa, or placenta accreta.[61] This technique involves the use of a large absorbable suture on a blunt straight needle. The needle is passed from the anterior to the posterior aspects of the uterus and back in the opposite directions, to form a square. The suture is tied firmly to provide compression to the bleeding surfaces.

Hysterectomy

The final surgical intervention for refractory bleeding caused by uterine atony is hysterectomy. Hysterectomy provides definitive therapy, and is required in the management of PPH in approximately 1 in 1000 deliveries.[67] The procedure should be reserved for cases in which other measures have failed, and the ACOG recommends that if hysterectomy is performed for uterine atony, there should be documentation of first attempting other therapies.[7]

SPECIAL SITUATIONS
Retained Placenta

When there is failure to spontaneously deliver the placenta within 30 minutes after birth, it is considered a retained placenta. This can occur in 0.5% to 3% of deliveries.[10]

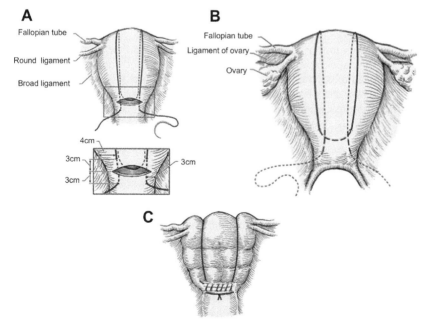

Fig. 8. (*A–C*) B-Lynch compression suture. (*From* Gabbe SG, Niebyl JR, Simpson JL. Obstetrics: normal and problem pregnancies. 4th edition. New York: Churchill Livingstone; 2002. p. 471; with permission.)

The most popular approach in this situation is an attempt at manual extraction of the placenta, which can be performed in the delivery room with proper pain control or, preferably, in the operating room under anesthesia. Although it has become common practice to administer prophylactic antibiotics to patients who require a manual extraction of a retained placenta after vaginal delivery, no data exist to support its effectiveness in preventing subsequent endometritis.[68] If manual removal is unsuccessful in controlling hemorrhage, a curettage with a 16-mm suction catheter or a larger blunt curette (banjo curette) can be used to remove remaining placental fragments or fetal membranes. Often, transabdominal ultrasound guidance is helpful in determining that the evacuation of tissue is complete.

Two alternative approaches to manual removal of a retained placenta include intraumbilical-vein injection of oxytocin and sublingual nitroglycerin. A large meta-analysis study has shown that injection of oxytocin into the intraumbilical vein has no clinically significant effect in preventing the need for manual extraction.[69] Sublingual nitroglycerin, however, may be effective, although it may cause hemodynamic changes in blood pressure and thus warrants more clinical trials on its safety for this use.[70]

Uterine Inversion

Uterine inversion is a life-threatening obstetric emergency that occurs when the uterine fundus collapses into the endometrial cavity. Its reported incidence ranges from 1 in 2000 to 23,000 deliveries.[71,72] The most common causes of a uterine inversion are excessive umbilical cord traction with a fundally attached placenta, and fundal pressure in the setting of a relaxed uterus (Crede maneuver).[73] Once diagnosed, a uterine inversion should elicit immediate intervention because of the high maternal mortality that results from hemorrhage and shock. Uterotonic agents should be discontinued promptly. A call for additional personnel, including anesthesiology, obstetric, and operating room staff, should be placed. Adequate intravenous access for maternal fluid resuscitation should be established. The obstetric provider should then immediately attempt to manually replace the inverted uterus in its normal position. This is best accomplished by placing a hand inside the vagina and pushing the fundus cephalad along the long axis of the vagina. Prompt intervention is important because the lower uterine segment and cervix contract over time, thus making manual replacement progressively more difficult.

When immediate uterine replacement is unsuccessful, pharmacologic agents should be given to relax the uterus. Manual replacement is then reattempted. The most common uterine relaxants used are terbutaline (0.25 mg intravenously or subcutaneously) and magnesium sulfate (4–6 g intravenously over 15–25 minutes). Nitroglycerin has also been shown to be an effective uterine relaxant at doses of 50 to 500 μg intravenously.[74] Furthermore, with its extremely short half-life, nitroglycerin may be advantageous in cases of severe hemorrhage and hemodynamic instability.[75]

When manual replacement is unsuccessful despite the aforementioned measures, the patient should be taken promptly to the operating room for surgical intervention.

Puerperal Hematomas

Because of the rich vascular supply of the pregnant uterus, vulva, and vagina, on occasion a blood vessel laceration may lead to the formation of a pelvic hematoma in the lower or upper genital tract. The most common locations for puerperal hematomas are the vulva, vaginal/paravaginal area, and retroperitoneum; they often present with pain within the first 24 hours of delivery.

Vulvar hematoma

Most vulvar hematomas result from injury to the branches of the pudendal artery that occur from episiotomies or spontaneous perineal lacerations. These vessels lie in the superficial fascia of the anterior and/or posterior pelvic triangle. Blood loss is tamponaded by Colle's fascia, the urogenital diaphragm, and the anal fascia (**Fig. 9**). Because of these fascial boundaries, the mass will extend to the skin and a visible hematoma will develop.

Vulvar hematomas usually present with rapid development of a severely painful, tense, compressible mass covered by skin with purplish discoloration.[76] The most common initial approach to a vulvar hematoma is conservative management (analgesia and application of cold packs). Most small (<5 cm), nonexpanding vulvar hematomas will resolve spontaneously with supportive care.[77] In cases of rapidly expanding vulvar hematomas resulting in hemodynamic changes or dropping hematocrit, surgical drainage is indicated.[13] A wide linear incision through the skin is recommended. Once the clot is evacuated, the dead space should be closed in layers with absorbable suture and a sterile pressure dressing applied. A transurethral Foley catheter should be placed until significant tissue edema subsides.

Vaginal hematoma

Vaginal hematomas result from injury to branches of the uterine artery that most often result from forceps deliveries, but may also occur with spontaneous vaginal deliveries. These hematomas accumulate above the pelvic diaphragm (**Fig. 10**). It is unusual for large amounts of blood to collect in this region, and protrusion of the hematoma into the vaginal-rectal area is common.[13] Consequently, vaginal hematomas often present with rectal pressure, and on physical examination a large mass protruding into the vagina is obvious.[78]

Conservative treatment is also recommended as the initial step for small (<5 cm), nonexpanding vaginal hematomas.[77] When surgical drainage is indicated, it should generally be performed under good anesthesia and lighting in an operating room. Unlike vulvar hematomas, the incision of a vaginal hematoma does not require closing; rather, a vaginal pack should be placed to tamponade the raw edges.[13] If bleeding persists, selective arterial embolization may be considered.

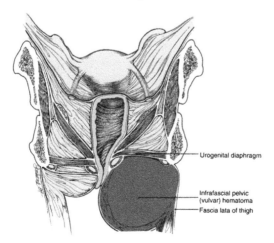

Urogenital diaphragm

Infrafascial pelvic (vulvar) hematoma

Fascia lata of thigh

Fig. 9. Vulvar hematoma fascial boundaries. (*From* Gabbe SG, Niebyl JR, Simpson JL. Obstetrics: normal and problem pregnancies. 4th edition. New York: Churchill Livingstone; 2002. p. 474; with permission.)

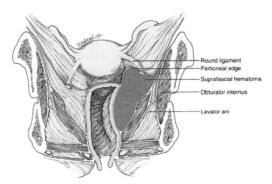

Fig. 10. Vaginal hematoma. (*From* Gabbe SG, Niebyl JR, Simpson JL. Obstetrics: normal and problem pregnancies. 4th edition. New York: Churchill Livingstone; 2002.)

Retroperitoneal hematoma

Although the least common puerperal hematoma, retroperitoneal hematomas are the most serious and life threatening. They are usually caused by injury to the branches of the hypogastric (ie, internal iliac) artery (**Fig. 11**). The most common childbirth-related causes are (1) laceration of a uterine artery during a cesarean delivery or uterine rupture and (2) extension of a paravaginal hematoma. Patients with retroperitoneal hematomas generally do not present with pain and are often asymptomatic initially. Rather, because of the significant amount of blood that can accumulate in the

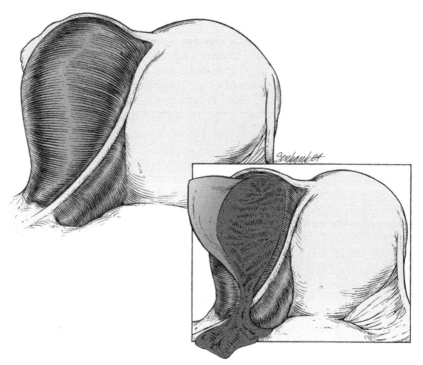

Fig. 11. Retroperitoneal hematoma. (*From* Gabbe SG, Niebyl JR, Simpson JL. Obstetrics: normal and problem pregnancies. 4th edition. New York: Churchill Livingstone; 2002. p. 476; with permission.)

retroperitoneal space, these patients often present with symptoms of hemodynamic instability from hemorrhage or shock. Treatment of a retroperitoneal hematoma requires either prompt surgical (incision and evacuation of hematoma) or angiographic (arterial ligation) intervention.

SIMULATION-BASED TRAINING FOR PPH

A small but growing body of literature has shown that designing a PPH protocol that involves training in a simulation-based setting with a multidisciplinary team may help optimize outcomes after PPH.[79–83] One study noted improvement in perinatal outcomes in terms of 5-minute Apgar scores and hypoxic-ischemic encephalopathy.[84] Several other studies showed an improvement of knowledge, practical skills, communication, and team performance in acute obstetric situations.[79] Running mock drills can also help identify the obstacles encountered and errors made in obstetric emergency settings that lead to delayed appropriate care.[85] The California Maternal Quality Care Collaborative has developed an excellent "Obstetric (OB) Hemorrhage Toolkit" as a resource for health care providers interested in initiating a standardized PPH protocol on their hospital's Labor & Delivery floor.[86]

SUMMARY

PPH is an obstetric emergency that all providers should be prepared for, because it is one of the most common complications after either vaginal or cesarean delivery. In managing PPH, one should remember the Four Ts mnemonic (Tone, Tissue, Trauma, Thrombin)[83] to aid in evaluating the possible etiology. Medical management should always be initiated before progressing to more aggressive interventions such as a laparotomy. If available, placement of a uterine tamponade balloon may prevent the necessity for surgical intervention. Also, if the patient is hemodynamically stable, arterial embolization is an option to consider. Active management of the third stage of labor can also prevent PPH and may, thus, be encouraged as the standard of practice. There is also a growing body of literature showing that the creation of a standardized PPH protocol that involves simulation-based training with a multidisciplinary team may help decrease maternal morbidity and improve perinatal outcomes.

REFERENCES

1. Kahn KS, Wojdyla D, Say L, et al. WHO analysis of causes of maternal death: a systematic review. Lancet 2006;367:1066–74.
2. Mous HA, Alfirevic Z. Treatment for primary postpartum haemorrhage. Cochrane Database Syst Rev 2003;1:CD003249.
3. Lu MC, Fridman M, Korst LM, et al. Variations in the incidence of postpartum hemorrhage across hospitals in California. Matern Child Health J 2005;9:297–306.
4. Andolina K, Daly S, Roberts N, et al. Objective measurement of blood loss at delivery: is it more than a guess? Am J Obstet Gynecol 1999;180:S69.
5. Stafford I, Dildy GA, Clark SL, et al. Visually estimated and calculated blood loss in vaginal and cesarean delivery. Am J Obstet Gynecol 2008;199:519.e1–7.
6. Combs CA, Murphy EL, Laros RK Jr. Factors associated with postpartum hemorrhage with vaginal birth. Obstet Gynecol 1991;77:69–76.
7. American College of Obstetricians, Gynecologists. American College of Obstetrics and Gynecology practice bulletin: clinical management guidelines for obstetrician-gynecologists number 76, October 2006: postpartum hemorrhage. Obstet Gynecol 2006;108:1039–47.

8. Stones RW, Paterson CM, Saunders NJ. Risk factors for major obstetric haemorrhage. Eur J Obstet Gynecol Reprod Biol 1993;48:15–8.

9. Christianson LM, Bovbjerg VE, McDavitt EC, et al. Risk factors for perineal injury during delivery. Am J Obstet Gynecol 2003;189:255–60.

10. Weeks AD, Mirembe FM. The retained placenta—new insights into an old problem. Eur J Obstet Gynecol Reprod Biol 2002;102:109–10.

11. Zelop CM, Harlow BL, Frigoletto FD Jr, et al. Emergency peripartum hysterectomy. Am J Obstet Gynecol 1993;168:1443–8.

12. Wu S, Kocherginsky M, Hibbard JU. Abnormal placentation: twenty-year analysis. Am J Obstet Gynecol 2005;192:1458–61.

13. Gabbe SG, Niebyl JR, Simpson JL. Obstetrics: normal and problem pregnancies. 4th edition. New York: Churchill Livingstone; 2002.

14. SI Clark, Koonings PP, Phelan JP. Placenta previa/accreta and prior cesarean section. Obstet Gynecol 1985;66:89–92.

15. Silver RM, Major H. Maternal coagulation disorders and postpartum hemorrhage. Clin Obstet Gynecol 2010;53:252–64.

16. Nichols WL, Hultin MB, James AH, et al. von Willebrand disease (VWD): evidence-based diagnosis and management guidelines, the National Heart, Lung, and Blood Institute (NHLBI) Expert Panel report (USA). Haemophilia 2008;14:171–232.

17. Kadir RA, Lee CA, Sabin CA, et al. Pregnancy in women with von Willebrand's disease or factor XI deficiency. Br J Obstet Gynaecol 1998;105:314–21.

18. Kadir RA, Economides DL, Braithwaite J, et al. The obstetric experience of carriers of haemophilia. Br J Obstet Gynaecol 1997;104:803–10.

19. Myers B, Pavord S, Kean L, et al. Pregnancy outcome in Factor XI deficiency: incidence of miscarriage, antenatal and postnatal haemorrhage in 33 women with Factor XI deficiency. BJOG 2007;114:643–6.

20. Richey ME, Gilstrap LC 3rd, Ramin SM. Management of disseminated intravascular coagulopathy. Clin Obstet Gynecol 1995;38:514–20.

21. Begley CM, Gyte GM, Murphy DJ, et al. Active versus expectant management for women in third stage of labour. Cochrane Database Syst Rev 2010;7:CD007412.

22. Soltani H, Hutchon DR, Poulose TA. Timing of prophylactic uterotonics for the third stage of labour after vaginal birth. Cochrane Database Syst Rev 2010;8: CD006173.

23. Anorlu RI, Maholwana B, Hofmeyr GJ. Methods of delivering the placenta at caesarean section. Cochrane Database Syst Rev 2008;3:CD004737.

24. Anderson J, Etches D, Smith D. Postpartum hemorrhage. In: Baxley E, editor. Advanced life support in obstetrics course syllabus. 4th edition. Leawood (KS): American Academy of Family Physicians; 2001.

25. Rajan PV, Wing DA. Postpartum hemorrhage: evidence-based medical interventions for prevention and treatment. Clin Obstet Gynecol 2010;53:165–81.

26. Jacobs AJ. Management of postpartum hemorrhage at vaginal delivery. Available at: www.uptodate.com. Accessed October 3, 2011.

27. Munn MB, Owen J, Vincent R, et al. Comparison of two oxytocin regimens to prevent uterine atony at cesarean delivery: a randomized controlled trial. Obstet Gynecol 2001;98:386–90.

28. Archer TL, Knape K, Liles D, et al. The hemodynamics of oxytocin and other vasoactive agents during neuraxial anesthesia for cesarean delivery: findings in six cases. Int J Obstet Anesth 2008;17:247–54.

29. Su LL, Chong YS, Sameul M. Oxytocin agonists for preventing postpartum haemorrhage. Cochrane Database Syst Rev 2007;3:CD005457.

30. Mosby's drug consult 2005. St Louis (MO): Mosby; 2005.
31. Lamont RF, Morgan DJ, Logue M, et al. A prospective randomised trial to compare the efficacy and safety of hemabate and syntometrine for the prevention of primary postpartum haemorrhage. Prostaglandins Other Lipid Mediat 2001;66: 203–10.
32. Oleen MA, Mariano JP. Controlling refractory atonic postpartum hemorrhage with Hemabate sterile solution. Am J Obstet Gynecol 1990;162:205–8.
33. Gulmezoglu AM, Forna F, Villar J. Prostaglandins for preventing postpartum hae-morrhage. Cochrane Database Syst Rev 2007;3:CD000494.
34. Hofmeyr GJ, Walraven G, Gulmezoglu AM, et al. Misoprostol to treat postpartum haemorrhage: a systematic review. BJOG 2005;112:547–53.
35. Chong YS, Chua S, Shen L, et al. Does the route of administration of misoprostol make a difference? The uterotonic effect and side effects of misoprostol given by different routes after vaginal delivery. Eur J Obstet Gynecol Reprod Biol 2004; 113:191–8.
36. Lumbiganon P, Villar J, Piaggio G, et al. Side effects of oral misoprostol during the first 24 hours after administration in the third stage of labour. BJOG 2002;109: 1222–6.
37. Dildy GA 3rd. Postpartum hemorrhage: new management options. Clin Obstet Gynecol 2002;45:330–44.
38. Carroli G, Belizan J. Episiotomy for vaginal birth. Cochrane Database Syst Rev 1999;3:CD000081.
39. Malhotra M, Sharma JB, Batra S, et al. Maternal and perinatal outcome in varying degrees of anemia. Int J Gynaecol Obstet 2002;79:93–100.
40. Duggal N, Mercado C, Daniels K, et al. Antibiotic prophylaxis for prevention of perineal wound complications: a randomized controlled trial. Obstet Gynecol 2008;111:1268–73.
41. Melamed N, Ben-Haroush A, Chen R, et al. Intrapartum cervical lacerations: char-acteristics, risk factors, and effects on subsequent pregnancies. Am J Obstet Gynecol 2009;200:388, e1–4.
42. Maier RC. Control of postpartum hemorrhage with uterine packing. Am J Obstet Gynecol 1993;169:317–21.
43. Bakri YN, Amri A, Abdul Jabbar F. Tamponade-balloon for obstetrical bleeding. Int J Gynaecol Obstet 2001;74:139–42.
44. Georgiou C. Balloon tamponade in the management of postpartum haemor-rhage: a review. BJOG 2009;116:748–57.
45. Doumouchtsis SK, Papageorghiou AT, Arulkumaran S. Systematic review of conservative management of postpartum hemorrhage: what to do when medical treatment fails. Obstet Gynecol Surv 2007;62:540–7.
46. Ganguli S, Stecker MS, Pyne D, et al. Uterine artery embolization in the treatment of postpartum uterine hemorrhage. J Vasc Interv Radiol 2001;22:169–76.
47. Barber JT Jr, Tressler TB, Willis GS, et al. Arteriovenous malformation identifica-tion after conservative management of placenta percreta with uterine artery embolization and adjunctive therapy. Am J Obstet Gynecol 2011;204(5):e4–8.
48. Sidhu HK, Prasad G, Jain V, et al. Pelvic artery embolization in the management of obstetric hemorrhage. Acta Obstet Gynecol Scand 2010;89:1096–9.
49. Ghai S, Rajan DK, Asch MR, et al. Efficacy of embolization in traumatic uterine vascular malformations. J Vasc Interv Radiol 2003;14:1401–8.
50. Ornan D, White R, Pollak J, et al. Pelvic embolization for intractable postpartum hemorrhage: long-term follow-up and implications for fertility. Obstet Gynecol 2003;102:904–10.

51. Wang H, Garmel S. Successful term pregnancy after bilateral uterine artery embolization for postpartum hemorrhage. Obstet Gynecol 2003;102:603–4.
52. Chauleur C, Fanget C, Tourne G, et al. Serious primary post-partum hemorrhage, arterial embolization and future fertility: a retrospective study of 46 cases. Hum Reprod 2008;23:1553–9.
53. Fiori O, Deux JF, Kambale JC, et al. Impact of pelvic arterial embolization for intractable postpartum hemorrhage on fertility. Am J Obstet Gynecol 2009;200. 384.e1–4.
54. Sentilhes L, Gromez A, Calvier E, et al. Fertility and pregnancy following pelvic arterial embolisation for postpartum haemorrhage. BJOG 2010;117:84–93.
55. Kirby JM, Kachura JR, Rajan DK. Arterial embolization for primary postpartum hemorrhage. J Vasc Interv Radiol 2009;20:1036–45.
56. Mousa HA, Walkinshaw S. Major postpartum haemorrhage. Curr Opin Obstet Gynecol 2001;13:595–603.
57. O'Learly JL, O'Leary JA. Uterine artery ligation in the control of intractable postpartum hemorrhage. Obstet Gynecol 1974;43:849–53.
58. Adrabbo F, Salah J. Stepwise uterine devascularization: a novel technique for management of uncontrolled postpartum hemorrhage with preservation of the uterus. Am J Obstet Gynecol 1984;171:694–700.
59. Evans S, McShane P. The efficacy of internal iliac artery ligation in obstetric hemorrhage. Surg Gynecol Obstet 1985;160:250–3.
60. B-Lynch C, Coker A, Lawal AH, et al. The B-Lynch surgical technique for the control of massive postpartum haemorrhage: an alternative to hysterectomy? Five cases reported. Br J Obstet Gynaecol 1997;104:372–5.
61. Cho JH, Jun HS, Lee CN. Hemostatic suturing technique for uterine bleeding during cesarean delivery. Obstet Gynecol 2000;96:129–31.
62. Price N, B-Lynch C. Technical description of the B-Lynch brace suture for treatment of massive postpartum hemorrhage and review of published cases. Int J Fertil Womens Med 2005;50:148–63.
63. Kayem G, Kurinczuk JJ, Alfirevic Z, et al. Uterine compression sutures for the management of severe postpartum hemorrhage. Obstet Gynecol 2011;117:14–20.
64. Baskett TF. Uterine compression sutures for postpartum hemorrhage: efficacy, morbidity, and subsequent pregnancy. Obstet Gynecol 2007;110:68–71.
65. Sentilhes L, Gromez A, Trichot C, et al. Fertility after B-Lynch suture and stepwise uterine devascularization. Fertil Steril 2009;91. 934.e5–9.
66. Tsitlakidis C, Alalade A, Danso D, et al. Ten year follow-up of the effect of the B-Lynch uterine compression suture for massive postpartum hemorrhage. Int J Fertil Womens Med 2006;51:262–5.
67. Habek D, Becarevic R. Emergency peripartum hysterectomy in a tertiary obstetric center: 8-year evaluation. Fetal Diagn Ther 2007;22:139–42.
68. Chongsomchai C, Lumbiganon P, Laopaiboon M. Prophylactic antibiotic for manual removal of retained placenta in vaginal birth. Cochrane Database Syst Rev 2006;2:CD004904.
69. Nardin JM, Weeks A, Carroli G. Umbilical vein injection for management of retained placenta. Cochrane Database Syst Rev 2011;5:CD001337.
70. Abdel-Aleem H, Abdel-Aleem MA, Shaaban OM. Tocolysis for management of retained placenta. Cochrane Database Syst Rev 2011;1:CD007708.
71. Baskett TF. Acute uterine inversion: a review of 40 cases. J Obstet Gynaecol Can 2002;24(12):953–6.
72. Shah-Hosseini R, Evrard JR. Puerperal uterine inversion. Obstet Gynecol 1989;73(4):567–70.

73. Lipitz S, Frenkel Y. Puerperal inversion of the uterus. Eur J Obstet Gynecol Reprod Biol 1988;27:271–4.

74. Smith GN, Brien JF. Use of nitroglycerin for uterine relaxation. Obstet Gynecol Surv 1998;53(9):559–65.

75. Dayane SS, Schwalbe SS. The use of small-dose intravenous nitroglycerin in a case of uterine inversion. Anesth Analg 1996;82(5):1091–3.

76. Zahn CM, Yeomans ER. Postpartum hemorrhage: placenta accreta, uterine inversion, and puerperal hematomas. Clin Obstet Gynecol 1990;33(3):422–31.

77. Zahn CM, Hankins GD, Yeomans ER. Vulvovaginal hematomas complicating delivery. Rationale for drainage of the hematoma cavity. J Reprod Med 1996; 41(8):569–74.

78. Guerriero S, Ajossa S, Bargellini R, et al. Puerperal vulvovaginal hematoma: sonographic findings with MRI correlation. J Clin Ultrasound 2004;32(8):415–8.

79. Merien AE, van de Ven J, Mol BW, et al. Multidisciplinary team training in a simulation setting for acute obstetric emergencies: a systematic review. Obstet Gynecol 2010;115(5):1021–31.

80. Skupski DW, Lowenwirt IP, Weinbaum FI, et al. Improving hospital systems for the care of women with major obstetric hemorrhage. Obstet Gynecol 2006;107(5): 977–83.

81. Fuchs KM, Miller RS, Berkowitz RL. Optimizing outcomes through protocols, multidisciplinary drills, and simulation. Semin Perinatol 2009;33(2):104–8.

82. Clark EA, Fisher J, Arafeh J, et al. Team training/simulation. Clin Obstet Gynecol 2010;53(1):265–77.

83. Advanced Life Support in Obstetrics (ALSO) Curriculum, American Academy of Family Physicians proprietary materials.

84. Draycott T, Sibanda T, Owen L, et al. Does training in obstetric emergencies improve neonatal outcome? BJOG 2006;113:177–82.

85. Maslovitz S, Barkai G, Lessing JB, et al. Recurrent obstetric management mistakes identified by simulation. Obstet Gynecol 2007;109:1295–300.

86. California maternal quality care collaborative (CMQCC): OB Hemorrhage Toolkit. Available at: http://www.cmqcc.org/ob_hemorrhage. Accessed October 25, 2010.

Intrapartum Care the Midwifery Way: A Review

Anita C. Jaynes, CNM*, Kathleen E. Scott, CNM

KEYWORDS

• Midwifery • Labor • Delivery • Birth • Obstetrics • Intrapartum

Many American women are interested in natural, normal, nonmedicalized birth, but they are unaware of midwifery services or none are available in their area. A family physician (FP) can fill this need by becoming comfortable and competent in providing care the midwifery way. The objective of this article is to introduce primary care physicians to some of the many intrapartum care concepts and techniques used by midwives that could be integrated into physician practice.

MIDWIFERY FOR THE TWENTY-FIRST CENTURY

The word midwife is derived from the middle English word "mid" meaning "with" and the old English word "wife" meaning "woman."[1] Therefore on the most basic level, the word has historically referred to a person who is "with woman" during childbirth. Because the "wife" in "midwife" refers to the pregnant woman and not to the birth attendant, a man can also be a midwife.

In this article, the word "midwife" refers to a Certified Nurse-Midwife (CNM) as defined by the American College of Nurse-Midwives (ACNM) and board-certified by the American Midwifery Certification Board (AMCB). A CNM is defined by ACNM as "an individual educated in the two disciplines of nursing and midwifery, who possesses evidence of certification according to the requirements of ACNM."[2] In general, a CNM holds a bachelor's degree in nursing, a master's degree in nurse-midwifery, and board certification. There are midwives in the United States who have other types of training and certification, for example, the Certified Professional Midwife (CPM). However, FPs are most likely to work with CNMs rather than CPMs in the hospital setting. Also, the American College of Obstetricians and Gynecologists (ACOG) endorses collaboration only with CNMs and not with other types of midwives.[3]

The authors have nothing to disclose.

Department of Obstetrics and Gynecology, University of Nebraska Medical Center, 983255 Nebraska Medical Center, Omaha, NE 68198-3255, USA

* Corresponding author.

E-mail address: ajaynes@unmc.edu

Prim Care Clin Office Pract 39 (2012) 189–206
doi:10.1016/j.pop.2011.12.001   primarycare.theclinics.com

A common misconception exists that midwifery is synonymous with home birth. In 2006, 96.7% of CNM births occurred in hospitals, 2.0% in birth centers, and 1.2% at home. Out-of-hospital births accounted for less than 1% of all births in the United States.[4]

MIDWIFERY VERSUS MEDICINE

Midwifery is not just a profession; it is a calling, a philosophy, and an approach to practice. Midwives view and respond to childbearing as a normal life event with not only physiologic but also psychological, interpersonal, and spiritual dimensions. The role of the midwife is to support the normalcy of this process, intervening only when necessary. However, sometimes normal is a difficult concept to define.

According to the World Health Organization (WHO) *Care in Normal Birth: Report of a Technical Working Group*:

> We define normal birth as spontaneous in onset, low-risk at the start of labor and remaining so throughout labor and delivery. The infant is born spontaneously in the vertex position between 37 and 42 weeks completed pregnancy. After birth mother and infant are in good condition.

However, as the labor and delivery of many high-risk pregnant women have a normal course, a number of the recommendations in this paper may also apply to the care of these women.[5]

Pregnant women are often told, "the most important thing is a healthy mother and a healthy baby." Although this is ultimately true, the significance of a birth experience that strengthens family bonds and is empowering, enriching, and fulfilling should not be discounted. The midwife's role is to "protect, support, and enhance *normal* childbearing and family formation."[1] As such, the midwife assumes that a woman can and will have a healthy and normal pregnancy and birth until proved otherwise. Midwives trust the normal birth process, and the ability of the woman's body and psyche to accomplish pregnancy and birth with minimal or no intervention. The midwife is vigilant in recognizing deviations from normal but she does not assume that the woman is an emergency waiting to happen. Midwifery care has been proved to decrease the use of medical interventions, pain medications, operative deliveries, and cesarean sections. According to the Cochrane review, midwifery-led care should be the standard for most women.[6]

By contrast, medical education trains physicians to diagnose and treat pathology. The WHO states that the diagnosis of "normal" can only be made in retrospect; nevertheless, 85% of births are normal.[5] However, in the medical model of childbirth, the use of technology and interventions that should be reserved for complicated cases has become a routine application for most laboring women, and normal, natural labor has been largely lost in American hospitals today. Use of epidural anesthesia, induction of labor, augmentation of labor with oxytocin, administration of intravenous (IV) fluids, continuous electronic fetal monitoring, amniotomy, and other interventions have become so commonplace that they are now considered normal.

According to the American Academy of Family Physicians (AAFP), "Family physicians ... because of their background and interactions with the family, are best qualified to serve as each patient's advocate in all health-related matters, including the appropriate use of consultants, health services, and community resources."[7] FPs are in a unique position to facilitate childbirth as both a normal physiologic process and a transformational experience in the lives of the mother and her entire family. Like the midwife, the FP generally cares for maternity patients who are considered normal or low risk while leaving those who are categorized as complicated or high risk to the purview of the obstetrician. In the opinion of the authors, it would be appropriate for the FP to consider approaching labor and birth from the midwifery point of view rather than through the lens of obstetrics.

CHOOSING OUR WORDS

Words are powerful and just as mighty as our actions. The words authors choose to describe pregnancy and birth convey their beliefs and attitudes, and subtly affect a woman's perspective as well.

Perhaps no word is more laden with meaning than "deliver" or "delivery." Hannah Hulme Hunter has referred to this as "The 'D' Word." A birth attendant, whether midwife or physician, can unthinkingly say, "I did a great delivery last night." Such a statement implies "doing to" rather than "being with" a woman and shifts the accomplishment from the mother to the care provider. It also suggests that the mother was a passive bystander in the process, with the active role being assumed by the birth attendant.[8]

Midwives prefer to attribute the achievement of birth to the person who did it: the mother. It is almost always possible to rephrase statements about deliveries to respect the fact that the woman gave birth to her baby, ideally with our minimal assistance. The following techniques describe some examples of the ways that midwives assist laboring women without intervening in their own innate ability to give birth.

1:1 SUPPORT AND THE ROLE OF THE DOULA

Continuous 1:1 support, beginning in early labor, results in better outcomes. The continuous presence of a trained support person is associated with fewer cesarean deliveries, fewer operative vaginal deliveries, less use of analgesia and anesthesia, and fewer Apgar scores less than 7.[9] Continuous support during childbirth also contributes to shorter labors and a higher level of satisfaction with the birth experience.[10,11] No adverse consequences of labor support have been identified.

Labor support can be categorized as physical, emotional, and informational. New mothers have been asked to articulate what kinds of support were helpful during labor. Physical support includes beneficial techniques to help cope with pain, such as application of heat or cold, caring touch such as massage, and the provision of simple comfort measures such as drinking water or pillows. Emotional support is described as words of encouragement, friendliness, and the ability to convey calm and a sense of security. Not leaving the woman alone can be considered labor support, although some women have expressed the desire to have time alone with their significant others or not to be "bothered," "observed," or "interrupted" while laboring. Women also appreciate being given information, explanations, and advice during labor while retaining the right to make decisions about the course of their care. They want to be informed about the progress of their labor and receive explanations of medical terminology, procedures, or anything that is unfamiliar. Supportive advice, for example, could include suggesting position changes every 20 to 30 minutes or recommending use of a birthing ball to facilitate progress in labor (**Fig. 1**). Finally, women want their support person to serve as their advocate during labor.[11,12]

Although the philosophy of the midwife is to be "with woman," the reality is that she might not always be able to provide continuous support. A CNM might be managing more than one woman in labor, she might be required to see clinic patients at the same time that she has someone laboring, or she might get called away from the labor room to triage a patient or to respond to pages and telephone calls. This is even truer of the

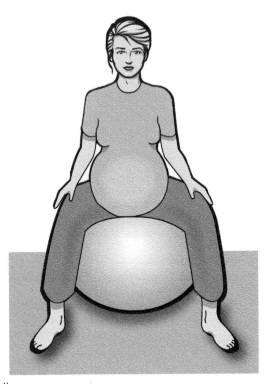

Fig. 1. Birthing ball.

physician. Labor nurses might have a greater opportunity to remain with a patient, but 1:1 nurse/patient ratios cannot always be expected or maintained. Therefore, the doula can fulfill an important role in providing labor support, improving outcomes, and enhancing the woman's satisfaction with her birth experience.

According to DONA International, "the word 'doula' comes from the ancient Greek meaning 'a woman who serves' and is now used to refer to a trained and experienced professional who provides continuous physical, emotional, and informational support to the mother before, during, and just after birth; or who provides emotional and practical support during the postpartum period."[12] Doula organizations provide formal training and certification to ensure competence and quality in those who call themselves doulas. A doula does not provide any medical, midwifery, or nursing care to her clients. The services of a doula have proved benefits and no evidence of any harm.[10–12]

ORAL INTAKE DURING LABOR

Standard hospital care during labor often requires IV hydration and limits oral intake to "sips and chips." The reasoning behind this policy has been that if the woman needed a cesarean delivery, it was important that she had an empty stomach to avoid aspiration while under anesthesia. This principle was introduced by Mendelson in 1946 and contradicted the previous standard of care that encouraged oral intake during labor. Despite decades of research to the contrary, restricting oral fluids and solid foods remains standard hospital practice today. In reality, the stomach is never truly empty because gastric acid production continues during periods of fasting.[13,14] Complications of anesthesia have become exceedingly rare events. Advances in anesthesia technique and the widespread use of regional rather than general anesthesia have reduced the risk of aspiration if anesthesia is required. As long ago as from 1994 to 1996, the rate of anesthesia-related maternal mortality in the United States, which includes complications other than aspiration, was quoted as 1.1 maternal deaths per million live births.[15] More recent studies from anesthesia have shown that consumption of food during labor is not harmful, although they did not find improvement in maternal or neonatal outcomes.[16,17]

Expecting normalcy rather than an emergency during labor means that food and oral fluids do not need to be restricted. Although no studies have been conducted on the nutritional needs of laboring women, it has been suggested that labor is comparable to continuous moderate aerobic exercise and may require a similar amount of energy.[13] A one-liter bag of D5LR contains 5000 g of dextrose. At a standard drip rate of 125 mL per hour, the laboring woman would receive 40 g of glucose or 160 calories per hour.

Most women will choose to consume less solid food, although they will continue to drink as labor progresses. Women report greater satisfaction with the childbirth experience when they have control over eating and drinking, and do not suffer the sense of deprivation that comes from being denied food or fluids. A sensible approach is to recommend soup, fruit, Popsicles, and other foods that are easily digestible, because of the stomach upset that often accompanies natural labor.

An ACOG Committee Opinion recommended that fasting was safer during labor and thus concluded that "there is insufficient evidence to address the safety of any particular fasting period for solids in obstetric patients" and therefore "solid foods should be avoided in laboring patients."[18] Unrestricted intake of food and fluids during labor is the norm in the United Kingdom, the Netherlands, and Australia. As long ago as 1998, it was reported that 33% of hospitals in the United Kingdom allowed intake of solid foods in labor, compared with less than 2% of hospital units in the United States,[16] and one can assume that those who give birth at home receive no IV hydration.

IV fluid replacement with solutions containing dextrose and normal saline or lactated Ringer's have not been shown to be superior to oral intake. Although it was believed that IV fluid would reduce ketosis in labor, this has not been proved, and in fact some experts believe that ketosis is a normal physiologic response to labor and has no harmful effects on the mother or fetus.[16,17,19] The Cochrane meta-analysis concluded that there was neither benefit nor harm in eating and drinking during labor for low-risk women, and therefore the practice of restricting oral intake is not justified.[14,19] Midwives believe that oral intake in labor is part of the natural process and should be standard practice for low-risk patients.

MONITORING OF THE FETAL HEART RATE

Because the fetus is not directly observable, ensuring well-being during labor poses a challenge. Electronic fetal heart rate monitoring (EFM) has become the standard method of evaluating fetal status, because it can be used to determine whether a fetus is well oxygenated. In 2003, birth-certificate data showed that EFM was used in 85.4% of births, making it the most frequently reported obstetric procedure.[20] EFM was introduced during the 1960s, without a complete understanding of fetal physiology and with very little research to support its efficacy. The goal of EFM was to detect fetal hypoxia early so that intervention could be implemented before asphyxia occurred and thus cerebral palsy could be prevented. However, experience with EFM has shown that although it has excellent sensitivity for identifying a fetus that is not compromised, it has poor predictive value for identifying a hypoxic fetus accurately. It is also recognized today that intrapartum hypoxia or asphyxia is not the cause of cerebral palsy.[21–23]

Implementation of EFM has resulted in a higher cesarean section rate, increased use of vacuum extractor or forceps, no reduction in perinatal mortality, and no reduction in the incidence of cerebral palsy. EFM results in a reduction in the risk of neonatal seizures, but has no effect on the rate of neonatal death. EFM is associated not only with a 59% reduction in the risk of fetal hypoxia but also with a 53% increase in cesarean deliveries and a 23% increase in operative vaginal deliveries.[24] Nevertheless, EFM is a form of technology that, once implemented, is seemingly impossible to abandon.

From the woman's point of view, continuous EFM confines her to bed and prevents her from ambulating, using hydrotherapy (as discussed later), or assuming a position or activity that causes an uninterpretable tracing. Telemetry monitoring is available in some institutions but may not be usable in all situations. Some women complain that the straps that hold the transducer and the tocodynanometer to the abdomen are tight and uncomfortable. Another criticism is that EFM shifts the focus of the care providers from the laboring woman to the "strip." EFM can be observed remotely and several tracings can be reviewed simultaneously. Fetal scalp electrodes and/or intrauterine pressure catheters are used for more precise monitoring, often resulting in increased diagnoses of fetal heart rate abnormalities or uterine dysfunction and, thus, more interventions.

For a more detailed discussion and review of EFM, the reader is referred to an article by Rodney and colleagues on this topic elsewhere in this issue.

Intermittent auscultation (IA) of the fetal heart rate by means of a hand-held Doppler or even a fetoscope is an appropriate alternative to continuous EFM in the low-risk patient (**Fig. 2**). A waterproof Doppler can be used if the patient is in a tub or shower (**Fig. 3**). As long ago as 1989, an ACOG technical bulletin concluded that "intermittent auscultation is equivalent to continuous EFM for the detection of fetal compromise and that no single method of monitoring is preferred over another in assessment of

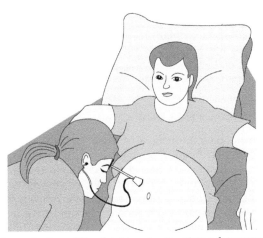

Fig. 2. Intermittent monitoring of the fetal heart rate using a fetoscope.

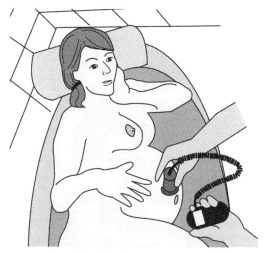

Fig. 3. Intermittent monitoring of the fetal heart rate using a waterproof Doppler.

the status of the fetus."[22] The US Preventive Services Task Force found that routine EFM for low-risk pregnancies was not recommended.[25]

To perform IA correctly, the examiner should auscultate the fetal heart rate before, during, and after a contraction, listening for the baseline rate, rhythm, accelerations, and decelerations. IA does not allow determination of fetal heart rate variability nor the types of decelerations; despite these limitations, randomized controlled trials comparing IA and EFM have found comparable outcomes.[21–25] From the clinician's point of view, EFM can be used briefly to confirm reassuring fetal status if IA raises a question regarding the baseline or decelerations.

There is no consensus regarding optimal time intervals for IA. ACNM has suggested every 15 to 30 minutes during active labor, every 15 minutes in the second stage of labor before expulsive efforts, and every 5 minutes while the woman is pushing.[26] Other organizations, including the Association of Women's Health, Obstetric, and Neonatal Nurses (AWHONN) and the ACOG, have proposed slight variations in the technique of IA. There is no research proving that one method is superior to any other.[20]

IA requires 1:1 care, which may not always be achievable. IA may increase patient satisfaction with the birth experience, but it is difficult to know whether this can be attributed to the method of monitoring itself or to the 1:1 attention. Differences in interpretation of the auscultated heart rate between examiners can be a problem; however, it is well known that interpretation of an EFM tracing does not always result in intraobserver agreement either.

At this time, both ACNM and ACOG consider IA an acceptable alternative to EFM in monitoring fetal status during normal labor.[22,26] Midwives continue to encourage wider acceptance and adoption of IA as the standard of care for low-risk women.

HYDROTHERAPY

Immersion in water during labor, including waterbirth, has strong proponents among midwives and patients. Hydrotherapy can be provided using a conventional bathtub, a whirlpool tub, or a special birthing tub or pool (**Fig. 4**). If none of these is available, a similar but less satisfactory result can be derived from a shower (**Fig. 5**).

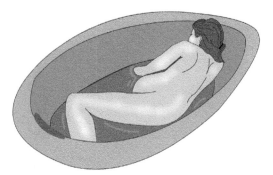

Fig. 4. Birthing tub for hydrotherapy in labor.

Hydrotherapy during labor provides relaxation, reduced anxiety, less need for analgesia, and a significantly shorter first stage of labor. Women report a high degree of satisfaction after laboring and, in some cases, giving birth in the water.[27]

Midwives' and patients' opinions are confirmed in part by the physiologic changes that occur as a result of hydrotherapy. Benfield and colleagues[27,28] found that immersion in water of adequate depth, defined as up to chest level, increased central blood

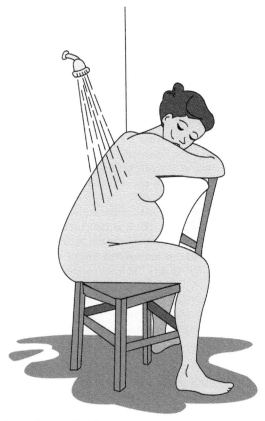

Fig. 5. Shower for hydrotherapy in labor.

volume because of the increase in hydrostatic pressure. This resulted in an increase in stroke volume, leading to greater cardiac output and a lower maternal heart rate. Water immersion also improved uterine contractility because of improved uteroplacental perfusion, and decreased the need for augmentation of labor. Immersion in water was found to decrease the circulating levels of cortisol and catecholamines, resulting in decreased anxiety and an improved ability to relax.

Opponents of hydrotherapy have focused on concern about adverse neonatal effects. However, in a study of 1600 waterbirths, Thoeni and colleagues[29] found no significant differences in arterial cord blood pH, base excess, and birth weight between the neonates born in water and those born conventionally. In addition, hydrotherapy has not been found to increase the risk of infection for the mother or the neonate, regardless of whether the membranes were intact or ruptured.

Adaptation of the neonate to extrauterine life is not compromised by being born into water. The diving reflex, which peaks at term, protects the newborn from aspiration pneumonia. The neonate will not take his or her first breaths until his or her face is exposed to air.[29]

The Cochrane review concluded that "there is no evidence of increased adverse effects to the fetus/neonate or woman from laboring in water or from waterbirth," although further research is needed.[30]

CARE OF THE PERINEUM

The incidence of perineal injury at the time of birth ranges from 40% to 85%, and about two-thirds of lacerations will require repair.[31] Reducing the incidence and severity of genital tract trauma at birth should be a shared responsibility between the mother and her birth attendant.

Prenatal perineal massage is a technique that can be performed at home by the mother, with the assistance of her partner if desired. The ACNM recommends starting perineal massage 6 weeks before the estimated date of delivery. The mother assumes a comfortable position and lubricates her thumbs with a lubricant such as vitamin E oil, almond oil, or a vegetable oil used for cooking such as olive oil. She then places her thumbs about 1 to 1.5 inches inside the vagina and presses down toward the anus until she feels a slight burning and stretching sensation. After that, she massages the lower vagina in a U-shaped movement. Performing prenatal perineal massage is recommended for 10 minutes once or twice daily (**Fig. 6**). Detailed instructions

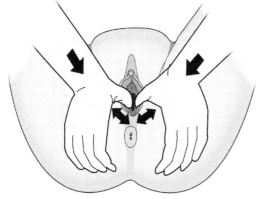

Fig. 6. Prenatal perineal massage.

including a diagram and a patient instruction sheet are available from the *Journal of Midwifery and Women's Health*.[32,33]

Improvement in perineal outcomes with perineal massage was seen particularly in primigravidae, women aged 30 and older, and women who had a prior episiotomy. Above all, results depended on women's compliance in performing massage at home; in other words, daily massage conferred more benefit than less frequent or sporadic massage.[31]

Although some women might ask about prenatal perineal massage, it will be a new concept for the majority. The prenatal care provider may choose to inform women about its possible benefits and to provide instructions on how to perform it.

At the time of birth, the midwife or physician can take several actions or "inactions" to help protect the maternal perineum. Fortunately, routine use of episiotomy has declined significantly. In 1999, the Cochrane review published recommendations for restricting the routine use of episiotomy that were endorsed by ACOG in 2006.[34] The episiotomy rate, which had already been decreasing, was subsequently studied by Frankmann and colleagues[35] and was found to have declined from 60.9% in 1979 to 24.5% in 2005. It is widely accepted that routine episiotomy confers no maternal or neonatal benefit, and increases the risk of third-degree and fourth-degree lacerations.[36]

However, the decrease in episiotomies has contributed to an increase in spontaneous lacerations, which shifts the birth attendant's management from episiotomy to techniques that protect the perineum. The positions of the practitioner's hands and maneuvers for the actual birth were extensively researched in the HOOP study, in which 5471 women were randomized to either hands-on or hands-poised approaches to crowning and emergence of the infant. There was no difference between the groups in the incidence of lacerations. The main outcome was a report of less perineal pain at 10 days postpartum in the hands-on group.[37] In a study by Mayerholfer and colleagues[38] of more than 1000 women, a hands-off approach was found to be safe and effective in preserving the perineum as opposed to handling the perineum and the infant's head as it emerged.

The mother's position at the time of birth can contribute significantly to not only perineal outcomes but also to maternal satisfaction. Upright, lateral, or positioning on hands and knees are all associated with less genital tract trauma (**Figs. 7** and **8**). Use of a modern birthing seat can help the woman to assume an upright and squatting position that increases the pelvic diameters and takes advantage of gravity.

Albers and colleagues[37] randomized 1200 women to compare a hands-off approach with warm compresses or massage with lubricant by the birth attendant

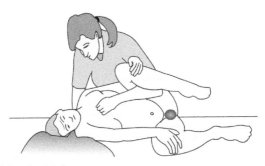

Fig. 7. Lateral position for birth.

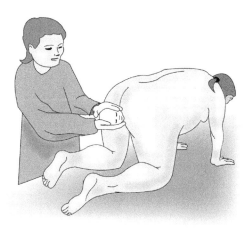

Fig. 8. Hands-and-knees position for birth.

during the late second stage of labor. The investigators concluded that there was no difference in outcomes. However, 75% of the requests to stop the intervention came from the women who were receiving the perineal massage, suggesting that this technique during labor is uncomfortable and unhelpful from the woman's point of view.

Albers and colleagues[37] concluded that the most important factors in protecting the perineum seem to be a reasonably comfortable mother, a slow and controlled expulsion of the infant, and shared responsibility for the outcome. Under normal circumstances, women should not be coached to push forcefully because the head is emerging. Rather, they should be encouraged to allow the head to pass slowly through the vaginal opening, grunting or nudging to advance the head, and giving birth to the head between contractions rather than with a contraction. The birth should be expedited by the use of forceful expulsive efforts only when fetal status is nonreassuring.

DELAYED CORD CLAMPING

Immediate clamping and cutting of the umbilical cord is standard practice in American hospitals today. A delay in clamping and cutting the cord has proven benefits for the neonate without adverse effects for the mother. Definitions of delayed cord clamping for research purposes have varied from 1 to 3 minutes. One guideline states that the birth attendant waits until the cord stops pulsating and becomes flaccid, indicating cessation of blood flow, a physiologic process that occurs within 4 to 5 minutes (**Fig. 9**).[39]

Active management of the third stage of labor consists of three interventions: administration of a uterotonic (usually oxytocin) with the birth of the anterior shoulder of the baby, clamping and cutting the umbilical cord (ideally within less than a minute), and applying controlled traction to the cord to facilitate delivery of the placenta. The purpose of active management of the third stage is to prevent postpartum hemorrhage, thus for maternal benefit. The Cochrane review of 11 trials showed no significant difference in hemorrhage between the early cord clamping and late cord clamping groups. The intervention that prevents hemorrhage is the administration of the uterotonic, not the management of the umbilical cord.[40]

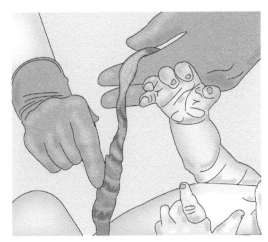

Fig. 9. Delayed cord clamping.

Those who advocate active management of the third stage for maternal benefit have not considered whether there is neonatal benefit or harm. A meta-analysis published in *JAMA* in 2007 concluded that delaying cord clamping for a minimum of 2 minutes in healthy term neonates is beneficial and that the benefits extend beyond the newborn period.[41]

Results of delayed cord clamping include higher hemoglobin and hematocrit levels as well as simply higher blood volume in neonates. Plasma bilirubin levels have been controversial, with some research showing an increase in jaundice requiring photo-therapy that was not found in other studies. Neonatal polycythemia was noted in infants with delayed cord clamping, but it was clinically insignificant and was associated with no adverse effects.[40,42]

Perhaps of even more interest is that the benefits of delayed cord clamping extend beyond the newborn period. Improved hematologic status of the newborn was found to decrease anemia at 3 months and to enrich iron stores and ferritin for as long as 6 months.[42,43] In the opinion of the authors, it is ironic that couples are choosing to bank umbilical cord blood for the future when in fact the baby could make use of it at the time of birth.

The Cochrane review concluded that delaying clamping of the cord for at least 2 to 3 minutes does not increase maternal hemorrhage and can improve the iron status of the neonate, although it does carry the risk of jaundice requiring phototherapy.[40] From the midwifery point of view, refraining from immediately clamping and cutting the cord is a physiologic and safe approach to management of the third stage of labor. The physician may find that parents are increasingly requesting delayed cord clamping as part of their birth plans.

APPROACHES TO LABOR PAIN

Epidural anesthesia has become routine in obstetric care, although many women neither need nor desire this intervention. Although epidurals are considered benign, they can have side effects such as poor progress in labor or fetal malpositioning because of lack of mobility or position changes, maternal hypotension reflected in a nonreassuring fetal heart tracing prompting intervention, and infection at the epidural site. A spinal headache is a common sequela of epidural anesthesia, which can be severe and debilitating for a new mother.[39]

Intrapartum fever is common with epidurals, although the mechanism remains unclear. In a study of 1004 laboring women, Gonen and colleagues[44] found that 11.8% who received epidural anesthesia became febrile compared with 0.2% who did not. It may be difficult to pinpoint epidural anesthesia as the cause of fever because the same group of women would be more likely to have other risk factors such as induction of labor, nulliparity, internal fetal monitoring, longer labor, longer duration of ruptured membranes, and more vaginal examinations during labor. After delivery, the placentas of 88% of the febrile women showed no evidence of infection and there was absence of infection in the neonates. Maternal fever rapidly resolved in 90% of the cases. The investigators concluded that thermoregulatory changes associated with epidurals, rather than infection, were the cause of most maternal fevers during labor. Nevertheless, intrapartum fever is usually presumed to be caused by infection, and often starts a cascade of interventions including antibiotic administration to the mother and infant, an evaluation of the infant for sepsis, and admission to the neonatal intensive care unit.

Although nurse-midwives working in hospitals do not deny IV analgesia or epidural anesthesia to laboring women, the midwifery philosophy and many women's birth plans favor an unmedicated birth. Women can assist in achieving this goal by participating in a childbirth preparation program that promotes natural birth.

The Lamaze method was introduced in France and focused on breathing, relaxation, continuous support from the father, and a specially trained nurse. Over the years, Lamaze has evolved from a specific set of techniques to a philosophy of childbirth preparation that no longer focuses on "the breathing."[45] Lamaze remains the best-known name in childbirth education, so much so that any childbirth class is often called "Lamaze."

Another well-known method is the Bradley Method of Husband-Coached Natural Childbirth. The Bradley method prepares couples to work as a team to achieve their objective of giving birth naturally. The Bradley method consists of a series of 12 classes and demands a serious commitment on the part of couples who wish to give birth naturally and without intervention.[46]

Use of self-hypnosis to prepare for birth has proved to be very successful in pain management for many women. The most recognized program of hypnosis education is HypnoBirthing, known as the Mongan Method. Self-hypnosis enables the woman to relax and remove the fear and tension that lead to an increased perception of pain.[47] Hypnosis classes and individual instruction in self-hypnosis are available as well as home study courses.

There has been no research to demonstrate that one method of childbirth education is superior to any other. The most important consideration seems to be that the pregnant woman finds an approach that appeals to her and conscientiously applies the principles and techniques that she has learned.

Many of the midwifery approaches that have already been presented in this article are useful in the management of pain. For example, immersion in water helps to relax the laboring woman and to relieve pain. Continuous labor support has been proved to reduce the need for analgesia or anesthesia. A doula, midwife, nurse, or well-prepared family members can provide comfort measures such as back rubs or the application of heat or cold in addition to words of encouragement. Frequent movement changes and positions that provide comfort can help to relieve pain. IA of the fetal heart rate allows the woman to assume positions of comfort and to move freely. Eating and drinking in labor, while not specifically pain-relief measures, give the woman energy and take away the feeling of deprivation or suffering that a forced fast engenders. Careful attention to the protection of the perineum can also reduce pain both during and after the birth.

Intradermal sterile water injections are a simple, safe, and easy-to-implement technique for reducing back pain. Anywhere from 15% to 74% of laboring women report back pain during labor. It is usually assumed to be caused by the occiput posterior fetal position, but can be caused by other factors such as asynclitism or the shape of the maternal pelvis.

To administer intradermal sterile water injections, the provider prepares 2 syringes with 25-gauge needles containing 0.5 to 1.0 mL of sterile water. Four sites on the lower back are identified: 1 over each posterior iliac spine and 2 others approximately 3 cm below and 1 cm medial to the sites first identified (**Fig. 10**). The injections initially cause intense stinging or burning for approximately 30 seconds. Administering the injections during a contraction or having 2 people give them simultaneously can help relieve the initial pain. Correct intradermal placement is confirmed by a wheal at each site.

Sterile water injections provide relief of back pain for anywhere from 45 minutes to 2 hours, but not relief from the pain of contractions or perineal pain. The mechanism of action of sterile water injections is unknown. It has been suggested that they cause a release of endorphins, or that they inhibit competing pain messages as in the gate control theory.[48,49]

Other pain management techniques have been reported in the literature, but there are insufficient data to recommend them. Also, they are not available in the typical hospital setting. Transcutaneous electrical nerve stimulation (TENS), acupuncture, chiropractic adjustments, and nitrous oxide are examples of modalities that are neither readily available nor widely studied.

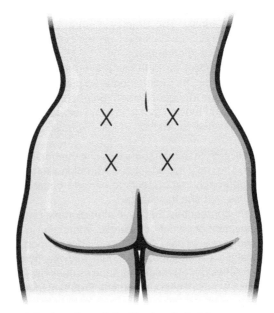

Fig. 10. Sterile water injections for relief of back pain in labor.

CHALLENGES TO PRACTICE CHANGE

There are challenges to practice change in institutions where the midwifery approach to birth is unfamiliar or not widely accepted.

Hospital policies such as routine establishment of an IV on admission, continuous electronic fetal monitoring, limitations on the use of a tub or shower, and restriction of food and fluids will need to be revised. A physician who serves on the planning committee for a new or remodeled labor unit can be influential in advocating for suitable hydrotherapy tubs, telemetry monitoring, equipment for IA, and a home-like atmosphere. Physicians can also advocate for the incorporation of midwifery and doula services if they are not already available.

Nurses who are only familiar with medicalized birth will need didactic education, skill development, and mentoring to learn how to care for a woman who desires a natural birth. Staff from a hospital or birthing center where midwifery care is well established could participate in a mentoring program or job exchange with the inexperienced nurses. Outside workshops including doula training could be offered, or midwives could be invited to the hospital to give in-house services. This staff development will require a commitment of time and money on the part of the hospital to expand the expertise of its nurses to fulfill the demand from some consumers for a natural birth. However, the benefit of satisfied patients in addition to better outcomes justifies the effort and expense.

To succeed in providing birth care the midwifery way, FPs will need to be personally convinced of its value. The scope of this article has allowed only a brief overview of midwifery; the authors hope that physicians will seek out their midwife colleagues to learn more tricks of the trade. Physicians who are accustomed to "doing something" will be challenged by a philosophy that emphasizes nonintervention. Holly Powell Kennedy, CNM, stated in her study of exemplary midwifery care that midwifery is the art of doing nothing—well.[50] There is ample evidence in the literature to support the safety and efficacy of a low-tech approach to the childbirth process. The challenge remains to educate oneself and then to influence hospital policies and personnel in settings where medicalized childbirth is the norm. Being able to fulfill the desire of women and their families for a natural, normal, safe, and fulfilling birth experience is the reward.

ACKNOWLEDGMENTS

The authors wish to thank Jack Kusler for creating the illustrations.

REFERENCES

1. Rooks J. Midwifery and childbirth in America. Philadelphia: Temple University Press; 1997.
2. American College of Nurse-Midwives. Definition of midwifery practice. Available at: http://www.midwife.org/ACNM/files/ccLibraryFiles/Filename/000000001385/CNM%20CM%20CPM%20ComparisonChart%20082511.pdf. Accessed April 5, 2001.
3. Statement of policy: midwifery education and certification. American College of Obstetricians and Gynecologists; 2007. Available at: http://www.acog.org/departments/perinatalHIV/sop0602.cfm. Updated June, 2004. Accessed March 1, 2011.
4. MacDorman M, Menacker F, Declercg E. Trends and characteristics of home and out-of-hospital births in the United States 1990-2006. Natl Vital Stat Rep 2010; 58(11):1–15.

5. World Health Organization. Care in normal birth: a practical guide. World Health Organization; 1996.
6. Hatem M, Sandall J, Devane D, et al. Midwife-led versus other models of care for childbearing women. Cochrane Database Syst Rev 2008;4:CD004667.
7. Family physician, definition. American Academy of Family Physicians; 2011. Available at: http://www.aafp.org/online/en/home/policy/policies/f/famphydef.html. Accessed March 1, 2011.
8. Hunter H. The "D" word. In: Wickham S, editor. Midwifery best practice. Edinburgh (United Kingdom): Elsevier Science Limited; 2003. p. 226–7.
9. Hodnett E, Gates S, Hofmeyr G, et al. Continuous support for women during childbirth. Cochrane Database Syst Rev 2007;3:CD003766.
10. Scott KD, Berkowitz G, Klaus M. A comparison of intermittent and continuous support during labor: a meta-analysis. Am J Obstet Gynecol 1999;180(5): 1054–9.
11. Bowers B. Mothers' experiences of labor support: exploration of qualitative research. J Obstet Gynecol Neonatal Nurs 2002;31(6):742–52.
12. DONA International. Available at: http://www.dona.org/mothers/index.php. Updated 2005. Accessed March 1, 2011.
13. American College of Nurse-Midwives. Clinical bulletin number 10: Providing oral nutrition to women in labor. J Midwifery Womens Health 2008;53(3): 276–83.
14. Singata M, Trammer J, Gyte G. Restricting oral fluid and food intake during labour. Cochrane Database Syst Rev 2010;1:CD003930.
15. Hawkins J. Maternal morbidity and mortality: anesthetic causes. Can J Anesth 2002;49(6):R1–5.
16. O'Sullivan G, Liu B, Shennan A. Oral intake during labor. Int Anesthesiol Clin 2007;45(1):133–47.
17. O'Sullivan G, Liu B, Hart D, et al. Effect of food intake during labour on obstetric outcome: randomised controlled trial. BMJ 2009;338:b784.
18. American College of Obstetricians and Gynecologists. Committee opinion: Oral intake during labor. Am J Obstet Gynecol 2009;114:714.
19. Toohill J, Soong B, Flenady V. Interventions for ketosis during labour. Cochrane Database Syst Rev 2008;3:CD004230.
20. Martin J, Hamilton P, Sutton J, et al. Births: final data for 2003. Natl Vital Stat Rep 2005;54(2):1–116.
21. Alfirevic Z, Devane D, Gyte G. Continuous cardiotocography (CTG) as a form of electronic fetal monitoring (EFM) for fetal assessment during labour. Cochrane Database Syst Rev 2006;3:CD006006.
22. American College of Obstetricians and Gynecologists. Practice bulletin 49: Intrapartum fetal heart rate monitoring: nomenclature, interpretation, and general management principles. Am J Obstet Gynecol 2009;106:1–11.
23. Barstow C, Gauer R, Jamieson B. Q/How does electronic fetal heart rate monitoring affect labor and delivery outcomes? J Fam Pract 2010;59(11): 653a–653b. Accessed April 4, 2011.
24. Vintzileos A, Nochimson D, Guzman E, et al. Intrapartum electronic fetal heart rate monitoring versus intermittent auscultation: a meta-analysis. Obstet Gynecol 1995;85(1):149–54.
25. Screening for intrapartum electronic fetal monitoring, topic page. U.S. Preventive Services Task Force. Available at: http://www.uspreventiveservicestaskforce.org/uspstf/uspsiefm.htm. Accessed April 5, 2011.

26. American College of Nurse-Midwives. Clinical bulletin: intermittent auscultation for intrapartum fetal heart rate surveillance. J Midwifery Womens Health 2010; 55(4):398–403.
27. Benfield R. Hydrotherapy in labor. J Nurs Scholarsh 2002;34(4):347–52.
28. Benfield R, Hortobagyi T, Tanner C, et al. The effects of hydrotherapy on anxiety, pain, neuroendocrine responses, and contraction dynamics during labor. Biol Res Nurs 2010;12(1):28–36.
29. Thoeni A, Zech N, Moroder L, et al. Review of 1600 water births. Does water birth increase the risk of neonatal infection? J Matern Fetal Neonatal Med 2005;17(5): 357–61.
30. Cluett E, Burns E. Immersion of water in labour and birth. Cochrane Database Syst Rev 2009;2:CD000111.
31. Albers L, Borders N. Minimizing genital tract trauma and related pain following spontaneous vaginal birth. J Midwifery Womens Health 2007;52(3):246–53.
32. American College of Nurse-Midwives (ACNM). Perineal massage in pregnancy. J Midwifery Womens Health 2005;50(1):63–4.
33. Beckmann M, Garrett A. Antenatal perineal massage for reducing perineal trauma. Cochrane Database Syst Rev 2006;1:CD005123.
34. American College of Obstetricians and Gynecologists. Practice bulletin: episiotomy. Am J Obstet Gynecol 2006;107(4):957–62.
35. Frankmann E, Wang L, Bunker C, et al. Episiotomy in the United States: has anything changed? Am J Obstet Gynecol 2009;200:573, e1–7.
36. Carroli G, Mignini L. Episiotomy for vaginal birth. Cochrane Database Syst Rev 2009;1:CD000081.
37. Albers L, Sedler K, Bedrick E, et al. Midwifery care measures in the second stage of labor and reduction of genital tract trauma at birth: a randomized trial. J Midwifery Womens Health 2005;50(5):365–72.
38. Mayerhofer K, Bodner-Adler B, Bodner K, et al. Traditional care of the perineum during birth. A prospective, randomized, multicenter study of 1,076 women. J Reprod Med 2002;47(6):477–82.
39. Varney H, Kriebs J, Gegor C. Varney's midwifery. 4th edition. Massachusetts: Jones and Bartlett; 2004.
40. McDonald S, Middleton P. Effect of timing of umbilical cord clamping of term infants on maternal and neonatal outcomes. Cochrane Database Syst Rev 2008;2:CD004074.
41. Hutton E, Hassan E. Late vs. early clamping of the umbilical cord in full-term neonates. JAMA 2007;297(11):1241–52.
42. Mercer J, Erickson-Owens D. Delayed cord clamping increases iron stores. Lancet 2006;367:1956–7.
43. Cernadas J, Carroli G, Pellegrini L, et al. The effect of timing of cord clamping on neonatal venous hematocrit values and clinical outcome at term: a randomized, controlled trial. Pediatrics 2006;117:e779–86.
44. Gonen R, Korobochka R, Degani S, et al. Association between epidural anesthesia and intrapartum fever. Am J Perinatol 2000;17(3):127–30.
45. Lamaze International. Available at: http://www.lamaze.org/. Updated 2010. Accessed April 9, 2011.
46. The Bradley method of husband coached natural childbirth. Available at: http://www.bradleybirth.com/. Updated 2011. Accessed April 9, 2011.
47. Hypnobirthing the Mongan method. Available at: http://www.hypnobirthing.com/. Update January 31, 2011. Accessed April 11, 2011.

48. Simkin P. Labor progress handbook. Oxford (United Kingdom): Blackwell; 2005.
49. Simkin P, Ohara M. Nonpharmacologic approaches to relieve labor pain and prevent suffering. Am J Obstet Gynecol 2002;186:s131–59.
50. Kennedy H. A model of exemplary midwifery practice: results of a Delphi study. J Midwifery Womens Health 2000;45(1):4–19.

Index

Note: Page numbers of article titles are in **boldface** type.

A

B

Prim Care Clin Office Pract 39 (2012) 207–219
doi:10.1016/S0095-4543(12)00009-7
0095-4543/12/$ – see front matter © 2012 Elsevier Inc. All rights reserved.

primarycare.theclinics.com

Moving?

Make sure your subscription moves with you!

To notify us of your new address, find your **Clinics Account Number** (located on your mailing label above your name), and contact customer service at:

Email: journalscustomerservice-usa@elsevier.com

800-654-2452 (subscribers in the U.S. & Canada)
314-447-8871 (subscribers outside of the U.S. & Canada)

Fax number: 314-447-8029

Elsevier Health Sciences Division
Subscription Customer Service
3251 Riverport Lane
Maryland Heights, MO 63043

*To ensure uninterrupted delivery of your subscription, please notify us at least 4 weeks in advance of move.

ELSEVIER

Printed and bound by CPI Group (UK) Ltd, Croydon, CR0 4YY

03/10/2024

01040445-0004